Clinical Manual of Emergency Psychiatry

Second Edition

Clinical Manual of Emergency Psychiatry

Second Edition

Edited by

Michelle B. Riba, M.D., M.S.

Divy Ravindranath, M.D., M.S.

Gerald Scott Winder, M.D.

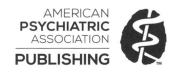

AMERICAN
PSYCHIATRIC
ASSOCIATION
PUBLISHING

If you wish to buy 50 or more copies of the same title, please go to www.appi.org/ specialdiscounts for more information.

Copyright © 2016 American Psychiatric Association Publishing
ALL RIGHTS RESERVED
Manufactured in the United States of America on acid-free paper
19   18   17   16   15   5   4   3   2   1
Second Edition
Typeset in Adobe's Formata and AGaramond.
American Psychiatric Association Publishing
1000 Wilson Boulevard
Arlington, VA 22209-3901
www.appi.org

Library of Congress Cataloging-in-Publication Data
Clinical manual of emergency psychiatry / edited by Michelle B. Riba, Divy Ravindranath, Gerald S. Winder. — Second edition.
    p. ; cm.
Includes bibliographical references and index.
ISBN 978-1-58562-507-9 (pbk. : alk. paper)
I. Riba, Michelle B., editor. II. Ravindranath, Divy, 1977– , editor. III. Winder, Gerald S., 1981– , editor. IV. American Psychiatric Association, issuing body.
    [DNLM: 1. Emergency Services, Psychiatric—methods. 2. Emergency Services, Psychiatric—organization & administration. 3. Mental Disorders—diagnosis. 4. Mental Disorders—therapy. WM 401]
    RC480.6
    616.89′025—dc23

                                                                        2015016059

British Library Cataloguing in Publication Data
A CIP record is available from the British Library.

Contents

List of Tables

List of Figures

Contributors

James Abelson, M.D., Ph.D.
Professor, Department of Psychiatry, University of Michigan, Ann Arbor, Michigan

Joshua Berezin, M.S., M.D.
Resident (PGY-3), Department of Psychiatry, New York University School of Medicine, New York, New York

James A. Bourgeois, O.D., M.D., F.A.P.M.
Clinical Professor and Interim Vice Chair of Clinical Affairs, Department of Psychiatry, University of California San Francisco School of Medicine, San Francisco, California

Philippe-Edouard Boursiquot, M.D.
Clinical Scholar, Department of Psychiatry and Behavioural Neurosciences, McMaster University, Hamilton, Ontario, Canada

Jennifer S. Brasch, M.D.
Associate Professor, Department of Psychiatry and Behavioural Neurosciences, McMaster University; Attending Psychiatrist, Concurrent Disorders Program, St. Joseph's Healthcare Hamilton, Ontario, Canada

Kirk J. Brower, M.D.
Professor, Department of Psychiatry, University of Michigan Medical School, Ann Arbor, Michigan

Nancy Byatt, D.O., M.B.A., F.A.P.M.
Assistant Professor of Psychiatry and Obstetrics and Gynecology, University of Massachusetts Medical School; Medical Director, Massachusetts Child Psychiatry Access Project for Moms (MCPAP for Moms); Attending Psychiatrist, Women's Mental Health and Psychosomatic Medicine, UMass Memorial Medical Center, Worcester, Massachusetts

Gregory W. Dalack, M.D.
Associate Professor; Chair and Associate Chair for Education and Academic Affairs, Department of Psychiatry, University of Michigan Health System, Ann Arbor, Michigan

Emily Deringer, M.D.
Attending Psychiatrist, Comprehensive Psychiatric Emergency Program, Bellevue Hospital; Assistant Professor, New York University School of Medicine, NYU Langone Medical Center, New York, New York

Charletta Dillard, M.D.
Resident Physician, Department of Psychiatry, Henry Ford Health System, Detroit, Michigan

Renee Garcia, M.D.
Clinical Assistant Professor of Psychiatry, Department of Psychiatry and Behavioral Sciences, Stanford University School of Medicine, Stanford, California

Rachel L. Glick, M.D.
Clinical Professor, Department of Psychiatry, University of Michigan Medical School, Ann Arbor, Michigan

Erick Hung, M.D.
Assistant Clinical Professor of Psychiatry, Department of Psychiatry, University of California—San Francisco, San Francisco, California

Monique James, M.D.
Resident Physician, Department of Psychiatry, University of California—San Francisco, San Francisco, California

B. Harrison Levine, M.D., M.P.H.
Private practice; formerly Assistant Professor, Department of Psychiatry, University of Colorado School of Medicine; Medical Director, Psychiatric Consultation Liaison and Emergency Services, Children's Hospital Colorado, Aurora, Colorado

Kishor Malavade, M.D.
Vice Chair for Acute Care Services, Department of Psychiatry, and Chief Medical Officer for Behavioral Health, Department of Population Health, Maimonides Medical Center, Brooklyn, New York

José R. Maldonado, M.D., F.A.P.M., F.A.C.F.E.
Associate Professor of Psychiatry, Internal Medicine, Surgery, Emergency Medicine, and Law; Medical Director, Psychosomatic Medicine Service; Director, Psychosomatic Medicine Fellowship Program, Stanford University School of Medicine, Stanford, California

Katherine Maloy, M.D.
Associate Director, Comprehensive Psychiatric Emergency Program, Bellevue Hospital; Clinical Assistant Professor, New York University School of Medicine, NYU Langone Medical Center, New York, New York

Tracy McCarthy, M.D.
Resident, Department of Psychiatry and Behavioral Sciences, University of California–Davis Medical Center, Sacramento, California

Adam D. Miller, M.D.
Clinical Instructor, Department of Psychiatry, University of Michigan Medical School, Ann Arbor, Michigan

Julia E. Najara, M.D.
Private practice; formerly Assistant Clinical Professor of Psychiatry, Columbia University; Director, Comprehensive Emergency Service, Pediatric Psychiatry Division, Morgan Stanley Children's Hospital of New York Presbyterian, New York, New York

Robert Neumar, M.D., Ph.D.
Professor and Chair, Department of Emergency Medicine, University of Michigan Health System, Ann Arbor, Michigan

Debra A. Pinals, M.D.
Director, Forensic Education, Law and Psychiatry Program; Associate Professor, Law and Psychiatry Program, Department of Psychiatry, University of Massachusetts Medical School, Worcester, Massachusetts

Ernest Poortinga, M.D.
Adjunct Clinical Assistant Professor of Psychiatry, University of Michigan Medical School; Forensic Psychiatry and Consulting Forensic Examiner, Center for Forensic Psychiatry, Saline, Michigan

Vasilis K. Pozios, M.D.
Assistant Medical Director, MHM Services, Inc., Michigan Department of Corrections, Lansing, Michigan

Divy Ravindranath, M.D., M.S.
Director, Psychiatry Consultation-Liaison Service and Mental Health Evaluation Clinic, VA Palo Alto Health Care System, Palo Alto, California; Clinical Assistant Professor (Affiliated), Department of Psychiatry, Stanford University School of Medicine, Stanford, California

Michelle B. Riba, M.D., M.S.
Professor of Psychiatry and Associate Chair for Integrated Medical and Psychiatric Services, Department of Psychiatry, University of Michigan; Associate Director, University of Michigan Comprehensive Depression Center, Ann Arbor, Michigan

Heather E. Schultz, M.D.
Clinical Instructor, Department of Psychiatry, University of Michigan Hospital and Health Systems, Ann Arbor, Michigan

Patricia Schwartz, M.D.
Psychiatrist, New York City Department of Health and Mental Hygiene (DOHMH) Assisted Outpatient Treatment (AOT), Long Island City, New York; Clinical Assistant Professor, Department of Psychiatry, New York University School of Medicine, New York, New York

Steven Storage, M.D.
Resident in Psychiatry, Stanford Hospital & Clinics, Stanford, California

Mary Weathers Case, M.D.
Attending Psychiatrist, New York University School of Medicine/Bellevue Hospital Center, New York, New York

Gerald Scott Winder, M.D.
Assistant Professor, Department of Psychiatry, University of Michigan Medical Center, Ann Arbor, Michigan

Disclosure of Competing Interests

The following contributors to this book have no competing interests to report:

James Abelson, M.D., Ph.D.
Joshua Berezin, M.S., M.D.
James A. Bourgeois, O.D., M.D., F.A.P.M.
Philippe-Edouard Boursiquot, M.D.
Jennifer S. Brasch, M.D.
Kirk J. Brower, M.D.
Nancy Byatt, D.O., M.B.A., F.A.P.M.
Gregory W. Dalack, M.D.
Emily Deringer, M.D.
Charletta Dillard, M.D.
Renee Garcia, M.D.
Rachel L. Glick, M.D.
Erick Hung, M.D.
Monique James, M.D.
B. Harrison Levine, M.D., M.P.H.
Kishor Malavade, M.D.

José R. Maldonado, M.D., F.A.P.M., F.A.C.F.E.
Katherine Maloy, M.D.
Tracy McCarthy, M.D.
Adam D. Miller, M.D.
Julia E. Najara, M.D.
Robert Neumar, M.D., Ph.D.
Debra A. Pinals, M.D.
Ernest Poortinga, M.D.
Vasilis K. Pozios, M.D.
Divy Ravindranath, M.D., M.S.
Michelle B. Riba, M.D., M.S.
Heather E. Schultz, M.D.
Patricia Schwartz, M.D.
Steven Storage, M.D.
Mary Weathers Case, M.D.
Gerald Scott Winder, M.D.

Foreword

Gregory W. Dalack, M.D.
Robert Neumar, M.D., Ph.D.

Medicine has entered an era of unprecedented and ever-increasing awareness of the frequent co-occurrence and impact of psychiatric disorders on both acute and chronic medical conditions. This is welcome news, and the health of the population will improve as psychiatric and other behavioral health care becomes better integrated into care delivery systems. The imperative, and the challenge, to do that may be greatest in the emergency department (ED) setting. The ED remains one of the most challenging and high-stakes settings in which to make assessments and provide clinical care. It is a critical support in times of crisis and an important launching point for many patients to initiate care of not only acute but also chronic conditions. This clinical manual is an important guide that will help you to carefully consider the complex situations that arise in patients presenting to the ED. The approach here is unique: Focused on clinical situations (as opposed to diagnostic categories), each chapter combines the insights of an accomplished psychiatry trainee with the sage advice of a senior practitioner in the field. This pairing provides a richly integrated perspective, which we trust will be useful to those in training as well as those supervising trainees.

At the end of each chapter are constructive "take-home" points that underscore broad themes pertinent to clinical care in the ED setting. We highlight these themes here:

- Pay attention to the chief complaint and think broadly about the clinical presentation as you develop a differential diagnosis and plan of care. Beware the temptation to assume that the patient with psychiatric symptoms could only have a primary psychiatric disorder. This is no more correct than assuming that all patients presenting with chest pain have cardiac disease. Many of the chapters in this manual emphasize the potential for "medical mimics" to cause the presenting complaints, including symptoms of anxiety, depression, psychosis, catatonia, and cognitive impairment. Indeed, the recognition that comorbid conditions are quite often present is critical to the complete assessment of patients presenting for care.
- Partner with your medical and nonmedical colleagues in the emergency setting to ascertain and understand the patient's presentation and available clinical information. Psychosocial stressors are often present, sometimes causing or exacerbating the crisis at hand. The information contained in this clinical manual underscores the important input often required from members of the team from social work, legal, or security staff in approaching cases where abuse, violence, or patient safety are at issue. Like the first edition, this book contains helpful guidance to assess the risk of violence in patients, consider the need for seclusion and restraint, and face the legal and ethical issues that arise in the emergency setting.

The psychiatric emergency service contact is an important link in the continuing chain of care. Thoughtful attention to developing an effective disposition and connecting the patient and family to care management and additional resources is key to addressing the presenting complaint and reducing the chances of a return visit, in crisis, to the emergency setting. This clinical manual emphasizes teachable moments, not only for patients and family members but also for trainees in the clinical setting.

The ED remains a frequent entry point into the health system and is a safe haven during an exacerbation of a chronic condition. The guidelines and approaches outlined in this book will help you tease out the complexities inherent in the often-complex clinical presentations by patients in crisis, allow you to make sense of the clinical situations you encounter, and guide you to advance your skills as clinician, educator, and lifelong learner. We wish you well in that journey.

Preface

One of the most challenging clinical settings in psychiatry is the psychiatric emergency department. Taking care of patients who are acutely ill in a timely manner takes incredible skill and ability. Making the incorrect assessment can have life-and-death implications. In addition, family members are very much a part of the clinical situation and are often themselves frightened and worried. Besides facing the acuity of the clinical issues, trainees working in this very difficult and high-stress setting at times have only backup supervision by phone rather than in-person oversight. Busy psychiatric emergency departments where first-year and second-year psychiatry residents are trying to quickly understand complicated clinical situations from patients who are quite ill makes for very challenging work indeed.

In this second edition, we have again sought to provide trainees and clinicians with an understanding and background of psychiatric emergency services in a format that can be easily read and highlighted. Each chapter was co-written by a trainee or junior faculty member as well as a senior faculty member at an academic medical center. We chose topics that are generally the most important and practical in any busy psychiatric emergency department and added chapters on increasingly important clinical topics, such as agitation. Case vignettes are also included to contextualize the information provided and allow readers to envision the applicable clinical scenario even if they are not actively seeing patients in the emergency department setting. Key points at the end of each chapter refine and summarize main ideas. This is not meant to be a textbook but rather a first pass at what psychiatrists often confront when working in this type of setting. Our hope was to make this a reader-friendly and useful clinical manual that reflects widespread practices in various academic centers and that can be read by trainees in many different disciplines.

With this in mind, we arranged many of the chapters by chief complaint (e.g., suicidal ideation) rather than by psychiatric diagnosis (e.g., borderline personality disorder). Many psychiatric conditions can result in the same psychiatric emergency. Moreover, the emergency department is one of the few arenas where patients do not arrive "prelabeled." Therefore, we felt that organizing the book based on chief complaints would give the reader the greatest opportunity to review the key points, as needed, just before seeing a patient.

We continue to appreciate the opportunity to have our respected colleagues participate in the writing and editing of this clinical manual. We hope that this second edition will inspire readers to strengthen and refine their clinical and teaching skills, thereby equipping them to provide excellent service and care to patients and families.

Michelle B. Riba, M.D., M.S.
Divy Ravindranath, M.D., M.S.
Gerald Scott Winder, M.D.

Acknowledgments

The volume editors extend their appreciation to the following faculty, residents, and fellows for their expert chapter reviews and editorial assistance:

- Lauren Edwards, M.D., Resident in Psychiatry, University of Michigan
- Peter Jackson, M.D., Resident in Psychiatry, University of Michigan
- Seth Knight, M.D., Resident in Psychiatry, University of Michigan
- Brianna Newhouse, M.D., Forensic Psychiatry Fellow, University of Michigan
- Scott Pekrul, M.D., Clinical Lecturer in Psychiatry, University of Michigan
- Zhenni Wang, M.D., Resident in Psychiatry, University of Michigan
- Shinji Yasugi, M.D., Child and Adolescent Psychiatry Fellow, University of Michigan

Drs. Riba, Ravindranath, and Winder also wish to express their sincere thanks and appreciation to Linda Gacioch, the administrative manager for this clinical manual. Linda did an excellent job of organizing and making sure that this project was done in a thoroughly professional and systematic manner. In addition, the volume editors appreciate the support and help of their colleagues at American Psychiatric Association Publishing.

1

Approach to Psychiatric Emergencies

Katherine Maloy, M.D.
Emily Deringer, M.D.
Kishor Malavade, M.D.

Although the vast majority of psychiatric practice takes place outside the hospital setting, patients with psychiatric or behavioral problems present to emergency departments (EDs) for a variety of reasons and in increasing numbers. According to a 2008 utilization study, uninsured patients with psychiatric disorders were more likely to have multiple ED visits and hospitalizations than insured patients (Baillargeon et al. 2008). Although national health care reform should increase access to psychiatric care, and in some cases increased insurance coverage has been shown to reduce utilization of hospital-based services (Meara et al. 2014), it is not clear that supply will meet the increase in demand for outpatient services. Patients in crisis will continue to require emergency evaluation, and the majority of these evaluations will occur in general ED settings. Patients who come to the ED solely for medical reasons can present with personality traits and maladaptive coping skills that may complicate their medical care. The aging of the population also increases demand by increasing prevalence of dementia and chronic medical illness (Walsh et al. 2008). EDs being overwhelmed with psychiatric patients is a problem receiving attention in the national media (Creswell 2013).

In all these situations, the role of the mental health clinician as consultant, liaison, educator, and detective can be crucial in facilitating appropriate care. The mental health clinician practicing in the ED setting must be adept at managing hospital systems issues, informed on medical illnesses and their psychiatric manifestations, skilled in conflict resolution, ethically and legally informed about responsibilities for patients' safety, and able to serve as a team leader who can direct staff in a crisis.

A General Approach to the Emergency Psychiatric Patient

Although hospital systems, police, and local mental health law vary by state and even individual hospital settings, an overall approach to the psychiatric emergency patient involves an understanding of systems and a focus on patient and clinician safety.

Understanding Health Care Systems

Psychiatrists and mental health workers, including psychologists, social workers, and psychiatric nurses, work in a variety of capacities within EDs. Trainees, including medical students or psychiatric residents, may also be involved in delivering emergency psychiatric care. To practice effectively, clinicians must know their role within the system in which they practice. Issues that commonly arise include admission privileges, follow-up planning, insurance issues, safety, medical care, available facilities at the ED or at affiliate hospitals, and supervision, particularly for trainees or nonphysician consultants. Every hospital has its own method of dividing responsibility and varying levels of support staff. The answer to the question "Who does what?" is determined primarily by the training of the clinician within the ED and the department's overall policy for handling psychiatric cases (Brown 2005). The settings of emergency psychiatric care delivery exist on a spectrum. In most community hospitals, the volume of psychiatric cases is not high enough to warrant dedicated psychiatric evaluation space or a comprehensive psychiatric evaluation team. Typically, in primary care and community-based centers, the mental health clinician acts as consultant to the ED. The facility may not have dedicated space for psychiatric evaluation and assessment, and the nursing and support staff may be less familiar with psychiatric issues (Woo et al. 2007). In facilities with more psychiatric cases, particularly in hospitals with active inpatient psychiatric services, EDs may set aside space or have more support services available for psychiatric emergencies, as advocated by the American Psychiatric Association (Allen et al. 2002). A true comprehensive psychiatric ED is most common in large, urban settings, which have a higher volume of psychiatric cases. For example, dedicated social work staff, psychiatrically trained nursing and support staff, a separate locked area, and the possibility of extended observation (up to 72 hours) are features of the Comprehensive Psychiatric Emergency Program in New York State. Variations on this model have developed across the country. Having a dedicated space with trained staff and support services for disposition, discharge, and transfer can also alleviate pressure on a busy medical ED.

Regardless of the system in which the clinician works, the same basic principles apply. The patient should receive as comprehensive an evaluation as possible, followed by a thorough disposition plan—whether admitted or discharged—in a setting that is safe and as therapeutic as possible.

Ensuring Safety

Evaluating patients who are acutely suicidal, agitated, disorganized, psychotic, or intoxicated is not uncommon when working in an emergency setting. Clinicians should consider their own safety and act to ensure the safety of the patient, the staff, and other patients in the area.

Hospital systems play a large role in how safety is achieved, so it is important for the clinician to know the particular challenges in his or her ED and to have a plan for ensuring patient and staff safety when a potentially dangerous situation arises. Predetermined, rehearsed safety plans are easier to execute in a crisis. EDs should establish policies regarding searching patients for weapons and specifying when and how to call for backup support if a patient becomes violent. Ideally, all patients should be searched prior to the interview. If a search is not performed routinely, the clinician should request a search or consider requesting that the patient change into a hospital gown or pajamas prior to the interview, thereby making it harder to conceal weapons or contraband. At the start of a shift, consultants—particularly those who work only occasionally in the ED—should introduce themselves to security staff so staff know whom to contact if backup support is needed. Even in facilities that have security cameras or panic buttons, it is helpful to notify staff prior to meeting with a patient so they can be ready to respond if a crisis situation arises. Particularly in the general ED, patients may require one-to-one observation to prevent elopement or self-harm, and precautions must be taken to remove potentially dangerous items from the area.

Approaching Agitated or Violent Patients

Asking staff how the patient has been behaving prior to the clinician's arrival can help the clinician tailor an initial approach. If the patient has been calm and cooperative, then the clinician may elect to interview the patient following the hospital's standard safety protocol. However, if the patient has been agitated, then additional precautions may be warranted prior to interviewing the patient.

Prior to initiating an encounter with an agitated patient, the clinician should first determine some key points about the patient, both through the clinician's own observation and by asking the staff for their input. Who is the patient, including his or her basic physical characteristics and presenting complaint? Is the patient upset about a specific issue, or psychotic and disorganized? What is the patient's behavior? Is he or she yelling? Throwing things? Making any specific threats? Finally, are there any indicators as to the etiology of the agitation, such as appearing ill, the smell of alcohol on the patient's breath, or obvious head trauma? In a setting where consultants are called in from another location, these are helpful questions to ask over the phone when taking the initial consult.

Once the nature of the situation is clear, the clinician can determine the environment in which to further assess the patient. For example, a higher degree of agitation may warrant interviewing the patient in a more public area than usual so that other staff members can monitor the interaction directly. Additionally, the clinician may request that security staff be present on standby in the ED to provide assistance rapidly if needed. Finally, the clinician may elect to begin the interaction with the patient by addressing the agitation directly rather than by trying to determine the chief complaint, the history of the presenting illness, and so forth. For example, the clinician may start by pointing out the level of agitation to the patient and then offering to help, or simply by asking what the patient thinks will help or what is bothering him or her. This may include an offer of a medication to calm the patient. Given that situations may not always be as they appear, the clinician should always err on the side of caution and containment of the patient in the least restrictive method possible. Time spent on verbal de-escalation is well spent because it can help prevent use of restraints or physical confrontation (Richmond et al. 2012).

Maintaining a calm demeanor goes a long way toward preventing escalation of agitation to violence. Many patients will resonate with the nonverbal communication of the clinician, and a clinician who is becoming more agitated may cause the patient to become more agitated as well (Flannery 2007). The clinician should be vigilant for signs of escalating tension, such as clenching fists, increased respiratory rate, threatening postures, or restlessness, and be ready to terminate an interview or interaction before a situation escalates, even if little information has been obtained. Clinicians should avoid provocative language or statements, listen actively and empathically, and offer clear choices (Richmond et al. 2012). Of course, maintaining such control in a difficult situation requires training and guidance, particularly for trainees, nonmedical staff, and medical staff without a psychiatric background.

General Rules for Approaching Agitated Patients

In encounters with agitated patients, the following general principles are helpful in maintaining safety and perhaps de-escalating the situation.

1. *Take charge and make a plan.* Staff members or other patients, meaning well, may try to intervene in various ways. This is confusing to the patient and can escalate the situation. The team leader should identify himself or herself as such and ask staff to follow his or her directions, delegating re-

sponsibility when appropriate. The team leader may not always be the person best suited to verbally interact with the patient, but the team leader should have the ultimate goal and plan in mind and be monitoring the situation as it proceeds. The team leader's role may involve discussing specific contingencies, such as elaborating what the next step will be if the patient does not calm down after specific interventions or a period of time.

2. *Keep a safe distance.* Crowding someone who is already upset is not generally a soothing tactic. An extra few feet of distance also gives time for escape if a patient does begin to strike out physically.

3. *Ask for backup.* Whether security should be present depends on the nature of the situation at hand. If the clinician is concerned that the patient may require a medication or restraints, other staff can be delegated to prepare these items, either before the patient is approached or while verbal interventions are ongoing.

4. *Provide an easy out.* People who are upset and confused generally want a way to resolve the issue rather than escalating it further. Providing a quick and safe alternative to further escalation allows the patient a way out. Giving in to a small, short-term demand may avoid a larger confrontation.

5. *Give clear instructions and set clear limits.* Specifically asking the patient to sit down in a certain place, lower his or her voice, put down the chair, and so on, is much more likely to yield a result than general directives to calm down, relax, or take it easy.

Dealing With Escalation

If a patient escalates to violence during an interview, the clinician's priority should always be his or her own safety. Escape is the first priority, followed by alerting other staff and then containment of the patient.

Particularly for trainees, who may feel that they are letting other staff down or appearing cowardly if they protect themselves, violent situations can provoke intense feelings of guilt or self-blame. Clinicians who are injured may feel that they provoked the attack or feel intense anger that is unfamiliar and difficult to reconcile with their values and ideals of what constitutes good patient care. Clinicians need to remember that they are also human beings, who exhibit a full range of normal human emotions in response to trauma. Clinicians are advised to seek support from friends, colleagues, or a mental health professional after a frightening incident. There is no one right answer regarding whether the clinician should press charges against an assaulting patient. Some hospitals may have policies in place to assist employees in this process, and it may be helpful to seek supervision—particularly if trainees are involved—in making this decision. Trainees, in particular, may find the decision about whether to press charges to be particularly stressful, and may benefit from supervisory guidance on this matter.

In the moment, an injury inflicted by a patient—even if not a deliberate attack, and even if not severe—can make it difficult to function effectively as a clinician. Having another team member take over and taking time out of the acute situation are warranted, if possible.

Etiologies of Agitation

After safety has been ensured, the overriding principle in addressing agitation is to rule out life-threatening medical causes. The assumption that a patient is suffering from a psychotic break as the result of schizophrenia could be fatal for a belligerent patient with hypoglycemia and diabetes or a patient experiencing delirium tremens. The process for assessment and management of agitation is discussed further in Chapter 7, "The Agitated Patient."

The Emergency Psychiatric Interview

The psychiatric interview of a patient in an emergency setting is unique. Compared with a typical outpatient psychiatric interview, the emergency interview is usually shorter and frequently less private, and its primary goals are to assess the patient's safety and determine the appropriate disposition, not to establish an ongoing therapeutic relationship. It can be complicated by the fact that the patient may be unwilling to cooperate and may not have been the person who decided that psychiatric intervention was indicated. Despite the compelling need to uncover complicating medical conditions and sources of collateral information, the interview need not be formulaic. Given that the clinician is trying to establish rapport and ask about intimate issues after only a brief interaction, the clinician should always be flexible enough to switch the topic when necessary, follow the patient's train of thought if indicated, and adapt to the patient's personality style (Manley 2004).

An important part of the assessment occurs before the clinician even enters the room with the patient. Before initiating contact with the patient, the clinician should always find out 1) the reason for seeing the patient, 2) basic available demographic information, and 3) the patient's behavior prior to the clinician's arrival. If possible, brief covert observation of the patient's behavior can also be extremely useful because it may reveal behavior that the patient will attempt to hide during the interview itself. Clinicians should always begin an interview by clearly introducing themselves, making the patient aware that they are conducting a psychiatric evaluation, and establishing a safe seating arrangement. It is also helpful to remind the patient that the purpose of the assessment is to figure out how best to help him or her in the given situation.

Components of the Interview

The components of an emergency psychiatric interview (Vergare et al. 2006) are similar to those of a more comprehensive diagnostic interview but necessarily focus more on immediate medical and safety risk factors and on the events immediately preceding the patient's arrival to the ED.

Patient Identification

The clinician first determines who the patient is and how he or she got to the ED. A brief sketch of the patient's demographics contextualizes the patient for the rest of the assessment. Knowledge of how the patient arrived (e.g., on his or her own, with family, with police) is helpful for understanding the patient's attitude toward treatment.

Chief Complaint

The clinician should then determine what the patient sees as the presenting problem.

History of Present Illness

A patient who is agitated, intoxicated, or psychotic may have difficulty clearly reconstructing how events unfolded before arriving at the ED. The patient may require specific redirection as to times, dates, events, and the chronology of symptoms, and the clinician may require data from collateral informants.

Past Psychiatric History

Information sought about the patient's past psychiatric history should include 1) prior hospitalizations, last hospitalization, and age at first hospitalization; 2) prior suicide attempts or self-harming behaviors; 3) prior episodes of violence or agitation; 4) prior trials of medications or therapies; and 5) history of arrests or incarceration. If there is a history of incarceration, it is useful to ask about psychiatric treatment during incarceration.

Substance Use History

In questioning a patient about his or her history of substance use, the clinician should start by asking about tobacco, which is generally the most socially acceptable. For each substance, a complete history should include the patient's 1) prior use or experimentation, 2) highest level of use, 3) longest sober period, and 4) current level of use. In addition to questioning about alcohol, marijuana, cocaine, and opiates, the clinician should ask about hallucinogens, inhalants, club drugs, and prescription drugs. The clinician should also screen for history of withdrawal symptoms (e.g., delirium tremens and seizures) and prior treatment history (e.g., rehabilitation, outpatient programs, Alcoholics Anonymous).

Medical History

The medical history should include questions about the patient's history of cardiac disease, hypertension, diabetes, epilepsy, head injury, hepatitis, cancer, and surgeries. A general reproductive history for women can also be helpful, specifically asking if the woman is menstruating regularly, is perimenopausal or postmenopausal, might be pregnant, or has undergone any reproductive surgeries. Because the Centers for Disease Control and Prevention (2006) has recommended that all adults be tested for HIV as a routine part of health maintenance, the clinician should routinely ask about HIV status. In at-risk populations, history of a positive purified protein derivative or QuantiFERON test or of tuberculosis diagnosis or treatment is also important in determining whether further evaluation by chest X ray or even respiratory isolation will be necessary.

Social Circumstances

In emergency presentations, instead of taking a detailed developmental history, the clinician should focus on painting a picture of the patient's current social circumstances. The following information is helpful for making disposition determinations: living situation, financial support, employment history, relocation history, social situation and supports, educational background, important developmental events, and legal/immigration status. More detailed developmental milestones may be warranted in the evaluation of children or adolescents.

Mental Status Examination

The mental status examination in the emergency psychiatric interview is similar to any other mental status examination, except that particular attention must be paid to documenting 1) active psychotic symptoms, 2) thoughts of self-injury or suicide and thoughts of harming others or homicide, 3) evidence of drug or alcohol intoxication, and 4) cognitive functioning.

Safety Alerts

Certain safety-related situations that may present during the emergency psychiatric interview should trigger more immediate action. These include the following:

- Children in the home or other persons for whom the patient is the primary caregiver (necessary to ascertain where these individuals are and who is caring for them, document this information carefully, and send authorities to retrieve anyone who is unsupervised while the patient is in the ED)
- Medical conditions requiring immediate treatment
- Active alcohol or benzodiazepine intoxication and withdrawal
- Active suicidal ideation with intent and plan
- Active violent ideation with intent and plan

Collateral Information

Collateral information can be helpful in forming a clear assessment in an emergency situation, and taking steps to obtain this information can be considered a standard of care when making determinations about safety and risk assessment. If possible, the clinician should obtain the patient's consent to talk to collateral informants. However, in an emergency situation, the clinician is permitted, even with existing Health Insurance Portability and Accountability Act (HIPAA) regulations, to contact collateral sources of information if demanded by the patient's emergency circumstances. Even though the clinician may obtain collateral information, the physician is still not permitted to unnecessarily share information about the patient without the patient's consent. (This point is discussed further in Chapter 12, "Legal and Ethical Issues in Emergency Psychiatry.") All attempts to gain information via contacting collateral sources should be carefully documented, including statements about why it was deemed necessary to contact the source and whether the contact was made with or without the patient's consent (U.S. Department of Health and Human Services Office for Civil Rights 2014).

Medical Clearance

The term *medical clearance* has entered into the medical parlance without a consensus about its definition. There is no way to rule out every possible medical illness a patient may have prior to admission to a psychiatric unit (Zun 2005). Therefore, the goal of the ED physician and/or mental health clinician should be to make a reasonable investigation into the possibility that the patient has an illness that 1) would be better treated in a medical setting (e.g., an infection requiring intravenous antibiotics, a stroke, myocardial infarction); 2) will cause the acute decompensation of the patient in the next few hours and thus requires a higher level of care (e.g., active alcohol withdrawal that is not responding to oral medication, a smoldering gastrointestinal bleed); 3) is causing the behavioral symptoms that brought the patient to the hospital in the first place and should be treated by something other than psychiatric medication (e.g., delirium due to an underlying infection, intracranial hemorrhage); or 4) is worsening the psychiatric process (e.g., untreated pain causing agitation; anemia-related fatigue and low energy causing deterioration of mood). This investigation is accomplished through a careful diagnostic interview, a careful physical examination, and a combination of screening lab tests and imaging studies.

The more that ED psychiatrists are able to retain familiarity with routine medical issues and communicate effectively with other services as needed, the more help they will be to their patients. Clinicians without medical training (psychologists, social workers, licensed mental health counselors) who are working in an ED will need to rely more heavily on the ED physician to assist with the differentiation of medical and psychiatric issues. However, familiarity with common medical comorbidities, the medical complications of substance withdrawal, and the differences between delirium and psychiatrically caused psychosis is crucial to a thorough evaluation.

Many hospital systems require that the psychiatrist admitting the patient to a psychiatric unit perform his or her own physical examination as part of the assessment. This examination can be particularly difficult with a patient who is agitated or psychotic, but it may reveal important information that can contribute to treatment decisions. Table 1–1 details the contents of a focused physical examination when seeking medical clearance for psychiatric evaluation, and Table 1–2 details relevant laboratory tests and studies that may be considered. Patients who are disorganized, catatonic, or thought-blocked may not report physical symptoms readily or may require more specific or concrete questions and an attentive physical examination to uncover injury or illness.

In summary, the examination of a psychiatric patient in the ED should be targeted toward finding occult medical processes that require treatment in a nonpsychiatric setting, are imminently life threatening, or are contributing to the psychiatric process (Guze and Love 2004).

Substance Abuse and Withdrawal Syndromes

Substance abuse accounts for many ED visits. Mental health clinicians are frequently called to evaluate patients who are acutely intoxicated or in withdrawal, both to assess their safety and to assist in determining a disposition.

The emergency assessment of substance abuse problems should focus on the immediate issues of safety, which include protecting the acutely intoxicated or withdrawing patient from harming self or others and making a decision about when the patient is safe to leave. Consultants may be asked to comment on a patient's capacity to refuse medical care when the patient is acutely intoxicated or in withdrawal.

Stigma about substance abuse can contribute to the difficulty of evaluating patients effectively in an emergency setting and can make it difficult for patients to obtain appropriate treatment. Clinicians may be inclined to con-

Table 1–1. Focused physical examination when seeking medical clearance for psychiatric evaluation

Area examined	What to look at	What to look for
General appearance	Weight, stature, grooming, level of distress, skin	Cachexia—suspicion of tuberculosis, cancer, HIV, malnutrition Obvious respiratory distress Obvious physical distress or agitation Grossly disheveled or malodorous patient Rashes—allergic or infectious illnesses
Head, ears, eyes, nose, throat	Mucous membranes, conjunctiva, pupils and eye movements, any discharge or lesions, evidence of trauma, dentition	Dry mucous membranes—dehydration Pupils and eye movements—focal neurological deficits, evidence of drug intoxication or withdrawal Scleral icterus—jaundice Proptosis—hyperthyroidism Bruises, lacerations—evidence of head or facial trauma Poor dentition—nutritional status, occult abscesses
Neck	Thyroid size, neck mobility	Thyromegaly—goiter, hyperthyroidism Neck rigidity—meningitis, encephalitis
Chest	Breath sounds, accessory muscle use, any evidence of trauma	Rales—congestive heart failure Rhonchi—pneumonia Chest trauma—emergent need for treatment of a wound; risk of future pneumonia from decreased chest expansion
Cardiovascular system	Heart sounds, peripheral pulses	Rate, rhythm, regularity of heartbeat Any absent peripheral pulses—vascular disease

Table 1–1.   Focused physical examination when seeking medical clearance for psychiatric evaluation *(continued)*

Area examined	What to look at	What to look for
Abdomen	Any palpable masses, liver size, scars, areas of tenderness	Hepatomegaly—undiagnosed liver disease Surgical scars Acute tenderness—acute pathology that needs to be addressed in emergency department
Back and spine	CVA tenderness, spinal curvature	Curvature—scoliosis or osteoporosis CVA tenderness—kidney infection or stones
Extremities	Movement, strength, range of motion	Any deficits, limps, or pain that might indicate occult neurological illness
Neurological system	Cranial nerves, strength, sensation, gait, reflexes	Any focal deficits indicating stroke or occult mass Festinating gait, rigidity—parkinsonism Tremors—parkinsonism, EPS Evidence of tardive dyskinesia Broad-based gait—hydrocephalus, tertiary syphilis

Note.   CVA=costovertebral angle; EPS=extrapyramidal symptoms.

Table 1–2. Common laboratory tests and studies when seeking medical clearance for psychiatric evaluation

Test	Abnormal results and their psychiatric implications
Complete blood count	Macrocytic anemia—vitamin B_{12}/folate deficiency, alcohol abuse Microcytic anemia—iron deficiency Normocytic—acute bleeding or chronic inflammatory disease Leukocytosis—acute infection Leukopenia—advanced HIV disease, immune suppression, leukemia Low platelets—side effect of valproate or carbamazepine, autoimmune thrombocytopenia
Basic metabolic panel	Elevated creatinine—renal failure Hyponatremia—potential side effect of SSRIs, particularly in elderly Hypernatremia—dehydration, renal failure Low potassium—risk of arrhythmia; may be due to diuretic use, bulimia, diarrhea High potassium—risk of arrhythmia; may be due to renal failure Low bicarbonate—acidosis; aspirin ingestion
Liver enzymes	Elevated ALT:AST ratio—alcohol abuse Elevated ALT and AST—liver failure due to multiple causes (e.g., drugs, acetaminophen ingestion, hepatitis)
Urinalysis	Urinary tract infection in elderly or sick patient can lead to severe delirium
Urine drug screen	Positive—detection of some common drugs of abuse (be aware of the substances of abuse that are *not* screened for in the institution's routine urine drug screen, as well as the reliability of the screen with regard to false positives and negatives)

Table 1–2.   Common laboratory tests and studies when seeking medical clearance for psychiatric evaluation *(continued)*

Test	Abnormal results and their psychiatric implications
Thyroid-stimulating hormone	Elevated—hypothyroidism leading to depression, cognitive changes Low—hyperthyroidism leading to manic-like symptoms, agitation
Vitamin B_{12}/folate	Low B_{12}—neurological changes, memory problems Low folate—evidence of general malnutrition; may be associated with depression, thromboembolic events Low B_{12} and folate are both often associated with alcohol abuse
Rapid plasma reagin	Latent syphilis—can lead to dementia, mood changes, neurological deficits
Chest X ray	Considered for homeless or incarcerated patients, any patients with risk factors for tuberculosis, and elderly patients—look for evidence of tuberculosis, occult masses, pneumonia
Head computed tomography	Occasionally used for screening for gross masses or bleeding in patients with altered mental status or new-onset psychosis Less sensitive than magnetic resonance imaging but less expensive, more accessible, and faster
Electroencephalography	If available acutely, can be used to look for nonconvulsive status epilepticus, evidence of metabolic encephalopathy (delirium)
Lumbar puncture	Indicated for any patient with new mental status changes, fever, and/or meningeal signs Look for evidence of viral or bacterial meningitis, encephalitis, bleeding, cryptococcal infection
Electrocardiogram	Important both for routine medical evaluation and for treatment planning Antipsychotics, methadone, and other medications can prolong the QTc interval

Note. ALT=alanine aminotransferase; AST=aspartate aminotransferase; SSRI=selective serotonin reuptake inhibitor.

sider patients who are intoxicated as less deserving of time or attention because they seemingly have brought the problem on themselves. In addition, if these patients are abusive or belligerent and being held against their will, providing appropriate care becomes even more difficult. Patients who return repeatedly with substance-related issues present an additional challenge because they may have exhausted their community resources and be seeking shelter in the ED. Despite the difficulties, intoxicated patients require close monitoring and are at greatly increased immediate risk of intentional or unintentional harm to themselves and others. (For more details on substance abuse in the psychiatric emergency setting, see Chapter 9, "Substance-Related Psychiatric Emergencies.")

Documentation

Whenever a patient is hospitalized or released, either voluntarily or involuntarily, one of the clinician's most important jobs is to provide clear and thorough documentation. ED documentation serves both to communicate to future and current providers and to show the reasoning and justification for the disposition decision. Thus, communication should be concise and clear but also should demonstrate that a thorough evaluation took place. In hospitals with electronic medical record systems, it may be possible to build templates or prompts that remind the clinician of the components of an evaluation, including the required items for billing purposes. Some electronic health records systems may incorporate standardized checklists or scales, but there is no good substitute for a well-written, concise note that reflects a thorough and well-reasoned formulation of the patient's presenting issues, history, risk factors, psychosocial context, and risk assessment.

Components of Documentation

Documentation for every psychiatric admission or release should include the following:

• The facts on which an assessment is based, including the sources of these facts, such as the patient, collateral informants, and laboratory tests and studies

- A risk assessment of the patient's chronic *and* immediate risk of danger to self and others (Jacobs et al. 2003)
- A reasoned argument for the decision that was made and against the alternative disposition
- In the case of admission, clear documentation of all evidence that proves the patient's dangerousness or inability to care for self and the manner in which this will be addressed by psychiatric admission
- In the case of discharge, clear documentation of the lack of imminent dangerousness or what contingencies are in place to minimize risk in the community, as well as follow-up recommendations

It is absolutely essential that the risk assessment be documented in a clear and coherent manner that justifies the decision regarding admission, discharge, or other treatment that has been made by the treating clinician. Readers of the assessment should not be left to deduce or infer the clinician's thought process.

Examples of Documentation of a Case Formulation

Case Example 1

Ms. A is a 34-year-old single white woman, employed and recently divorced, with a history of alcohol dependence and depressive episodes. She was brought to the ED by emergency medical services after she called 911 reporting that she had taken an overdose of alcohol, diazepam, and painkillers. After medical stabilization, she was referred for psychiatric evaluation. Ms. A currently denies that she was intending to harm herself and maintains that she accidentally ingested these medications. She does not remember calling 911 for help and denies any current depressive symptoms. Collateral information from her ex-husband as well as a close friend reveals that the divorce resulted in the loss of custody of her children and that she has been absent from work and drinking more heavily since. Despite Ms. A's assertions of her safety, it is evident that she is at high risk of harming herself in the near future, given the potential lethality of her ingestion, her lack of insight into the dangerousness of her behavior, and reports of her decreasing ability to function. In addition, losing custody of her children is likely to have increased her risk of suicidal behavior due to feelings of guilt. She has minimal support in the community and no current psychiatric care. Due to these risks, she will be admitted for 72-hour observation for improvement in her mood, undergo supportive and group psychotherapy, and be monitored for withdrawal from alcohol and benzodiazepines. Plans for aftercare will be made before her release.

Case Example 2

Mr. B, a 55-year-old single white man with no formal psychiatric history, was recently released from a brief jail stay for domestic violence. He presented to the ED after his mother called 911 stating that he was "acting crazy" and smashing items in her home. The patient was agitated on arrival but has maintained behavioral control since then and has shown no evidence of aggression or agitation. He admits to "having problems with my temper" and using cocaine earlier in the day. He is currently staying with his mother since his arrest for domestic violence. He admits to having angry feelings toward his ex-girlfriend who filed charges, and states that if he knew where she was staying, he would probably "knock some sense into her." However, he evidences no symptoms of mental illness and has a clear and coherent thought process. He is fully aware of the legal implications and risks of assaulting his ex-girlfriend. He declined referral to substance abuse treatment. Despite Mr. B's assertions of violent ideation, he does not demonstrate symptoms of a mental illness at this time and does not warrant psychiatric hospitalization. Prior to his release, the precinct in his ex-girlfriend's neighborhood was warned of his impending release. She has not been notified because she has entered a domestic violence shelter and her family does not know her location. In addition, staff spoke with the patient's mother and advised her to call police if her son's behavior escalated and to take steps to ensure her own safety.

Special Situations

Telephone Emergencies

EDs frequently receive calls from people in the community seeking medical advice. When these calls are of a psychiatric nature, they may be directed to the consulting mental health clinician or routed to the psychiatric ED. Calls cover a wide range of questions, including issues of medications, side effects, and drug use. The clinician should try to help to the degree that he or she can. Patients should always be assured that they can come to the ED for further evaluation of their complaint and encouraged to contact their personal physician or mental health clinician for further assistance. When phone calls involve threats of violence or self-harm, the clinician should attempt to remain on the line with the patient, be supportive, and try to obtain as much information as possible about the patient's location. If the patient refuses to reveal his or her identity or location, the clinician should notify other ED staff to contact the police so that they can attempt to trace the call, although in the age of cell phones, tracing can be difficult. If a clinician is concerned about the safety of the caller, notifying police and asking them to visit the caller to check on him or her is the safest option.

Sexual Assault

Although many sexual assault victims never seek treatment, some victims may request a psychiatric consultation, ED staff may request a psychiatric consultation when concerned that a rape victim may be suicidal or otherwise psychiatrically compromised by the event, or a patient may reveal an assault while being evaluated for another psychiatric issue. Clinicians should ensure that all appropriate medical, legal, and counseling services are made available to the patient. The hospital's social work department can be helpful for finding appropriate services available in the victim's area. Patients who have experienced rape or sexual traumatization should be offered the opportunity for a full physical examination by a clinician trained in evidence collection, even if they do not want to press charges at that time. Women should be offered prophylactic contraception to prevent pregnancy, and all patients should be counseled about and offered prophylaxis for sexually transmitted diseases and HIV. Patients may not wish to report the incident but should be offered the opportunity to do so, and whenever possible they should be assisted by a rape crisis counselor or victim's advocate during this process. When patients are considered "mentally ill" by the report takers, the stigma attached to psychiatric diagnosis may cause more difficulty in the accurate reporting of assaults. The mental health clinician may have to assume more of an advocacy role in assisting the patient to make a report if the patient wishes to do so. However, it is important to focus on acute psychiatric issues and treatment, and avoid acting as a police investigator.

Domestic Violence

Emergency psychiatric clinicians may be involved in the evaluation of a patient reporting domestic violence. Counseling or advocacy services, legal services, physical examinations if indicated, and psychiatric follow-up should be made available to patients affected by domestic violence. An adult reporting domestic violence is not required to report the events to the police. However, if children in the home are at risk as a result of the violence, the clinician may be mandated by state law to report suspected child abuse. The clinician should avoid giving patients any pamphlets or fliers that are obviously about domestic violence because these materials can lead to escalation if discovered. Leaving the abuser is not always immediately possible or indicated for a victim; however, the victim should be encouraged to make a "safety plan" for how to leave the home safely when he or she is ready. Victims sometimes require multiple tries before they successfully leave a violent situation. Once again, social work services should also be involved.

If the clinician suspects that a patient is unable to make a reasoned decision about his or her own safety due to mental illness, the clinician can arrange for psychiatric admission or make a report to adult protective services. For example, a woman with severe psychosis may not be able to organize herself to get out of an abusive situation and therefore may be deemed unable to care for herself.

Abuse and Neglect

In almost all states, physicians are mandated to report suspected child abuse. If a clinician has a reasonable suspicion that a child is being abused, neglected, or mistreated by a caregiver, the clinician should inform the appropriate agency of the suspicion. If a patient with dependent children is to be admitted to the hospital, efforts should be made to contact someone who can care for the children during the hospitalization to avoid referral to child protective services. Information about children's exposure to violence, drug abuse, or neglect may be uncovered during evaluation of a parent or family member. These suspicions must be reported, and mandated reporting in such cases is an exception to patient confidentiality rules.

Abuse of elders or dependent adults (i.e., those with intellectual or other disabilities who are dependent for care on another person) may be either reported by the patient or revealed by a caregiver during an evaluation. The aging of the population has led to increased burden on families to provide caregiving that may exhaust their resources. Nonjudgmental questioning of caregivers is a good strategy for uncovering abusive or potentially abusive situations. Many chronically mentally ill patients are also cared for by family members, who may not be able to provide a safe environment. Consultation with hospital social work departments can be helpful in all cases in which abuse or neglect is suspected.

The "Frequent Flyer"

Some patients present repeatedly to the ED with psychiatric or medical complaints, to the point that they become known to staff as "frequent flyers." The stereotype of the frequent ED utilizer, particularly in urban areas, is a homeless individual who uses substances and uses the ED in lieu of other shelter alternatives. However, one study found that frequent users of medical ED services could not be so easily characterized (LaCalle and Rabin 2010). Targeted case management to provide access to housing and outpatient services has had some positive results in some systems (Abello et al. 2012). A perception that a particular patient is overusing ED services can certainly provide significant problems for the staff's ability to continue to provide consistent care, and the psychiatric consultant may be called on to help uncover the cause of or "fix" the problem of even a nonpsychiatric frequent presenter. There are no simple answers in these cases, but providing empathic support to burned-out staff members may be an unofficial role of the ED consultant in helping to manage these patients.

The Patient in Legal Custody

Patients in legal custody are brought to an emergency setting for psychiatric evaluation for a variety of reasons, including evaluation for suicidality, behavioral problems, treatment or prevention of withdrawal, or the need for a recommendation for psychiatric observation or treatment while in custody. Prior to interviewing the patient, the clinician should consider several key points that will determine what kind of interview takes place, whether any assessment is even indicated, and what question is being asked by those seeking the patient evaluation. Most important, the clinician needs to remember that patients do not surrender their right to doctor-patient confidentiality simply because they are under arrest or serving a jail or prison term (U.S. Department of Health and Human Services 2004). The clinician should ask the officers escorting the patient to delineate the patient's current legal status; to state the charges against the patient, so that the clinician can determine whether the patient understands the charges; and to explain why the patient is being brought for evaluation. If the patient is released from the ED, the officers should know where the patient will go next—that is, to court, to jail, or to the community. The officers can also provide information about the patient's behavior while he or she was in custody. The patient should be interviewed without the police present, but precautions should be taken to maintain safety.

The nature of the evaluation is determined by the question being asked, but the following general points are helpful when interviewing any patient in custody:

- Set the frame with the patient, which involves notifying the patient of his or her right to confidentiality and explaining the purpose of the assessment. Patients under arrest may refuse to answer questions out of concern that records can be subpoenaed, which can indeed occur.
- Clarify the evaluator's role and the parameters of the evaluation. An emergency evaluation for treatment should not have bearing on whether charges are pressed or dropped, and patients should understand the limits of the clinician's influence.
- Inform the patient not to make statements during the interview about his or her guilt or innocence regarding the charges, because the medical record could be subpoenaed.
- Document the interview thoroughly in the medical record, particularly noting the patient's risk of causing injury to self or others while in custody and any recommendations to the officers or the court for special precautions while the patient is in custody.

The Patient Who Does Not Speak English or Who Requires Sign Language Interpretation

All hospitals are required to provide interpretation services for patients who do not speak English or who are deaf or hard of hearing. For language interpretation, the best available option may be use of phone interpreter services, which can offer the widest range of languages. If ED staff speak the patient's language, they can also be useful, but they should have been trained and certified as fluent in the language used. It is *never* acceptable to rely entirely on a family member or friend who is accompanying the patient; this practice violates patient confidentiality and may prohibit the patient from making a full and honest accounting of his or her situation. If absolutely no other option is available, then it is better to at least get some information from the friend or family member, but more appropriate alternatives should be sought. Hospitals have been and can be sued for not providing appropriate language interpretation services or interpreter services for people who are deaf and hard of hearing. Sign language interpretation via video relay may be an option that is more readily available, particularly for after-hours assessments.

The Pregnant Patient

Pregnancy should be suspected in women of reproductive age until proved otherwise by laboratory testing. The range of what is considered reproductive age is vast, so liberal use of β-human chorionic gonadotropin testing is advised to avoid missing a pregnancy.

Safety data on the use of psychiatric medication in pregnant patients are limited to case reports and population surveillance; therefore, more data are available about older medications (Menon 2008). According to the American College of Obstetricians and Gynecologists (ACOG Committee on Practice Bulletins—Obstetrics 2008), it is better practice to treat pregnant women for their psychiatric problems with medication, if indicated, than to not treat, because the risk of teratogenicity due to psychiatric medication is smaller than the known risk of low birth weight and other complications from having an untreated psychiatric illness during pregnancy. In the ED, discovery of a pregnancy can influence multiple areas of the patient's psychiatric care but should not preclude appropriate treatment, including treatment of agitation if indicated (Ladavac et al. 2007).

For many women, discovery of a pregnancy may be an unexpected or unpleasant surprise and therefore may complicate whatever crisis brought them into the ED in the first place. The following are considerations for the pregnant psychiatric patient in the ED:

* *Disposition planning.* Concerns include providing obstetric gynecological care as part of discharge planning, increased risk of suicide after discovery of an unplanned pregnancy, and referral to appropriate services.

- *Pharmacotherapy.* The clinician should make an informed choice of psychotropic medication based on risks and benefits, clearly document the thought process involved in either prescribing or refraining from prescribing medication, and document the discussion of these risks and benefits with the patient.
- *Restraint.* Safe restraint becomes more complicated as a pregnancy progresses and should be avoided if possible. Patients in advanced stages of pregnancy should not be restrained on their back due to compromised blood flow through the vena cava.

The legal and ethical issues surrounding pregnancy in psychiatric patients are complicated. Patients with psychosis or severe psychiatric illness do not automatically surrender their right to reproductive choices, including choosing to terminate or continue a pregnancy, choosing to use or not use contraception, and so forth. The most appropriate option for dealing with pregnancy in the psychiatric patient is to treat the patient first, because optimizing her physical and psychiatric health allows the patient to be in the best position to make decisions regarding her pregnancy and overall health.

Disposition

In most systems, there are essentially two disposition options: admission to an inpatient psychiatric unit or discharge to outpatient care. Some systems have worked toward developing alternatives such as crisis respite centers, facilitating referral to sober living or substance abuse residential treatment, or short-term crisis center stabilization. Depending on the medical system, the clinician performing the mental health evaluation may be responsible for recommending and/or facilitating the disposition merited by the patient's condition.

Disposition to inpatient treatment may involve transfer from the ED to a medical ward, to a psychiatric ward, or to a ward with hybrid medical-psychiatric expertise. In general, ED providers will feel comfortable with the steps needed to transfer the patient to a medical ward. However, the mental health clinician may be needed to provide recommendations for initial workup and management of the patient's mental health condition and, as needed, to assist with ensuring ongoing mental health comanagement on arrival to the medical ward. For example, the mental health clinician may be asked for medication recommendations to manage agitation in delirium. Clear documentation will help facilitate a clean handoff of the patient to the next set of treatment providers.

Disposition to inpatient psychiatry or a hybrid ward may be more complicated in certain systems of medical care. Some EDs are attached to hospitals with these services. Other EDs may have no access to such services, and patients in need may have to transfer elsewhere to receive the inpatient care they need. Even hospitals with inpatient psychiatric services can fill up, and transfer will be required. Depending on the system of medical care, the mental health clinician performing the ED evaluation may also be required to investigate local hospitals for available inpatient resources, contact health insurance or other third-party payers to obtain permission to transfer the patient to an available ward, and/or contact the receiving hospital to secure authorization for admission to the psychiatry ward. This process can take time, contributing to boarding delays in the ED. The mental health clinician may also be responsible for comanagement of the boarded patient in the ED, including ongoing management of the patient's mental health conditions, provision for basic needs such as food and grooming, and ensuring that the patient does not abscond in the process. At times, the patient's presenting mental health crisis, such as psychosis induced by cocaine intoxication, may resolve during the boarding period. Therefore, the mental health clinician should also perform periodic reevaluation of the patient with regard to ongoing need for hospitalization and document findings accordingly. There may be pressure from medical ED providers to alleviate crowding, and trainees in particular should be carefully supervised around liaising with the ED in these cases. In high-volume systems, the availability of a short-term stabilization unit can help unburden the ED by providing treatment and disposition for patients expected to stabilize quickly, while saving scarce inpatient beds for those most likely to require a longer period of hospitalization. Hospitals that utilize mobile crisis teams may be able to provide support in the community and bridging treatment that can also provide a way to safely defer inpatient admission.

Disposition to outpatient treatment will require some thought from the mental health clinician about how to keep the patient stable until the case can be picked up by the outpatient providers. In some circumstances, this will be easy, as in the case of a patient who is already well established with an outpatient provider and has a prescheduled appointment in the coming few days. In this circumstance, the mental health clinician will only have to consider how to temporarily resolve the presenting crisis. Did the patient present because he was out of medications? If so, it may be appropriate to prescribe a small bridging supply of medications to cover until the outpatient appointment. Did the patient present because of a life stressor contributing to suicidal thoughts that have since resolved? If so, then the mental health clinician may brainstorm solutions to the crisis with the patient and consider developing a temporary suicide safety plan with the patient to keep her safe until the follow-up appointment. If a patient seen in the ED already has established outpatient care, notifying that provider of the ED visit is essential to effective coordination of care. Every effort should be made to contact and conference with the outpatient provider prior to determining a disposition and course of action.

When outpatient care is not readily available—whether due to insurance issues, wait times for appointments, or lack of availability of a specific type of care (e.g., dual-diagnosis programs, dialectical behavior therapy or partial hospital programs)—disposition becomes more complicated. In creating a disposition plan, the clinician should take into account the patient's available resources, including social support, housing, financial resources to pay for care or prescriptions, and accessibility of the recommended treatment. At times, inpatient admission is unavoidable when adequate support or a high enough level of outpatient care is not immediately available.

Needless to say, availability of rapid follow-up provides for lower-risk discharges, and some hospital systems have developed techniques for providing short-term follow-up until a connection can be made with someone who will serve as the patient's ongoing outpatient treater. These techniques include centralized scheduling available through the ED, telephone or postcard follow-up from the ED to help the patient stay on track, and bridging appointments in the ED. As mentioned earlier in this chapter (see "A General Approach to the Emergency Psychiatric Patient"), some EDs have access to a comprehensive psychiatric emergency program, which can provide temporary wrap-around services to help patients through crises and avoid inpatient treatment.

At times, disposition is the most challenging piece of an ED encounter. Nevertheless, safe disposition is necessary to ensure that the process for nuanced assessment is more than an academic exercise. The best advice is to work with what the medical system gives and keep track of ways in which the medical system can be improved so that each patient encounter gives an opportunity to improve both the patient's crisis and the approach to future crises of similar patients.

Conclusion

Emergency psychiatry is a developing field, providing an opportunity for exposure to a vast array of patients and situations. Clinicians in this practice need to have skills in consultation-liaison psychiatry, crisis management, brief psychotherapy, and risk assessment, as well as a broad knowledge of medicine, hospital and health care systems, and general psychiatry. To best direct the care of patients, the mental health clinician working in the ED must view patients as individuals, as part of their social environment, and as part of the health care system.

Key Clinical Points

- Clinicians should consider their personal safety first. Clinicians should be aware of the protocols in the emergency department in which they are working, the environment in which they will be seeing patients, and patient factors that may lead to violent escalation.

- Assessment should focus on the patient's safety. Critical questions to consider are whether the patient's presentation is due to a medical condition better treated by a different clinician and whether the patient can adequately maintain his or her safety and the safety of others in the current outpatient setting.

- All emergency department encounters should be documented in the medical record, with sufficient detail that the reader of the documentation can understand the factors that went into the assessment and disposition of the patient.

References

Abello A Jr, Brieger B, Dear K, et al: Care plan program reduces the number of visits for challenging psychiatric patients in the ED. Am J Emerg Med 30(7):1061–1067, 2012 22030183

ACOG Committee on Practice Bulletins—Obstetrics: ACOG Practice Bulletin: Clinical management guidelines for obstetrician-gynecologists number 92, April 2008 (replaces practice bulletin number 87, November 2007). Use of psychiatric medications during pregnancy and lactation. Obstet Gynecol 111(4):1001–1020, 2008 18378767

Allen MA, Forster P, Zealberg J, et al: American Psychiatric Association Task Force on Psychiatric Emergency Services: Report and recommendations regarding psychiatric emergency and crisis services: a review and model program descriptions. August 2002. Available at: http://www.psychiatry.org/File%20Library/Learn/Archives/tfr2002_EmergencyCrisis.pdf. Accessed March 17, 2015.

Baillargeon J, Thomas CR, Williams B, et al: Medical emergency department utilization patterns among uninsured patients with psychiatric disorders. Psychiatr Serv 59(7):808–811, 2008 18587001

Brown JF: Emergency department psychiatric consultation arrangements. Health Care Manage Rev 30(3):251–261, 2005 16093891

Centers for Disease Control and Prevention: Revised Recommendations for HIV Testing of Adults, Adolescents, and Pregnant Women in Health-Care Settings. MMWR Morbidity and Mortality Weekly Report Recommendations and Reports (Vol 55, No RR14), September 22, 2006. Available at: http://www.cdc.gov/mmwr/PDF/rr/rr5514.pdf. Accessed December 18, 2014.

Creswell J: ER costs for mentally ill soar, hospitals seek better way. New York Times, December 2, 2013. Available at: http://www.nytimes.com/2013/12/26/health/er-costs-for-mentally-ill-soar-and-hospitals-seek-better-way.html?pagewanted=all&_r=0. Accessed December 18, 2014.

Flannery RB Jr: Precipitants to psychiatric patient assaults: review of findings, 2004–2006, with implications for EMS and other health care providers. Int J Emerg Ment Health 9(1):5–11, 2007 17523371

Guze BH, Love MJ: Medical assessment and laboratory testing in psychiatry, in Kaplan and Sadock's Comprehensive Textbook of Psychiatry. Edited by Sadock BJ, Sadock VA. Philadelphia, PA, Lippincott Williams & Wilkins, 2004, pp 916–928

Jacobs DG, Baldessarini RJ, Conwell Y, et al; American Psychiatric Association Work Group on Suicidal Behaviors: Practice guideline for the assessment and treatment of patients with suicidal behaviors. Washington, DC, American Psychiatric Association, 2003

LaCalle E, Rabin E: Frequent users of emergency departments: the myths, the data and the policy implications. Ann Emerg Med 56(1):42–48, 2010

Ladavac AS, Dubin WR, Ning A, et al: Emergency management of agitation in pregnancy. Gen Hosp Psychiatry 29(1):39–41, 2007 17189743

Manley M: Interviewing techniques with the difficult patient, in Kaplan and Sadock's Comprehensive Textbook of Psychiatry. Edited by Sadock BJ, Sadock VA. Philadelphia, PA, Lippincott Williams & Wilkins, 2004, pp 904–907

Meara E, Golberstein E, Zaha R, et al: Use of hospital-based services among young adults with behavioral health diagnoses before and after health insurance expansions. JAMA Psychiatry 71(4):404–411, 2014 24554245

Menon SJ: Psychotropic medication during pregnancy and lactation. Arch Gynecol Obstet 277(1):1–13, 2008 17710428

Richmond JS, Berlin JS, Fishkind AB, et al: Verbal de-escalation of the agitated patient: consensus statement of the American Association for Emergency Psychiatry Project BETA De-escalation Workgroup. West J Emerg Med 13(1):17–25, 2012 22461917

U.S. Department of Health and Human Services: Health information privacy: When does the privacy rule allow covered entities to disclose protected health information to law enforcement officials? July 23, 2004. Available at: http://www.hhs.gov/ocr/privacy/hipaa/faq/disclosures_for_law_enforcement_purposes/505.html. Accessed March 17, 2015.

U.S. Department of Health and Human Services Office for Civil Rights: Bulletin: HIPAA privacy in emergency situations. November 2014. Available at: http://www.hhs.gov/ocr/privacy/hipaa/understanding/special/emergency/emergency-situations.pdf. Accessed March 17, 2015.

Vergare M, Binder R, Cook I, et al.; Work Group on Psychiatric Evaluation: Practice guideline for the psychiatric evaluation of adults, 2nd edition. June 2006. Available at: http://psychiatryonline.org/pb/assets/raw/sitewide/practice_guidelines/guidelines/psychevaladults.pdf. Accessed March 17, 2015.

Walsh PG, Currier G, Shah MN, et al: Psychiatric emergency services for the U.S. elderly: 2008 and beyond. Am J Geriatr Psychiatry 16(9):706–717, 2008 18757766

Woo BK, Chan VT, Ghobrial N, et al: Comparison of two models for delivery of services in psychiatric emergencies. Gen Hosp Psychiatry 29(6):489–491, 2007 18022041

Zun LS: Evidence-based evaluation of psychiatric patients. J Emerg Med 28(1):35–39, 2005 15657002

Suggested Readings

Allen MA, Forster P, Zealberg J, et al: American Psychiatric Association Task Force on Psychiatric Emergency Services: Report and recommendations regarding psychiatric emergency and crisis services: a review and model program descriptions. August 2002. Available at: http://www.psychiatry.org/File%20Library/Learn/Archives/tfr2002_EmergencyCrisis.pdf. Accessed March 17, 2015.

Dubin WR, Lion JR (eds): Clinician Safety (APA Task Force Report 33). Washington, DC, American Psychiatric Association, 1993

Manley M: Interviewing techniques with the difficult patient, in Kaplan and Sadock's Comprehensive Textbook of Psychiatry. Edited by Sadock BJ, Sadock VA. Philadelphia, PA, Lippincott Williams & Wilkins, 2004, pp 904–907

2

Suicide Risk Assessment and Management

José R. Maldonado, M.D., F.A.P.M., F.A.C.F.E.

Renee Garcia, M.D.

Epidemiology

One of the most important and difficult tasks in emergency psychiatry is the assessment and management of suicide. The term *suicide* means a fatal self-inflicted destructive act with explicit or inferred intent to die.

According to the World Health Organization (2014), global suicide rates have increased 60% over the past 45 years, and now more than 800,000 people die from suicide every year—roughly one death every 40 seconds. It is estimated that there are 10–40 nonfatal suicide attempts for every completed suicide among adults 18 years and older in the United States, and this figure is even higher among youth ages 15–24 years, for whom estimates indicate 100–200 attempts for every completed suicide (Centers for Disease Control and Prevention 2012a). In 2009, the number of deaths from suicide surpassed the number of deaths from motor vehicle crashes in the United States (Rockett et al. 2012). Current global estimates indicate that 650,000 people per year receive emergency treatment after a suicide attempt (World Health Organization 2014).

Suicide rates vary based on factors such as race/ethnicity, gender, and age (Figure 2–1) (Centers for Disease Control and Prevention 2011a; National Institute of Mental Health 2009). The statistics in the United States are staggering. In 2012, suicide was the tenth leading cause of death for all age groups, the third among people ages 15–24 years, the second among people ages 25–34 years, the fourth among people ages 35–54 years, and the eighth among people ages 55–64 years (Centers for Disease Control and Prevention 2012a). Each year since 2001, more than 30,000 people have died by suicide in the United States (0.01% of population) (Centers for Disease Control and Prevention 2012b). The latest estimates for the United States indicate that 38,364 suicides occurred in 2010, which averages out to 105 suicides each day (Centers for Disease Control and Prevention 2012a). That number is more than twice the number of patients who die as a result of complications related to HIV/AIDS, and suicides now outnumber homicides by three to two (Centers for Disease Control and Prevention 2012b). In the United States, suicide is estimated to cost $34.6 billion per year in lost income alone (Centers for Disease Control and Prevention 2012b).

Psychoneurobiology of Suicide

Genetic Influences

Studies have demonstrated that a family history of suicide increases an individual's risk of suicide (Roy 1983; Wender et al. 1986), even independent of psychiatric diagnosis (Brent et al. 1988).

Biological and Neurochemical Influences

Serotonin transmission is thought to be deficient in suicidal depressed patients. First, cerebrospinal fluid serotonin precursor concentrations have been observed to be lower in suicidal depressed patients compared with nonsuicidal depressed patients (Bellivier et al. 2000; Mann et al. 1996). Additionally, the ventrolateral subnucleus of the dorsal raphe nucleus is known to have serotonin 1A receptors, but some postmortem studies of depressed suicidal in-

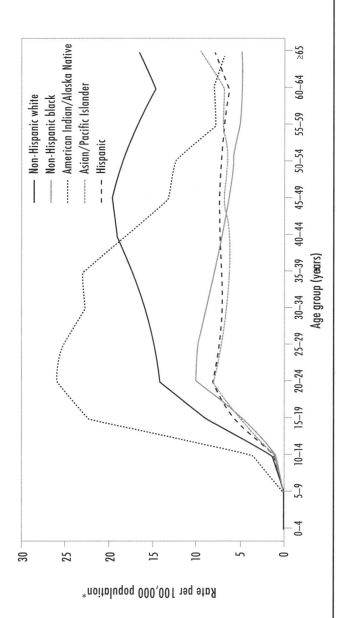

Figure 2–1.   Suicide rates, by race/ethnicity and age group—United States, National Vital Statistics System, 1999–2007. *Unadjusted (crude) death rates per 100,000 population.

Source.   Reprinted from Centers for Disease Control and Prevention: "Health Disparities and Inequalities Report—United States, 2011." *MMWR Morbidity and Mortality Weekly Report* 60 (Suppl):56–59, January 14, 2011. Available at: http://www.cdc.gov/mmwr/pdf/other/su6001.pdf. Accessed May 18, 2015.

dividuals have demonstrated decreased activity in the dorsal raphe nucleus (Stockmeier 1997). This finding indicates that the severity of serotonin deficiency is more pronounced in individuals who make planned, highly lethal attempts (Gos et al. 2007).

In contrast, other research suggests that compared with control subjects without psychiatric disorders, suicide victims have an increased number of serotonergic neurons (Underwood et al. 1999). For example, the activity of dorsal raphe neurons in suicide completers has been found to be at least the same as in nonpsychiatric controls or higher than in nonsuicidal deceased people with mood disorders (Bielau et al. 2005). Because up to 70% of the human dorsal raphe neurons are serotonergic, this result clearly challenges the assumption of a hypoactive serotonergic system in individuals with affective illness *who kill themselves*. This hypothesis does not negate the long-standing belief that depressed patients may indeed experience a serotonin deficit but instead suggests that the subset of patients who experience increased activation of the serotonergic system may be at higher risk of suicide attempts (Bielau et al. 2005). Most postmortem studies have been conducted in depressed patients who were receiving treatment with antidepressant agents, which may be associated with increased serotonin levels. Despite the likelihood that medication-induced activation of serotonergic neurons will over the long term have beneficial effects on the course of affective illness in the majority of depressed patients, it is conceivable that the medication's serotonergic activation may in the short term contribute to an increased risk of suicidal behavior in a subgroup of mood disorder patients. If this hypothesis were true, it could explain why it is difficult to determine the effect of antidepressants on suicide completion. Finally, some studies suggest that suicidality may be associated with altered cell plasticity in key frontolimbic areas, implicating multiple neuromodulatory systems (e.g., GABAergic, serotonergic, noradrenergic, and glutamatergic pathways) (Ernst et al. 2009; Hercher et al. 2009).

Life Events

Various life events have been identified as affecting the threshold for suicidal behavior. These include marital isolation (Crawford et al. 2010), parental loss through death before age 11 years (You et al. 2014), and a childhood history of physical and sexual abuse (Turecki et al. 2012).

Hopelessness

Studies have found that hopelessness is a key variable linking depression to suicidal behavior (Beck 1986) and is a predictor of completed suicide (Fawcett et al. 1987). In separate studies over a 10-year period, hopelessness and pessimism were the factors that best predicted suicide risk in patients admitted with major depressive disorder (Beck et al. 1985; Bulik et al. 1990; Galfalvy et al. 2006).

Low Self-Esteem

A variable closely related to hopelessness is low self-esteem. Among patients with recurrent major depressive disorder but without personality disorders, patients who reported "feeling like a failure" were significantly more likely to have made a suicide attempt (Bulik et al. 1990).

Clinical and Comorbidity Influences

Comorbid conditions that increase the risk of attempted suicide include alcohol abuse, substance abuse, and Cluster B personality disorders (Cornelius et al. 1995). Of note, patients with comorbid major depression and borderline personality disorder were more likely to make multiple suicide attempts, and those attempts were no less medically damaging than were those of depressed patients without borderline personality disorder (Corbitt et al. 1996).

Presentation

Four types of suicide cases are commonly encountered in the emergency department (ED):

1. Patients who report suicidal ideation
2. Patients who just survived a suicide attempt
3. Patients presenting with other, usually somatic complaints but in whom suicidal thoughts are discovered during a comprehensive evaluation
4. Patients who deny suicidal ideation but whose behavior (or family's report) suggests suicidal potential or risk

Foreseeability of Suicide

The concept of *imminent suicide* imposes an illusory time frame on an unpredictable act (Pokorny 1983). Suicide is typically impulsive in nature. As such, many patients remain uncertain to the last moment, with little premeditation, and are often ambivalent about dying (Cornelius et al. 1996). Following interviews with survivors of jumps off the Golden Gate Bridge, Friend (2003) reported that "survivors often regret their decision in midair, if not before" (p. 50). However, when patients do make the final decision to act on their suicidal plans, they may wait for an opportune time to act (e.g., when spouse or family members are absent).

According to Pokorny (1983), clinicians' attempts to identify specific subjects who will eventually commit suicide have been mostly unsuccessful, despite the use of individual assessment items, factor scores, and a series of discriminant functions. Pokorny concluded that "although we may reconstruct causal chains and motives after the fact, we do not possess the tools to predict particular suicides before the fact" (p. 257). No short-term risk factors have been identified to determine when, or even if, a patient will attempt or complete suicide (Simon 2006). In fact, commonly used criteria for approving hospitalization for potentially suicidal patients have not proved predictive of future attempts (Hall et al. 1999). For example, contrary to common belief, the presence of a suicide note or of a specific plan has not been associated with the seriousness of the current suicide attempt or the severity of future attempts (Hall et al. 1999).

Risk Factors

It is essential that an adequate, individualized suicide assessment be performed so that the clinician is able identify, treat, and manage acute, patient-specific risk factors (Simon 2006). Table 2–1 summarizes factors associated with an increased risk of suicide. Even though risk factors are not predictive, they are still positively correlated with subsequent suicide attempts and/or completion. Clinicians need to recognize the utility and limitations of the available risk assessments and understand that although clinicians cannot foresee whether a patient will commit suicide, they can identify risk factors known to be associated with increased risk of suicide.

Table 2–1. Factors associated with an increased risk of suicide

History of previous suicide attempts or threats

The strongest single factor predictive of suicide is prior history of attempted suicide.

Psychiatric disorders

Psychiatric illness is a strong predictor of suicide.

More than 90% of suicide attempters and 95% of suicide completers have a mental disorder.

Severity of the psychiatric illness is associated with suicide risk.

The psychiatric disorders most commonly associated with suicide include depression, bipolar disorder, alcoholism or other substance-related disorders, schizophrenia, personality disorders, anxiety disorders, and delirium.

Co-occurrence of an anxiety disorder (either primary or comorbid) with any other psychiatric disorder increases (two times) the risk of suicide attempts. The risk is highest with comorbid depression and anxiety.

Symptoms of psychosis (delusions, command auditory hallucinations, paranoia) may increase suicide risk regardless of diagnosis.

Hopelessness and impulsivity

These symptoms are strongly associated with suicide.

Adverse childhood experiences

Both childhood abuse and other adverse childhood experiences appear to increase the risk of suicide in adults.

Family history and genetics

The risk of suicide increases in patients with a family history of suicide.

Age, gender, and race/ethnicity

The risk of suicide increases with age; however, young adults attempt suicide more often than do older adults.

Females attempt suicide three times more frequently than males, but males die by suicide four times more often and represent 79% of all U.S. suicides.

American Indians/Alaska Natives and non-Hispanic whites have the highest suicide rates among ethnic groups in the United States, followed by Asian/Pacific Islanders, Hispanics, and non-Hispanic blacks.

Rates of attempted suicide are higher among young Hispanic females compared with young black or white females.

Suicide is the second leading cause of death among American Indians/Alaska Natives ages 15–34 years (2.5 times higher than national average).

Table 2–1. Factors associated with an increased risk of suicide *(continued)*

Marital status

The highest suicide risk occurs among those never married, followed in descending order of risk by widowed, separated, or divorced; married without children; and married with children.

Occupation

Unemployed and unskilled patients are at higher risk for suicide than are those who are employed and skilled.

Health status

Suicide risk increases with physical illness such as chronic pain, recent surgery, and chronic or terminal disease.

Antidepressant medication use

These medications potentially increase the risk of suicide (see Table 2–2).

History of violence

A history of violence against others predicts violence against self.

Other factors

The risk of suicide increases with accessibility to weapons, especially firearms.

Risk also increases in patients who live alone, have lost a loved one, or have experienced a failed relationship within 1 year.

The anniversary of a significant relationship loss is also a time of increased risk.

Previous Attempts

The most important predictor of a suicide attempt is a personal past history of a suicide attempt. The acute suicide risk in patients with mood disorders has been reported to be 12% in those who have had a previous attempt compared with 2% in those without a prior suicide attempt, and the long-term risk is 15% in previous attempters compared with 5% in nonattempters (Nordström et al. 1995). Among individuals who died by suicide, 19.8% had a history of prior attempts, 28.3% disclosed their intent before dying, and 33.1% left a suicide note (Goldsmith et al. 2002). Following a suicide attempt, the risk of another attempt in the next year is 12%–30%, whereas the risk of completed suicide is 1%–3% (Vaiva et al. 2006). In general, suicide attempts predict a 10%–30% risk of suicide occurrence over 10 years (Fawcett 2001).

Mental Illness

Almost all psychiatric disorders are associated with an increased risk of suicide (Goldsmith et al. 2002), and more than 90% of suicides in the United States are associated with mental illness (Mościcki 2001). The severity of psychiatric illness is also associated with risk of suicide (Claassen et al. 2007).

- *Depressive disorders:* Of individuals who completed suicide, 30%–90% had depressive disorders (Lönnqvist 2000). The incidence of completed suicide in major depression has been estimated at 15% (Guze and Robins 1970). The first 3 months after onset of a major depressive episode and the first 5 years after the lifetime onset of a depressive disorder represented the highest risk periods for attempted suicide (Malone et al. 1995). The lifetime prevalence of nonfatal suicide attempts has been estimated at 3%–5% in the general U.S. population and as high as 16% in community samples with a diagnosis of major depressive disorder (Claassen et al. 2007). Over one-third of patients who receive treatment in the ED for a suicide attempt carry a diagnosis of major depressive disorder at the time of the attempt (Claassen et al. 2007).
- *Bipolar disorder:* Five percent of individuals who completed suicide had bipolar disorder (Lönnqvist 2000).
- *Anxiety disorders:* The presence of anxiety symptoms (not necessarily a disorder) is associated with a twofold increase in likelihood of reporting suicidality (Diefenbach et al. 2009; Thibodeau et al. 2013). Up to 79% of patients reported severe anxiety and/or agitation in the week before suicide (Busch et al. 2003). Anxiety is an immediate risk factor that is potentially modifiable (Fawcett 2001).
- *Psychosis:* Estimates are that 5%–13% of patients with schizophrenia commit suicide (Altamura et al. 2007). Suicide attempts by patients with schizophrenia are more likely to be lethal and violent (Altamura et al. 2007).
- *Personality disorders:* Although suicidal behavior is a more persistent feature among patients with personality disorders, their clinical characteristics at the time of a suicide attempt may not differ from those of individuals without personality disorders (Suominen et al. 2000).

- *Substance use disorders:* Substance abuse, either as a primary disorder or as a comorbid condition with another psychiatric disorder, increases the risk of attempted and completed suicide (Szanto et al. 2007). A family history of alcoholism is associated with an increased risk of suicidality; in fact, there is a familial clustering of alcoholism, depression, and suicide (Makhija and Sher 2007). Most subjects reported drinking more heavily than usual on the day of their suicide attempt. Recent suicidal behavior is associated with recent heavy drinking (≥70 drinks per week) and with a greater number of drinks per drinking day (Cornelius et al. 1996). According to the National Violent Death Reporting System, 33.3% of suicide decedents tested positive for alcohol (i.e., blood alcohol level≥0.08 g/dL), 23.0% for antidepressants, and 20.8% for opiates (e.g., heroin and prescription opiates) (Centers for Disease Control and Prevention 2011b).
- *Violence:* Suicide threats and attempts were significantly associated with violence in both males and females with schizophrenia (Witt et al. 2014).
- *Multiple factors:* Baseline suicidal ideation has been associated with greater depressive severity, childhood neglect, childhood abuse, early major depressive disorder onset, greater psychiatric comorbidity, and worse functioning and quality of life (Zisook et al. 2009), implying that many individuals who attempt suicide are simultaneously subject to multiple risk factors.

Regardless of the increased risk of suicide in individuals with mental disorders, the clinician needs to remember that about 28%–30% of the U.S. population suffers from some form or mental disorder but that more than 95% of individuals with mental illness do not complete suicide (Ahmedani et al. 2014; Bakst et al. 2014; Conwell et al. 1996; Gray et al. 2014; Harris and Barraclough 1997; Lin et al. 2014; O'Hare et al. 2014; Page et al. 2014; Roberts and Lamont 2014).

Family History

The risk of suicide increases in patients with a family history of suicide (Qin et al. 2002). In fact, having a first-degree relative who committed suicide increases the risk sixfold (Goldsmith et al. 2002).

Age

The prevalence of suicidal thoughts, planning, and attempts is higher among individuals ages 18–29 years than among older individuals (Centers for Disease Control and Prevention 2011b). Suicide accounts for 20% of all deaths annually among individuals ages 15–24 years (Centers for Disease Control and Prevention 2012a). In a 2011 nationally representative sample of ninth through twelfth graders, 15.8% reported that they had seriously considered attempting suicide during the 12 months preceding the survey; 12.8% reported that they had made a plan about how they would attempt suicide; 7.8% reported that they had attempted suicide one or more times; and 2.4% reported that they had made a suicide attempt that resulted in an injury, poisoning, or an overdose that required medical attention (Centers for Disease Control and Prevention 2012c). Suicide rates are highest for females ages 45–54 years and for males ages 75 years and older (Centers for Disease Control and Prevention 2012a).

Gender

Males are four times more likely to complete suicide than females and represent 79% of suicides in the United States (Centers for Disease Control and Prevention 2012a, 2012b). Females, however, are more likely to have suicidal thoughts and attempts. Common themes among both genders include professional (15.9% male, 10.0% female), financial (14.0% male, 12.0% female), criminal-legal (10.6% male, 5.3% female), and intimate-partner (33.0% male, 25.0% female) problems (Centers for Disease Control and Prevention 2012b).

Race/Ethnicity

In 2007, American Indians/Alaska Natives (14.6%) and non-Hispanic whites (14.4%) had the highest suicide rates among ethnic groups in the United States. Rates among Asian/Pacific Islanders (6.2%), Hispanics (5.4%), and non-Hispanic blacks (5.1%) were much lower and were roughly equivalent (Centers for Disease Control and Prevention 2011a).

Among students in high school (i.e., grades 9–12), more Hispanic females (13.5%) than black females (8.8%) or white females (7.9%) reported attempting suicide in the past year (Centers for Disease Control and Prevention 2012c). The suicide rate among American Indians/Alaska Natives ages 15–34 years (31 per 100,000) is 2.5 times higher than the national average for that age group (12.2 per 100,000) (Centers for Disease Control and Prevention 2012a; see also Figure 2–1).

Suicide Method

The risk of completed suicide is three times greater among individuals with access to firearms than among individuals without available firearms (Anglemyer et al. 2014). Of suicides in the United States, firearms accounted for 51.8%, asphyxiation (e.g., hanging, strangulation, suffocation) for 24.7%, and poisoning for 17.2% (Centers for Disease Control and Prevention 2012b). Among males, the most commonly used method is a firearm (56.7%), followed by some form of asphyxiation (25.3%), whereas among females, poison (36.9%) is the method most often used, followed by firearms (33.8%) (Centers for Disease Control and Prevention 2012b, 2012c).

Social Factors

Intimate-partner problems (31.4%), a crisis in the preceding 2 weeks (26.6%), physical health problems (21.0%), professional problems (14.6%), or financial problems (13.8%) were most often encountered as acute stressors among individuals who died by suicide (Centers for Disease Control and Prevention 2012b; Heikkinen et al. 1995).

Marital Status

Married persons ages 25 years and older have the lowest rate of suicide, at 11.1 per 100,000 (U.S. Department of Health and Human Services 2014). Rates are 23.0, 30.8, and 32.1 per 100,000 population (age adjusted) for never married, divorced, and widowed persons, respectively (U.S. Department of Health and Human Services 2014).

Occupation

Individuals who are unemployed and unskilled are at higher risk of suicide than are those who are employed and skilled; also, a recent sense of failure may lead to higher risk (Platt 1984). Physicians may be at increased risk of suicide, with the rate of suicide among female physicians being higher than that among male physicians (Simon 2006). A 2004 analysis in *The American*

Journal of Psychiatry found that male doctors were 1.41 times more likely to commit suicide than other men; the statistic for female doctors was significantly higher (Schernhammer and Colditz 2004).

Health Status

Chronic physical illness has also been reported to contribute to suicide risk (Juurlink et al. 2004; Kontaxakis et al. 1988). Various medical conditions have been named as contributors to suicide, with high suicide prevalence rates among people with central nervous system disorders, such as Parkinson's disease (Kostić et al. 2010), Huntington's disease (Hubers et al. 2012), motor neuron disease (Bak et al. 1994), epilepsy (Andrijić et al 2014), and multiple sclerosis (Viner et al. 2014). Similarly, higher suicide rates have been described for other chronic or fatal illnesses, including cancer (Costantini et al. 2014; de la Grandmaison et al. 2014), chronic pain (Racine et al. 2014), fibromyalgia (Triñanes et al. 2015), and AIDS (Cooperman and Simoni 2005).

Geography

The suicide rate in metropolitan areas (11.5 per 100,000) is lower than that in nonmetropolitan areas (15.4 per 100,000) (U.S. Department of Health and Human Services 2014).

Media

News coverage has been shown to increase the likelihood of suicide in vulnerable individuals, with the magnitude of the increase being related to the amount, duration, and prominence of coverage. Additional risk is noted when news stories explicitly describe the suicide method and use dramatic or graphic headlines or images (National Institute of Mental Health 2012).

Antidepressant Medication Use

Some evidence suggests that antidepressant agents can, in rare instances, induce or exacerbate suicidal tendencies, and multiple clinical mechanisms have been proposed (Table 2–2) (Courtet et al. 2014; Teicher et al. 1993). One of the problems with the early treatment of depression is the time lag experienced between initiation of treatment and the time when the medication begins to impart its therapeutic effects; patients who already feel pessimistic about the possibility of getting better with medication are then faced with a period of no improvement. The additional burden of side effects may also lead to increased risk. Some researchers have found that during the first month of therapy, selective serotonin reuptake inhibitor (SSRI) antidepressants have been associated with a nearly fivefold higher risk of completed suicide than other antidepressants, and that suicides of a violent nature were distinctly more common during SSRI therapy (Courtet et al. 2014; Juurlink et al. 2006). Although some authors suggest that treatment-emergent suicidal ideation is associated with the severity of the depressive episode and a poor response to antidepressant treatment (Zisook et al. 2009), others suggest that the emergence of suicidality after initiation of antidepressant therapy may be a surrogate for the lack of improvement of depression (Courtet et al. 2014). Notably, even though the U.S. Food and Drug Administration (2009) has issued warnings about the possible increased risk of suicidal behavior in children, adolescents, and young adults taking antidepressants, subsequent studies have found a significant reduction in the risk of suicidal behavior when antidepressants are used judiciously (Leon et al. 2011; Seemüller et al. 2009; Stone et al. 2009). Similarly, other studies have found an age-dependent decline in suicide rates for depressed patients receiving antidepressant therapy. In fact, a 2% (3% for women) decline in suicide rate for those ages 80 and older has been found (Erlangsen and Conwell 2014). These findings heighten the need for the clinician to monitor the patient closely and to have an adequate rapport with the patient. Thus, it is important to balance the well-known beneficial effects of these agents on psychopathology (e.g., anxiety, panic, obsessive-compulsive symptoms) against potential adverse effects, including suicidal ideation and behavior.

Protective Factors

Factors that have been associated with a decreased risk of suicide include the following:

- Family cohesiveness
- Parenthood
- Pregnancy
- Religious affiliation
- Social support

Table 2–2.   Proposed mechanisms of antidepressant-related suicidality

Energizing depressed patients to act on preexisting suicidal ideation

Paradoxically worsening depressive symptoms

Inducing akathisia or incipient anxiety, worsening the patient's self-destructive or aggressive impulses

Inducing panic attacks

Causing medication-induced mania or switch into mania or mixed states, in patients with undiagnosed bipolar disorder

Interfering with the normal sleep-wake cycle, either by producing severe insomnia or by interfering with sleep architecture

Inducing obsessional or ruminative states

Leading to mental status changes, by exacerbating or inducing electroencephalographic changes or other neurological disturbances

Causing disinhibition and acting-out behavior

Causing an acute confusional state (e.g., delirium) as a result of excess medication or as an adverse effect (especially true of agents with high anticholinergic activity, or in combination with other agents)

Causing serotonin syndrome

Causing serotonin withdrawal states either in the case of nonadherent patients or when an inducer is added to the patient's pharmacological regimen (especially in the case of agents with a short half-life)

Increasing the level of frustration and hopelessness after a failed response to antidepressant treatment

Warning Signs

Suicide is associated with a tetrad of warning signs (Glickman 1981; Menninger 1985):

1. The wish to die (as a way to end suffering or facilitate a reunion with lost loved ones)
2. The wish to kill (the aim to cause the destruction of others, as well as oneself)
3. The wish to be killed (a form of reaction formation—i.e., "I don't hate you; you hate me")

4. The wish to be rescued (a sign of ambivalence; a desire to prove they are loved and desired)

The following signs are often present in suicidal patients. There may be an additional increase in risk if the behavior is new, if it has increased or worsened, or if it seems related to a painful event, loss, or change.

- Talking about wanting to die or to kill oneself
- Looking for a way to kill oneself (e.g., searching online suicide sites, buying a gun)
- Talking about feeling hopeless or having no reason to live
- Talking about feeling trapped or in unbearable pain (physical or emotional)
- Talking about being a burden to others
- Unwillingness to provide enough information for clinician to assess suicide risk
- Increasing use of alcohol or drugs
- Acting anxious or agitated
- Behaving recklessly
- Sleeping too little or too much
- Withdrawing or isolating oneself
- Showing rage or talking about seeking revenge
- Displaying extreme mood swings

Assessment

Although it is impossible to accurately predict suicide, it is clinically necessary to conduct an adequate suicide risk assessment. Clinically meaningful detection and treatment of suicidal patients most frequently occurs in the primary care setting or in the ED. A comprehensive assessment for suicidal behaviors or ideation should take into consideration the risk factors and warning signs listed in the preceding section. Table 2–3 lists the components of a suicide assessment. It is important to know that even though patients may be reluctant to discuss their suicidal ideation, they will generally respond truthfully, if asked (Michel 2000).

Table 2–3.   Components of a suicide assessment

1. Conduct a thorough psychiatric evaluation
    a. Identify specific psychiatric signs and symptoms
    b. Assess past suicidal behavior, including intent of self-injurious acts
    c. Review past treatment history and treatment relationships
    d. Identify familial history of suicide, mental illness, and dysfunction
    e. Identify current psychosocial situation and nature of crisis
    f. Identify patient's psychological strengths and vulnerabilities
2. Inquire about suicidal thoughts, plans, and behaviors
    a. Elicit the presence or absence of suicidal ideation
    b. Elicit the presence or absence of a suicide plan
    c. Assess the degree of suicidality, including suicidal intent and lethality of plan
    d. Understand the relevance and limitations of suicide assessment scales
3. Establish a diagnosis
4. Estimate the suicide risk
5. Develop and administer a treatment plan
6. Determine the most appropriate treatment setting
7. Provide education to patient and family
8. Monitor the patient's psychiatric status and response to treatment
9. Obtain consultation, if indicated
10. Reassess safety and suicide risk
11. Ensure adequate documentation and risk management
    a. Detail general risk management plan and document issues specific to suicide
    b. Limit the use of suicide contracts
    c. Communicate with pertinent parties, especially patients' clinicians and significant others
    d. Implement mental health interventions for surviving family and friends after suicide

Management

Not all suicides can be prevented, but many can by implementing a number of measures directed at identifying suicidal ideation and addressing the factors contributing to the patient's emotional distress. It is helpful to conceptualize suicide management strategies in terms of primary prevention, treatment interventions, and secondary prevention.

Primary Prevention

Psychoeducation and Training of Health Care Workers

Over 75% of patients who committed suicide had contact with primary care providers within the year of their death, but only one-third had contact with mental health services (Luoma et al. 2002). Therefore, caregivers should be trained in the recognition of conditions associated with high suicidal behavior, risk factors, warning signs, and basic knowledge of intervention modalities. This is particularly true of front-line care providers, such as primary care physicians and nurse practitioners, as well as emergency personnel and first responders. It is important to remember that about half of all suicide victims seek medical care in the 3 months prior to their death, yet only 12% received adequate doses of antidepressant medications (Isacsson et al. 1994). Educational programs for primary care physicians have been shown to increase antidepressant prescriptions and decrease suicide rates (Rihmer et al. 1995; Rutz et al. 1995).

Diagnosing and Treating People With Mental Disorders

A thorough history of current and past psychiatric symptoms is necessary for the purpose of identifying any existing psychiatric illnesses so that appropriate treatment and/or therapies can be initiated.

Addressing Substance Use Disorders

Management of substance abuse and alcoholism is pertinent to primary prevention of suicide.

Reducing Access to the Means of Suicide

Reduction of access to lethal methods (e.g., gun control or reduction of carbon monoxide content in natural gas) is of paramount importance. Clinicians can intervene by inquiring about the presence of firearms at home, as well as stored medications or other lethal substances, and these should be removed from the home. Multiple U.S. studies have demonstrated that access to firearms is associated with increased suicide risk (Harvard School of Public Health 2014) and that depressed and/or psychotic patients are more likely to attempt suicide with a firearm (Shenassa et al. 2000). According to the Centers for Disease Control and Prevention (2012b), 81,328 Americans died in gun suicides and accidents in the 4-year period between 2009 and 2012. Notably, 85% of attempted suicides with a gun result in fatalities versus 4% of attempted suicides by all other methods (Harvard School of Public Health 2014). To put matters in context, in 2010 there were 31,076 gun-related deaths in the United States; of these, 606 were unintentional shootings, 11,078 were homicides, and 19,392 were suicides (Law Center to Prevent Gun Violence 2012). It is important to remember that federal law categorically excludes some people with mental illness from accessing firearms and may require that physicians report those patients (Gun Control Act of 1968).

Treatment Interventions

Risk Reduction Through Hospitalization

Individuals at high risk of imminent suicide should be hospitalized.

1. Key issues regarding imminent suicide risk are intent and means, severity of psychiatric illness, the presence of psychosis or hopelessness, a lack of personal resources, and older age among men (Hirschfeld 2001).
2. Because interrupting a suicide has been proved effective, psychiatric holds are useful. The substantive criteria for civil commitment of a patient require the presence of a mental illness and dangerousness to self or others (Simon 2006). Legally, the term *gravely disabled* may be subsumed under dangerousness to self. A study that followed suicide attempters who were stopped from jumping off the Golden Gate Bridge (*N*=515) demonstrated that during the 25-year follow-up period, 94% of the would-be suicides were either still alive or had died of natural causes (Friend 2003; Hirschfeld 2001). A matched sample of nonbridge suicide attempters admitted to a local psychiatric hospital revealed a similar fate; at the end of the study, 89% of patients were still alive or had died of natural causes, 6%–11% had died of other violent causes, and only 5%–7% had died from suicide (Seiden 1978). These findings suggest that "suicidal behavior is crisis-oriented and acute in nature; if you can get a suicidal person through his crisis, chances are extremely good that he won't kill himself later" (Seiden 1978, p. 12), thus providing further support for the use of psychiatric holds.
3. The psychiatric hospitalization should allow for a more extended period of observation by trained personnel from the inpatient psychiatric multi-

disciplinary team and assist in achieving a more accurate diagnosis, which should help in designing a more definitive treatment plan.

4. Once hospitalized, the patient should be closely monitored, and reasonable precautions must be taken to ensure the patient's safety at all times, especially during the first few days (Hirschfeld 2001). One-to-one sitter supervision should be used, if needed, to ensure the patient's safety. This is particularly necessary in case the patient is admitted to a medical floor for stabilization after a suicide attempt. Table 2–4 presents recommendations for ensuring a patient's safety during the hospital admission.

5. Voluntary admission should first be offered, but if this is turned down, further assessment is required to determine the potential need for an involuntary hospitalization. Every state in United States has enacted legislation that allows for the involuntary hospitalization of any patient who has been deemed to be a danger to self (i.e., suicidal) or others (i.e., homicidal) or to be gravely disabled as a result of a mental illness (e.g., a mental disorder that renders the person unable to secure food, clothing, and shelter). Additional legal authorization for involuntary administration of psychotropic medications for patients refusing psychiatric treatment may be required.

Close Monitoring But No Hospitalization

When patients have elevated but not imminent suicide risk, they can be discharged home with close observation by family or friends.

1. This is not a viable option for patients who lack a support structure, those who are too unstable or psychotic, or those who have already exhibited dangerous or self-injurious behavior.

2. If a patient is to be discharged home, all potential lethal means must have been removed or secured. These include firearms, medications, and other potential methods to commit suicide.

3. Involvement of family, friends, or other support systems is imperative. This may include the patient's therapists or outpatient psychiatrist.

4. A patient's reluctance regarding clinical contact with care providers or support system is cause for concern and may highlight problems with safety. In this case, hospitalization may be necessary.

Table 2–4.   Important considerations in the management of suicidal patients

1.   A postsuicidal patient should be considered at extremely high suicide risk during the acute hospitalization. The following steps are recommended:

   a.   Initiate or continue involuntary psychiatric hold.

   b.   Initiate or continue 1:1 sitter supervision at all times, even when family members are visiting.

   c.   Never leave patient alone.

   d.   Maintain visual monitoring (e.g., "line of sight") at all times, even to go to the bathroom.

2.   Objects that may be used for self-harm should be removed from the room.

   a.   Do not provide sharp objects (e.g., metal or plastic forks or knifes) under any circumstances. If need be, cut patient's food and provide only a plastic spoon. Some patients may be provided only "finger food" (e.g., sandwich) due to risk of self-harm.

   b.   Remove all long and flexible objects that patients may use for harming themselves or others via strangulation, including call buttons, telephone cords, loose sheets, intravenous lines, shoe laces, and electrical cords.

3.   If possible, obtain collateral information from family members and clinicians.

4.   Ideally, transfer patient to room on the ground floor, where there is less risk of harm if patient were to jump out of a window.

5.   Provide close psychiatric follow-up:

   a.   Ensure appropriate hand-off of all suicidal and dangerous patients.

   b.   Conduct ongoing safety evaluation and close monitoring.

   c.   When patient is medically stable, transfer to an appropriate inpatient psychiatric facility for further assessment and treatment.

   d.   Directly communicate all recommendations and the importance of closely following them to the patient's primary medical team or emergency department physician, the unit nurse manager, and the patient's nurse.

5.   Despite the extensive use of safety contracts in clinical practice, there is little evidence that such contracts actually reduce suicide (Goldsmith et al. 2002). Clinically, a patient's agreement to "contract for safety" means little; however, a patient's unwillingness to "contract for safety" should be an indication that the patient may not be safe in an outpatient setting and that hospitalization may be necessary.

Initiating Pharmacotherapy if Indicated

Psychopharmacological treatment should be initiated (or restarted in nonadherent patients), especially in those with acute agitation or a newly identified mental disorder. It is important to educate the patient regarding the lag between medication initiation and symptom relief, the possibility of adverse effects, and the risk of sudden discontinuation of pharmacological agents (e.g., serotonin, benzodiazepines), as well as to advise the patient what to do if adverse drug reactions emerge.

Secondary Prevention

Identification of High-Risk Patients

Important risk factors are discussed in the "Risk Factors" section earlier in this chapter and summarized in Table 2–1.

Close Follow-Up and Ongoing Prevention of Suicide

Adequate treatment of any underlying psychiatric disorder through pharmacological agents, psychotherapy, and family interventions is essential. Patients should be discharged with a treatment plan, which includes appropriate referral for follow-up; close monitoring of mental status and response to pharmacological treatment, including potential adverse effects; and involvement of family members and/or significant others, if appropriate and with the patient's consent, to enhance the odds of treatment success. Regularly scheduled office visits may improve the patient's medication continuation by providing the opportunity for the clinician to monitor side effects, adjust doses as necessary, and discuss the rationale for continuing medication despite symptom improvement.

Development of a Suicide Prevention Action Plan

If the patient already has a suicide prevention action plan, the clinician should review it with the patient; if the patient does not yet have one, the clinician should assist the patient in starting to develop one. A number of suicide prevention plans are available that may serve as guides for the clinician in developing a plan (one example is in Table 2–5). The goal of this plan is to help guide the patient, or those within the patent's support structure, through difficult moments of crisis.

Table 2–5.   Suicide prevention plan of action

It is best to develop your safety plan with consultation from your mental health provider to ensure that all elements have been covered. He or she may also help you identify triggers and coping mechanisms and strategies. The basic components of the safety plan are as follows:

1. Develop a list of all the reasons why your life is worth living.

   a. It is difficult to create this list during a crisis, so prepare well in advance.

   b. Recruit the assistance of your therapist, family members, and other loved ones to create and perfect this list.

   c. Update as needed.

2. Be proactive about taking care of yourself and looking after your physical health.

   a. Exercise regularly, eat a well-balanced and nutritional diet, establish a regular sleep-wake cycle, and avoid mind-altering substances.

3. Seek help immediately if you are abusing any substances (e.g., alcohol, marijuana, cocaine, "speed," painkillers, benzodiazepines).

   a. You may need to discuss openly with your mental health professional, enter an inpatient treatment program, or seek an outpatient resource (such as Alcoholics Anonymous or Narcotics Anonymous).

   b. The use of substances may increase your risk of acting out in a time of crisis.

4. Develop a mental fitness plan.

   a. Consider meditation (e.g., mindfulness meditation), compassion training, self-hypnosis, and progressive relaxation.

5. Be aware of triggers and recognize your warning signs (e.g., personal situations, thoughts, images, thinking styles, mood, behavior) that usually signal a potential suicidal crisis.

6. Know your limits:

   a. Do not wait until you have reached that limit before taking appropriate action.

   b. Before you reach the "point of no return," walk away from stressful situations.

   c. Know when to ask for help.

   d. Know when it is best to be alone but also when it would be safer for you to be with others.

Table 2–5.   Suicide prevention plan of action *(continued)*

7. Protect yourself.

    a. Make your environment safe and as harm-proof as possible; no guns, knives, or other lethal weapons should be kept in your personal space.

    b. You may need to ask family members, friends, or even law enforcement to remove and safely store weapons.

    c. You should only keep the medications you need; do not hoard medications, because doing so creates too much of a temptation.

    d. Most suicide attempts are impulsive—the best defense against such behavior is to not have access to ways to harm yourself.

8. Develop a list of personal coping strategies and design a way to employ them without needing to contact another person.

    a. This list usually includes a predetermined set of activities that help patients take their minds off their problems and prevent suicidal ideation from escalating.

    b. Activities can be either physical (e.g., take a walk, exercise, do yoga, draw or paint, write in a journal) or mental (e.g., meditate, perform self-hypnosis, listen to music).

    c. Do not wait until the last minute to implement coping skills. It is always better to prevent than to try to remediate.

9. Develop a contact list of reliable external resources—that is, members of your personal support team whom you can call upon, if needed.

    a. Involve them if your personal coping strategies are not sufficient to assist you through a crisis.

    b. These people should include only individuals you know will be unconditionally supportive in a moment of need and may include, for example, family members, friends, neighbors, a life coach, members of a support group, or a 12-step program sponsor.

10. If your personal support team members are not available or helpful, consider escalating to the next level:

    a. Consider whether it may be prudent to go to the emergency room or local clinic.

    b. Recruit the assistance of your mental health team.

    c. Develop a list of available mental health professionals (e.g., counselor, case manager, therapist) and professional agencies (e.g., local mental health clinic, emergency department, crisis hotline) that could assist in a time of crisis.

    d. This list must be developed beforehand, and the contact numbers must be kept updated. The middle of a crisis is no time to try to figure out where or whom to call.

Table 2–5. Suicide prevention plan of action *(continued)*

11. Use your resources wisely.

    a. It is difficult for members of your support team to assist you if they do not know what is happening.

    b. Share the following with your support team members:

        i. The list of your contact numbers

        ii. A list of warning signs, to help them identify when you are in need of assistance

        iii. Your safety plan (with a list of members of your support team and mental health team)

        iv. The number of the National Suicide Prevention Lifeline (1-800-273-TALK [8255])

12. Your safety plan should be a living document.

    a. It should change, adapt, and grow with you.

    b. Regularly review and modify your safety plan as your circumstances change (e.g., you may need new contact numbers if you move to a different neighborhood or community).

    c. Take it seriously, but at the same time experiment and be creative—after all, we are talking about your life.

13. If everything else fails, call 911 or go to the nearest emergency room.

Provision of Contact Information

Important types of resources that can be provided to patients with current or a past history of suicidal ideation include outpatient mental health referrals and crisis/suicide hotline information. The National Suicide Prevention Lifeline is a toll-free number (1-800-273-TALK [8255]), available 24 hours a day, 7 days a week, that routes to the closest crisis center and is manned by trained crisis workers. The "Suicide-Related Resources" section at the end of this chapter provides additional information.

Psychoeducation

An educational campaign should be directed at patients, their families, and physicians, with the objective of improving the psychiatric (e.g., antidepressant, mood-stabilizing, and/or antipsychotic) treatment they are receiving.

Responsible Media Reporting

General public education programs as well as broader public health initiatives can be rather effective at decreasing suicide risk factors. Covering suicide carefully can change public misperceptions and correct myths, which can encourage help seeking by those who are vulnerable or at risk (National Institute of Mental Health 2012). Responsible media coverage would do the following:

1. Inform the audience without sensationalizing the suicide.
2. Use school, work, or family photographs, rather than graphic images of incidents.
3. Keep details of the suicide to a minimum.
4. Use the reporting opportunity to educate the population about the warning signs of impending suicide, provide tips as to what a person should do if he or she suspects that someone may be suicidal, and provide information regarding assistance (e.g., suicide hotline number, crisis intervention contact information).

Key Clinical Points

- Suicide risk assessment is one of the most important and difficult tasks in emergency psychiatry.

- The U.S. suicide rate for men was four times higher than the rate for women.

- The majority of suicides completed in the United States are accomplished with firearms.

- Although early identification of presuicidal patients is possible, the data indicate that recognition, management, and treatment are suboptimal.

- More than 75% of patients who committed suicide had contact with primary care providers within the year of their death. Despite some reluctance, most patients will generally tell their physicians about suicidality, if asked.

- Suicide risk assessments include a determination of the degree of suicidal ideation, with special attention to the presence of hopelessness, impulsivity, ideation, plan, and intent.

- Major risk factors for suicide include a prior suicide attempt, a family history of suicide, and the presence of a psychiatric disorder, hopelessness, impulsivity, or an alcohol or other substance use disorder.

- The strongest single factor predictive of suicide is prior history of attempted suicide.

- Hopelessness is strongly associated with suicide. Any patient who conveys a sense of hopelessness must be questioned about possible suicidality.

- No risk factor has adequate specificity or sensitivity for predicting suicide; however, all clinicians should be knowledgeable about the risk factors associated with suicide.

- Anxiety disorders more than double the risk of suicide attempts.

- All suicide threats should be taken seriously and considered to be deserving of a full suicide risk assessment.

References

Ahmedani BK, Simon GE, Stewart C, et al: Health care contacts in the year before suicide death. J Gen Intern Med 29(6):870–877, 2014 24567199

Altamura AC, Bobo WV, Meltzer HY: Factors affecting outcome in schizophrenia and their relevance for psychopharmacological treatment. Int Clin Psychopharmacol 22(5):249–267, 2007 17690594

Andrijić NL, Alajbegović A, Zec SL, et al: Suicidal ideation and thoughts of death in epilepsy patients. Psychiatr Danub 26(1):52–55, 2014 24608152

Anglemyer A, Horvath T, Rutherford G: The accessibility of firearms and risk for suicide and homicide victimization among household members: a systematic review and meta-analysis. Ann Intern Med 160(2):101–110, 2014 24592495

Bak S, Stenager EN, Stenager E, et al: Suicide in patients with motor neuron disease. Behav Neurol 7(3):181–184, 1994 24487334

Bakst S, Braun T, Hirshberg R, et al: Characteristics of suicide completers with a psychiatric diagnosis before death: a postmortem study of 98 cases. Psychiatry Res 220(1–2):556–563, 2014 25091231

Beck AT: Hopelessness as a predictor of eventual suicide. Ann N Y Acad Sci 487:90–96, 1986 3471167

Beck AT, Steer RA, Kovacs M, et al: Hopelessness and eventual suicide: a 10-year prospective study of patients hospitalized with suicidal ideation. Am J Psychiatry 142(5):559–563, 1985 3985195

Bellivier F, Szöke A, Henry C, et al: Possible association between serotonin transporter gene polymorphism and violent suicidal behavior in mood disorders. Biol Psychiatry 48(4):319–322, 2000 10960164

Bielau H, Mawrin C, Krell D, et al: Differences in activation of the dorsal raphe nucleus depending on performance of suicide. Brain Res 1039(1–2):43–52, 2005 15781045

Brent DA, Perper JA, Goldstein CE, et al: Risk factors for adolescent suicide: a comparison of adolescent suicide victims with suicidal inpatients. Arch Gen Psychiatry 45(6):581–588, 1988 3377645

Bulik CM, Carpenter LL, Kupfer DJ, et al: Features associated with suicide attempts in recurrent major depression. J Affect Disord 18(1):29–37, 1990 2136867

Busch KA, Fawcett J, Jacobs DG: Clinical correlates of inpatient suicide. J Clin Psychiatry 64(1):14–19, 2003 12590618

Centers for Disease Control and Prevention: Health disparities and inequalities report—United States, 2011. MMWR Morb Mortal Wkly Rep 60 (suppl):1–116, January 14, 2011a. Available at: http://www.cdc.gov/mmwr/pdf/other/su6001.pdf. Accessed May 18, 2015.

Centers for Disease Control and Prevention: Suicidal thoughts and behaviors among adults aged ≥18 years—United States, 2008–2009. MMWR Surveill Summ 60(No. SS-13):1–22, October 21, 2011b. Available at: http://www.cdc.gov/mmwr/preview/mmwrhtml/ss6013a1.htm?s_cid= ss6013a1_e. Accessed December 18, 2014.

Centers for Disease Control and Prevention: Suicide facts at a glance: 2012. 2012a. Available at: http://www.cdc.gov/violenceprevention/pdf/Suicide-DataSheet-a.pdf. Accessed December 18, 2014.

Centers for Disease Control and Prevention: Injury Prevention and Control; Data and Statistics (Web-based Injury Statistics Query and Reporting System [WISQARS])—National Violent Death Reporting System: Violent Deaths 2003–2012. 2012b. Available at: http://www.cdc.gov/injury/wisqars/nvdrs.html. Accessed December 18, 2014.

Centers for Disease Control and Prevention: Youth risk behavior surveillance—United States, 2011. MMWR Surveill Summ 61(No. SS-4):1–162, June 8, 2012c. Available at: http://www.cdc.gov/mmwr/pdf/ss/ss6104.pdf. Accessed December 18, 2014.

Centers for Disease Control and Prevention: Suicide among adults aged 35–64 years—United States, 1999–2010. MMWR Morb Mortal Wkly Rep 62(17):321–325, May 3, 2013. Available at: http://www.cdc.gov/mmwr/preview/mmwrhtml/mm6217a1.htm?s_cid=mm6217a1_w. Accessed December 18, 2014.

Claassen CA, Trivedi MH, Rush AJ, et al: Clinical differences among depressed patients with and without a history of suicide attempts: findings from the STAR*D trial. J Affect Disord 97(1-3):77–84, 2007 16824617

Conwell Y, Duberstein PR, Cox C, et al: Relationships of age and Axis I diagnoses in victims of completed suicide: a psychological autopsy study. Am J Psychiatry 153(8):1001–1008, 1996 8678167

Cooperman NA, Simoni JM: Suicidal ideation and attempted suicide among women living with HIV/AIDS. J Behav Med 28(2):149–156, 2005 15957570

Corbitt EM, Malone KM, Haas GL, et al: Suicidal behavior in patients with major depression and comorbid personality disorders. J Affect Disord 39(1):61–72, 1996 8835655

Cornelius JR, Salloum IM, Mezzich J, et al: Disproportionate suicidality in patients with comorbid major depression and alcoholism. Am J Psychiatry 152(3):358–364, 1995 7864260

Cornelius JR, Salloum IM, Day NL, et al: Patterns of suicidality and alcohol use in alcoholics with major depression. Alcohol Clin Exp Res 20(8):1451–1455, 1996 8947324

Costantini A, Pompili M, Innamorati M, et al: Psychiatric pathology and suicide risk in patients with cancer. J Psychosoc Oncol 32(4):383–395, 2014 24797891

Courtet P, Jaussent I, Lopez-Castroman J, et al: Poor response to antidepressants predicts new suicidal ideas and behavior in depressed outpatients. Eur Neuropsychopharmacol 24(10):1650–1658, 2014 25112546

Crawford MJ, Kuforiji B, Ghosh P: The impact of social context on socio-demographic risk factors for suicide: a synthesis of data from case-control studies. J Epidemiol Community Health 64(6):530–534, 2010 19828511

de la Grandmaison GL, Watier L, Cavard S, et al: Are suicide rates higher in the cancer population? An investigation using forensic autopsy data. Med Hypotheses 82(1):16–19, 2014 24257413

Diefenbach GJ, Woolley SB, Goethe JW: The association between self-reported anxiety symptoms and suicidality. J Nerv Ment Dis 197(2):92–97, 2009 19214043

Erlangsen A, Conwell Y: Age-related response to redeemed antidepressants measured by completed suicide in older adults: a nationwide cohort study. Am J Geriatr Psychiatry 22(1):25–33, 2014 23567434

Ernst C, Mechawar N, Turecki G: Suicide neurobiology. Prog Neurobiol 89(4):315–333, 2009 19766697

Fawcett J: Treating impulsivity and anxiety in the suicidal patient. Ann N Y Acad Sci 932:94–102, discussion 102–105, 2001 11411193

Fawcett J, Scheftner W, Clark D, et al: Clinical predictors of suicide in patients with major affective disorders: a controlled prospective study. Am J Psychiatry 144(1):35–40, 1987 3799837

Friend T: Jumpers: the fatal grandeur of the Golden Gate Bridge. The New Yorker, October 13, 2003, pp 48–59

Galfalvy H, Oquendo MA, Carballo JJ, et al: Clinical predictors of suicidal acts after major depression in bipolar disorder: a prospective study. Bipolar Disord 8(5 Pt 2):586–595, 2006 17042832

Glickman L: The phenomenon of suicide, in Understanding Human Behavior in Health and Illness. Edited by Simons RC, Pardes H. Baltimore, MD, Williams & Wilkins, 1981, pp 640–651

Goldsmith SK, Pellmar TC, Kleinman AM, et al (eds): Reducing Suicide: A National Imperative. Washington, DC, National Academies Press, 2002

Gos T, Krell D, Brisch R, et al: The changes of AgNOR parameters of anterior cingulate pyramidal neurons are region-specific in suicidal and non-suicidal depressive patients. World J Biol Psychiatry 8(4):245–255, 2007 17853258

Gray D, Coon H, McGlade E, et al: Comparative analysis of suicide, accidental, and undetermined cause of death classification. Suicide Life Threat Behav 44(3):304–316, 2014 25057525

Gun Control Act of 1968, Pub. L. No. 90-168 in 18 U.S.C.: Crimes and Criminal Procedure, 1968

Guze SB, Robins E: Suicide and primary affective disorders. Br J Psychiatry 117(539):437–438, 1970 5481206

Hall RC, Platt DE, Hall RC: Suicide risk assessment: a review of risk factors for suicide in 100 patients who made severe suicide attempts: evaluation of suicide risk in a time of managed care. Psychosomatics 40(1):18–27, 1999 9989117

Harris EC, Barraclough B: Suicide as an outcome for mental disorders: a meta-analysis. Br J Psychiatry 170:205–228, 1997 9229027

Harvard School of Public Health: Firearm access is a risk factor for suicide. Means Matter 2014. Available at: http://www.hsph.harvard.edu/means-matter/means-matter/risk. Accessed December 19, 2014.

Heikkinen ME, Isometsä ET, Marttunen MJ, et al: Social factors in suicide. Br J Psychiatry 167(6):747–753, 1995 8829741

Hercher C, Turecki G, Mechawar N: Through the looking glass: examining neuroanatomical evidence for cellular alterations in major depression. J Psychiatr Res 43(11):947–961, 2009 19233384

Hirschfeld RM: When to hospitalize patients at risk for suicide. Ann N Y Acad Sci 932:188–196, discussion 196–199, 2001 11411186

Hubers AA, Reedeker N, Giltay EJ, et al: Suicidality in Huntington's disease. J Affect Disord 136(3):550–557, 2012 22119091

Isacsson G, Bergman U, Rich CL: Antidepressants, depression and suicide: an analysis of the San Diego study. J Affect Disord 32(4):277–286, 1994 7897092

Juurlink DN, Herrmann N, Szalai JP, et al: Medical illness and the risk of suicide in the elderly. Arch Intern Med 164(11):1179–1184, 2004 15197042

Juurlink DN, Mamdani MM, Kopp A, et al: The risk of suicide with selective serotonin reuptake inhibitors in the elderly. Am J Psychiatry 163(5):813–821, 2006 16648321

Kontaxakis VP, Christodoulou GN, Mavreas VG, et al: Attempted suicide in psychiatric outpatients with concurrent physical illness. Psychother Psychosom 50(4):201–206, 1988 3269554

Kostić VS, Pekmezović T, Tomić A, et al: Suicide and suicidal ideation in Parkinson's disease. J Neurol Sci 289(1–2):40–43, 2010 19737673

Law Center to Prevent Gun Violence: Introduction to gun violence statistics. Gun Violence Statistics November 18, 2012. Available at: http://smartgunlaws.org/category/gun-studies-statistics/gun-violence-statistics/. Accessed December 19, 2014.

Leon AC, Solomon DA, Li C, et al: Antidepressants and risks of suicide and suicide attempts: a 27-year observational study. J Clin Psychiatry 72(5):580–586, 2011 21658345

Lin CJ, Lu HC, Sun FJ, et al: The characteristics, management, and aftercare of patients with suicide attempts who attended the emergency department of a general hospital in northern Taiwan. J Chin Med Assoc 77(6):317–324, 2014 24726674

Lönnqvist JK: Psychiatric aspects of suicidal behaviour: depression, in The International Handbook of Suicide and Attempted Suicide. Edited by Hawton K, Heeringen K. Chichester, UK, Wiley, 2000, pp 107–120

Luoma JB, Martin CE, Pearson JL: Contact with mental health and primary care providers before suicide: a review of the evidence. Am J Psychiatry 159(6):909–916, 2002 12042175

Makhija N, Sher L: Childhood abuse, adult alcohol use disorders and suicidal behaviour. QJM 100(5):305–309, 2007 17449874

Malone KM, Haas GL, Sweeney JA, et al: Major depression and the risk of attempted suicide. J Affect Disord 34(3):173–185, 1995 7560545

Mann JJ, Malone KM, Sweeney JA, et al: Attempted suicide characteristics and cerebrospinal fluid amine metabolites in depressed inpatients. Neuropsychopharmacology 15(6):576–586, 1996 8946432

Menninger K: Man Against Himself. New York, Harcourt Brace Jovanovich, 1985

Michel K: Suicide prevention and primary care, in The International Handbook of Suicide and Attempted Suicide. Edited by Hawton K, Heeringen K. Chichester, UK, Wiley, 2000, pp 661–674

Mościcki E: Epidemiology of completed and attempted suicide: toward a framework for prevention. Clinical Neuroscience Research 1(5):310–323, 2001

National Institute of Mental Health: 1999–2007 trends in suicide rate. 2009. Available at: http://www.nimh.nih.gov/health/statistics/suicide/index.shtml. Accessed December 19, 2014.

National Institute of Mental Health: Recommendations for reporting on suicide. 2012. Available at: http://reportingonsuicide.org/Recommendations2012.pdf. Accessed December 19, 2014.

Nordström P, Asberg M, Aberg-Wistedt A, et al: Attempted suicide predicts suicide risk in mood disorders. Acta Psychiatr Scand 92(5):345–350, 1995 8619338

O'Hare T, Shen C, Sherrer M: Lifetime trauma and suicide attempts in people with severe mental illness. Community Ment Health J 50(6):673–680, 2014 24282033

Page A, Morrell S, Hobbs C, et al: Suicide in young adults: psychiatric and socio-economic factors from a case-control study. BMC Psychiatry 14:68, 2014 24597482

Platt S: Unemployment and suicidal behaviour: a review of the literature. Soc Sci Med 19(2):93–115, 1984 6382623

Pokorny AD: Prediction of suicide in psychiatric patients. Report of a prospective study. Arch Gen Psychiatry 40(3):249–257, 1983 6830404

Qin P, Agerbo E, Mortensen PB: Suicide risk in relation to family history of completed suicide and psychiatric disorders: a nested case-control study based on longitudinal registers. Lancet 360(9340):1126–1130, 2002 12387960

Racine M, Choinière M, Nielson WR: Predictors of suicidal ideation in chronic pain patients: an exploratory study. Clin J Pain 30(5):371–378, 2014 23887336

Rihmer Z, Rutz W, Pihlgren H: Depression and suicide on Gotland: an intensive study of all suicides before and after a depression-training programme for general practitioners. J Affect Disord 35(4):147–152, 1995 8749979

Roberts M, Lamont E: Suicide: an existentialist reconceptualization. J Psychiatr Ment Health Nurs 21(10):873–878, 2014 24796698

Rockett IR, Regier MD, Kapusta ND, et al: Leading causes of unintentional and intentional injury mortality: United States, 2000–2009. Am J Public Health 102(11):e84–e92, 2012 22994256

Roy A: Family history of suicide. Arch Gen Psychiatry 40(9):971–974, 1983 6615160

Rutz W, von Knorring L, Pihlgren H, et al: Prevention of male suicides: lessons from Gotland study. Lancet 345(8948):524, 1995 7861901

Schernhammer ES, Colditz GA: Suicide rates among physicians: a quantitative and gender assessment (meta-analysis). Am J Psychiatry 161(12):2295–2302, 2004 15569903

Seemüller F, Riedel M, Obermeier M, et al: The controversial link between antidepressants and suicidality risks in adults: data from a naturalistic study on a large sample of in-patients with a major depressive episode. Int J Neuropsychopharmacol 12(2):181–189, 2009 18662490

Seiden RH: Where are they now? A follow-up study of suicide attempters from the Golden Gate Bridge. Suicide Life Threat Behav 8(4):203–216, 1978 217131

Shenassa E, Catlin S, Buka S: Gun availability, psychopathology, and risk of death from suicide attempt by gun. Ann Epidemiol 10(7):482, 2000 11018434

Simon RI: Imminent suicide: the illusion of short-term prediction. Suicide Life Threat Behav 36(3):296–301, 2006 16805657

Stockmeier CA: Neurobiology of serotonin in depression and suicide. Ann N Y Acad Sci 836:220–232, 1997 9616801

Stone M, Laughren T, Jones ML, et al: Risk of suicidality in clinical trials of antidepressants in adults: analysis of proprietary data submitted to U.S. Food and Drug Administration. BMJ 339:b2880, 2009 19671933

Suominen KH, Isometsä ET, Henriksson MM, et al: Suicide attempts and personality disorder. Acta Psychiatr Scand 102(2):118–125, 2000 10937784

Szanto K, Kalmar S, Hendin H, et al: A suicide prevention program in a region with a very high suicide rate. Arch Gen Psychiatry 64(8):914–920, 2007 17679636

Teicher MH, Glod CA, Cole JO: Antidepressant drugs and the emergence of suicidal tendencies. Drug Saf 8(3):186–212, 1993 8452661

Thibodeau MA, Welch PG, Sareen J, et al: Anxiety disorders are independently associated with suicide ideation and attempts: propensity score matching in two epidemiological samples. Depress Anxiety 30(10):947–954, 2013 24108489

Triñanes Y, González-Villar A, Gómez-Perretta C, et al: Suicidality in chronic pain: predictors of suicidal ideation in fibromyalgia. Pain Pract 15(4):323–332, 2015 24690160

Turecki G, Ernst C, Jollant F, et al: The neurodevelopmental origins of suicidal behavior. Trends Neurosci 35(1):14–23, 2012 22177979

Underwood MD, Khaibulina AA, Ellis SP, et al: Morphometry of the dorsal raphe nucleus serotonergic neurons in suicide victims. Biol Psychiatry 46(4):473–483, 1999 10459396

U.S. Department of Health and Human Services: Healthy People 2020. 2014. Available at: http://www.healthypeople.gov/2020/LHI/mentalHealth.aspx?tab=data. Accessed December 19, 2014.

U.S. Food and Drug Administration: Labeling change request letter for antidepressant medications. 2009. Available at: http://www.fda.gov/Drugs/DrugSafety/InformationbyDrugClass/ucm096352.htm. Accessed December 19, 2014.

Vaiva G, Vaiva G, Ducrocq F, et al: Effect of telephone contact on further suicide attempts in patients discharged from an emergency department: randomised controlled study. BMJ 332(7552):1241–1245, 2006 16735333

Viner R, Patten SB, Berzins S, et al: Prevalence and risk factors for suicidal ideation in a multiple sclerosis population. J Psychosom Res 76(4):312–316, 2014 24630182

Wender PH, Kety SS, Rosenthal D, et al: Psychiatric disorders in the biological and adoptive families of adopted individuals with affective disorders. Arch Gen Psychiatry 43(10):923–929, 1986 3753159

Witt K, Hawton K, Fazel S: The relationship between suicide and violence in schizophrenia: analysis of the Clinical Antipsychotic Trials of Intervention Effectiveness (CATIE) dataset. Schizophr Res 154(1–3):61–67, 2014 24581550

World Health Organization: Mental Health: Suicide Data. 2014. Available at: http://www.who.int/mental_health/prevention/suicide/suicideprevent/en/. Accessed December 19, 2014.

You Z, Chen M, Yang S, et al: Childhood adversity, recent life stressors and suicidal behavior in Chinese college students. PLoS ONE 9(3):e86672, 2014 24681891

Zisook S, Trivedi MH, Warden D, et al: Clinical correlates of the worsening or emergence of suicidal ideation during SSRI treatment of depression: an examination of citalopram in the STAR*D study. J Affect Disord 117(1-2):63–73, 2009 19217668

Suicide-Related Resources

Action Alliance for Suicide Prevention—http://actionallianceforsuicideprevention.org

After an Attempt: A Guide for Medical Providers in the Emergency Department Taking Care of Suicide Attempt Survivors—http://store.samhsa.gov/home

After an Attempt: A Guide for Taking Care of Your Family Member After Treatment in the Emergency Department—http://store.samhsa.gov/home

After a Suicide: Recommendations for Religious Services and Other Public Memorial Observances—http://www.sprc.org/sites/sprc.org/files/library/aftersuicide.pdf

American Association of Suicidology—http://www.suicidology.org/home

American Foundation for Suicide Prevention—http://www.afsp.org

Assessment of Suicidal Risk Using the Columbia Suicide Severity Rating Scale (C-SSRS)—http://zerosuicide.actionallianceforsuicideprevention.org/sites/zerosuicide.actionallianceforsuicideprevention.org/files/cssrs_web/course.htm

Best Practices Registry (a collaborative project of the Suicide Prevention Resource Center and the American Foundation for Suicide Prevention, funded by the Substance Abuse and Mental Health Services Administration)—http://www.sprc.org/bpr

Charting the Future of Suicide Prevention: A 2010 Progress Review of the National Strategy and Recommendations for the Decade Ahead—http://www.sprc.org

Columbia Suicide Severity Rating Scale (C-SSRS)—http://cssrs.columbia.edu

How to Report Suicidal Users on Facebook—https://www.suicidepreventionlifeline.org/App_Files/Media/PDF/How%20to%20Report%20Suicidal%20Users%20on%20Facebook.pdf

The Jason Foundation (provides educational programs and seminars for the awareness and prevention of youth suicide)—http://jasonfoundation.com

The Jed Foundation (focuses on understanding the underlying causes of suicide and producing effective prevention programs, information, and interventions for college and university campuses nationwide)—http://www.jedfoundation.org

Lifeline Crisis Chat (a service of the National Suicide Prevention Lifeline in partnership with CONTACT USA)—http://www.crisischat.org

The Link Counseling Center: Suicide Prevention and Aftercare (dedicated to reaching out to those affected by suicide and connecting them to resources)—http://thelink.org/nrc.htm

National Council for Suicide Prevention (a coalition of eight national organizations working to prevent suicide; its mission is to advance suicide prevention through leadership, advocacy, and a collective voice)—http://www.ncsponline.org

National Organization for People of Color Against Suicide—http://www.nopcas.org

National Suicide Prevention Lifeline (1-800-273-TALK [8255])—http://www.suicidepreventionlifeline.org

NYC Guide to Suicide Prevention, Services and Resources—http://samaritansnyc.org/nyc-resource-guide

Patient Safety Plan Template—http://www.sprc.org/sites/sprc.org/files/SafetyPlanTemplate.pdf

The Relationship Between Bullying and Suicide: What We Know and What It Means for Schools—http://www.cdc.gov/violenceprevention/pdf/bullying-suicide-translation-final-a.pdf

Safe and Effective Messaging for Suicide Prevention—http://www.sprc.org/sites/sprc.org/files/library/SafeMessagingrevised.pdf

Safety Planning Intervention for Suicidal Individuals—http://zerosuicide.actionalliance forsuicideprevention.org/sites/zerosuicide.actionallianceforsuicideprevention.org/ files/sp/course.htm

Samaritans USA (a coalition of 11 nonprofit, nonreligious Samaritans suicide prevention centers in the United States; its primary purpose is to further the group's principles of befriending people who are depressed, in crisis, and suicidal as practiced on or through the volunteer-staffed crisis response hotlines, public education programs, and suicide survivor support groups)—http://www.samaritansusa.org

Saving Lives in New York: Suicide Prevention and Public Health—http://www.omh. ny.gov/omhweb/savinglives

Self-Help for Suicidal Feelings (downloadable tip sheet)—http://www.suicide-line.org.au/content/uploads/self-help_for_suicidal_feelings.pdf

Social Media Guidelines for Mental Health Promotion and Suicide Prevention—http:// www.eiconline.org/teamup/wp-content/files/teamup-mental-health-social-media-guidelines.pdf

Suicide Awareness Voices of Education (SAVE) (a national nonprofit agency whose mission is to prevent suicide through public awareness and education, reduce stigma, and serve as a resource for those touched by suicide)—http://www.save.org

Suicide Prevention Contract: Contracting for Comfort—http://www.psychiatrictimes. com/blogs/couch-crisis/suicide-prevention-contract-contracting-comfort#st-hash.1UkUaFgC.dpuf

Suicide Prevention Education and Awareness Kit (SPEAK)—http://www.omh.ny.gov/ omhweb/speak

Suicide Prevention Resource Center—http://www.sprc.org/sites/sprc.org/files/library/ SafetyPlanningGuide.pdf

Training Institute for Suicide Assessment and Clinical Interviewing—http:// www.suicideassessment.com

Yellow Ribbon Suicide Prevention Program (teaches about the internal nature of depression and loneliness)—http://yellowribbon.org

Youth Suicide Prevention School-Based Guide—http://theguide.fmhi.usf.edu

3

Violence Risk Assessment

Vasilis K. Pozios, M.D.
Charletta Dillard, M.D.
Ernest Poortinga, M.D.

Case Example

Mr. G is a 21-year-old single, unemployed white man with a history of schizoaffective disorder and alcohol use disorder. He was first diagnosed with schizoaffective disorder 6 months earlier when he was psychiatrically hospitalized after dropping out of college. Mr. G's mother brought him to the psychiatric emergency service because she had become increasingly concerned about his paranoid ideation. Mr. G's mother reported that her son believed that a former female classmate, with whom Mr. G has been infatuated, was taunting him via social media. Through repeated interrogation, Mr. G stated that he had been sending threatening e-mails to this woman because she was "psychically castrating" him through photographs posted to her social media account. While in the emergency department (ED), the patient said he wanted to kill the woman. He also reported that he had been bingeing on alcohol and had been nonadherent with risperidone and valproic acid since his hospitalization. The patient's father, with whom Mr. G lives, was contacted by telephone for corroborating information. The father stated that he was concerned about Mr. G's increasing social isolation. Mr. G's father reported that when he had attempted to remove his handgun from the home, he discovered it was missing. A search of the patient's vehicle revealed a loaded handgun in the glove compartment.

Psychiatric treatment in an emergency setting is one of the more challenging aspects of the practice of psychiatry. Whether services are provided in standard EDs or in a designated psychiatric emergency service, the setting is usually complex, and the provider is typically managing several emergency situations at one time. Also, clinicians in the emergency setting may face external pressures from various sources; for example, insurance companies may exert pressures to avoid patient hospitalization. Needless to say, even in the best of situations, clinicians can overlook subtle clues and make mistakes.

Emergency psychiatrists provide an undeniably fundamental service in medicine: maintaining the safety of the patient and protecting the patient from harm (self-inflicted or otherwise). Unlike other emergency medicine practitioners, however, the ED psychiatrist is more commonly charged with the responsibility of supporting the safety not only of the patient but, indirectly, of others as well (usually those with whom no doctor-patient relationship exists). This responsibility—exemplified in the case of Mr. G, in which the psychiatric emergency service clinician was asked to assess a patient's dangerousness to others—raises the importance of assessment and management of the potentially violent patient.

Our goal in this chapter is to describe strategies that the busy emergency psychiatrist and resident psychiatrist can use to assess the short-term risk of violence in an orderly and standardized manner. Recognizing the absence of a foolproof method of predicting the perpetration of violent acts upon others, we present accepted clinical methods of assessing risk in the context of landmark legal cases in which such methods have been highlighted. A continuum of violence risk assessment methods exists; included among them are actuarial instruments used to predict long-term violence risk (Monahan and Skeem 2014). Structured risk assessment methods based on the use of actuarial instruments largely fall outside the scope of this text because of our focus on psychiatric emergency situations and related short-term violence risk. Ultimately, it is the duty of the individual clinician to determine what combination of assessment strategies best serves his or her duties in the determination of violence risk assessment.

Violence and Mental Illness

To better understand the potential of patient violence, one needs to study the culture of violence that exists in the United States in the early twenty-first century. Studies have consistently shown that violent acts are directly related to low social class, low IQ and education levels, and employment and residential instability (Mercy et al. 2002; Office of the Surgeon General et al. 2001). Statistics have also demonstrated that violent acts in the United States are at an all-time low. Since 1994, the rate of violent crimes (defined by the FBI as "murder and nonnegligent manslaughter, rape, robbery, and aggravated assault") has declined, reaching the lowest level ever recorded in 2013 (U.S. Department of Justice, Federal Bureau of Investigation 2014).

Perceptions with regard to the part played by mental illness in the perpetration of violence on others are similarly misinformed. According to Appelbaum (2008), only 3%–5% of the risk of violence in the United States can be attributed to mental illnesses. Indeed, the effects of substance-related and personality disorders far outweigh the role played by other mental illnesses (e.g., schizophrenia, major depression) alone; individuals with these other mental illnesses are far more likely to be victims than perpetrators of violent crimes.

Why does the popular perception of those with mental illnesses as violent predators persist? According to *Mental Health: A Report of the Surgeon General* (Satcher 1999), one series of surveys found that selective media reporting reinforced the public's stereotypes linking violence and mental illness, and encouraged people to distance themselves from those with mental disorders. The portrayal of persons with mental illness on television and in film may consciously or subconsciously influence the treatment of persons with mental illness who are in the custody of law enforcement (and who often wind up in a psychiatric emergency service). Media portrayals may also influence the decisions of practitioners regarding the clinical treatment of persons with mental illness, especially those who are homeless or are otherwise in situations of compromise; homeless persons with mental illness commit 35 times more crimes than persons with mental illnesses who are not homeless (Martell et al. 1995).

Although the entertainment industry is making more responsible efforts to accurately depict the risk of violence from persons with mental illness, it is the duty of psychiatrists to determine the context in which the potential risk of violence posed by their patients exists, and to make efforts to appropriately assess that risk. Certainly, some mental disorders and symptoms of mental illnesses can contribute more to the risk of violence than others. Command auditory hallucinations are perhaps the most common cause for concern with regard to risk of violence attributable to a specific symptom, whereas disturbing visual hallucinations, irritability secondary to mania, and hopelessness secondary to depression can all contribute to a patient's potentially becoming violent (Appelbaum 2008). A paranoid patient may seek to "preemptively strike" targets who, in the patient's mind, are plotting to do him or her harm (Resnick 2009). All of these symptoms are exacerbated by the disinhibiting effects of substance abuse, which is more common among people with mental disorders (Appelbaum 2008).

The bottom line is this: Persons with mental illness are not violent most of the time, and those with tendencies toward violence are not always violent. Given this understanding, how does one accurately and reliably perform an assessment of risk of violence in an emergency setting?

Clinical Assessment of Risk of Violence

The clinical assessment of violence risk in the emergency setting is a challenging endeavor. In the best of circumstances, a clear account of the incident leading to the patient's presentation to the ED is given, a chart containing the patient's medical and psychiatric history is available for review, and a family member or other third-party source of information is present for corroboration.

Psychiatrists are intimately familiar with safety evaluations for risk of self-harm. The same thorough approach should be applied to the evaluation of risk of violence toward others. The risk assessment should comprise a standardized survey of the most important risk factors that contribute to an increased risk of violence. A more probing investigation can then be pursued if certain red flags are raised in the initial investigation.

We encourage ED mental health professionals to follow the example of several psychiatry residency training programs and utilize a structured professional judgment tool, such as the Historical Clinical Risk Management–20, Version 3 (HCR-20V3; Douglas et al. 2013), as a guide to important risk factors (McNiel et al. 2003, 2008; Wong et al. 2012). A structured professional judgment tool, also called a guided clinical approach, differs from an actuarial approach in that the former does not estimate the likelihood of future violence and does not provide a cutoff score at which intervention must occur. Instead, the judgment tool is used to develop a risk formulation or a conceptualization of the roots of a person's problems with the goal of intervention (Douglas et al. 2013).

The HCR-20V3 divides 20 risk factors into historical, clinical, and risk management categories (Table 3–1). All of these factors should be considered by the clinician before generating a final short-term violence risk assessment. Some factors may receive more weight than others. For instance, specific psychiatric symptoms may warrant increased scrutiny. Several researchers have demonstrated that psychotic symptoms that override one's sense of self-control and are threatening to one's safety (e.g., delusions in which patients believe that people are seeking to harm them or that outside forces are controlling their minds) have higher correlations with violence than psychotic symptoms without these characteristics (Link and Stueve 1994; Monahan 1996). If the patient is deemed to pose an imminent threat of violence in the short term, the clinician must take action, usually by initiating commitment proceedings. The data collected in this assessment, as well as the treatment plan, should be documented in writing, for continuity of care and legal purposes.

Legal Precedents for Violence Risk Assessment

Despite efforts to standardize the evaluation process through the development and refinement of actuarial instruments, no psychiatrist can state with certainty that he or she can accurately predict violent acts perpetrated by psychiatric patients. The courts, however, have decided otherwise, and negligence to dutifully determine risk of violence can result in malpractice and liability.

None of the cases identified as landmarks by the American Academy of Psychiatry and the Law involve risk assessment in the ED. Legal opinions,

Table 3–1.   Risk factors from the Historical Clinical Risk Management–20, Version 3 (HCR-20V3)

Historical

1. Violence: Does the patient have a history of any actual, attempted, or threatened physical harm of another person?

2. History of other antisocial behavior

3. History of problems with relationships

4. History of problems with employment

5. History of problems with substance use

6. History of problems with major mental disorder

7. History of problems with personality disorder

8. History of problems with traumatic experiences

9. History of problems with violent attitudes

10. History of problems with treatment or supervision response

Clinical

1. Recent problems with insight

2. Recent problems with ideation or intent

3. Recent problems with symptoms of major mental disorder

4. Recent problems with instability

5. Recent problems with treatment or supervision response

Risk management

1. Future problems with professional services and plans

2. Future problems with living situation

3. Future problems with personal support

4. Future problems with treatment or supervision response

5. Future problems with stress or coping

Source.   Douglas et al. 2013.

however, seldom differentiate between the standard of care expected in a physician's office and the standard of care expected in the ED. Therefore, useful information can be gleaned from legal opinions rendered about hospital and outpatient cases. Applicable landmark cases are often referred to as "duty to protect" cases and are summarized here.

Tarasoff

Tarasoff I

Mr. Poddar felt distraught when he learned that Ms. Tarasoff, a fellow University of California at Berkeley student who kissed him on New Year's Eve, did not consider their relationship to be serious and had kissed other men. He informed his university psychologist that he intended to get a gun and harm Ms. Tarasoff. The psychologist gave written and oral alerts to campus police, who interviewed Mr. Poddar and decided that he was not dangerous. Mr. Poddar stalked, stabbed, and shot Ms. Tarasoff, whose parents then sued the university and the psychologist. The trial and appeals courts both dismissed the case. In *Tarasoff v. Regents of the University of California* (1974), the California Supreme Court disagreed and ruled that the "doctor bears a duty to use reasonable care to give threatened persons such warnings as are essential to avert foreseeable danger arising from the patient's condition. The protective privilege ends where the public peril begins."

Tarasoff II

The university and the psychologist petitioned for and were granted a new hearing, so the California Supreme Court heard the case again. The following is a direct quote from the *Tarasoff* (1976) decision:

> When a therapist determines, or pursuant to the standards of his profession should determine, that his patient presents a serious danger of violence to another, he incurs an obligation to use reasonable care to protect the intended victim against such danger. The discharge of this duty may require the therapist to take one or more of various steps, depending upon the nature of the case. Thus it may call for him to warn the intended victim or others likely to apprise the victim of the danger, to notify the police, or to take whatever other steps are reasonably necessary under the circumstances.

Many states have since passed statutes to address therapist obligations in cases of potential violence. We recommend that mental health personnel become familiar with the applicable statute in their state.

Tarasoff Progeny

Jablonski by Pahls v. United States (1983)

Mr. Jablonski threatened the mother (Ms. Pahls) of his live-in girlfriend (Ms. Kimball) with a sharp object and attempted to rape her. He voluntarily went to the Loma Linda Veterans Administration (VA) Hospital, where he was evaluated by a psychiatrist as an outpatient. Although police gave the hospital information about Mr. Jablonski's previous obscene phone calls and malicious property damage, this information apparently was not passed on to the psychiatrist. During the psychiatric interview, Mr. Jablonski revealed that he had served 5 years in prison for the rape of his then-wife and also discussed the more recent attempted rape of Ms. Pahls. Mr. Jablonski mentioned that he had received psychiatric treatment previously but refused to sign a release of information or even to state where the treatment took place. The psychiatrist diagnosed Mr. Jablonski with antisocial personality disorder and offered voluntary hospitalization for dangerousness. Mr. Jablonski refused, and the psychiatrist planned to see him again in 2 weeks. In a separate meeting after the diagnostic interview, the psychiatrist advised Ms. Kimball to leave Mr. Jablonski but gave her no other warning. Ms. Kimball indeed moved out of the shared apartment 2 days later but continued to see Mr. Jablonski.

Four days after the first appointment, Mr. Jablonski was seen by the psychiatrist and his supervisor at the request of Ms. Pahls. The psychiatrists agreed that Mr. Jablonski was dangerous but not committable. He was given a prescription for diazepam and was asked to come back in 3 days; Ms. Kimball was again told to stay away from Mr. Jablonski. One day before the scheduled appointment, Ms. Kimball returned to Mr. Jablonski's apartment to get diapers, and he murdered her. The victim's family sued the VA, and the district court found malpractice based on 1) failure to adequately warn the victim, 2) failure to obtain old medical records, and 3) failure to record or transmit the information from police.

The court of appeals affirmed the decision and suggested that the Loma Linda VA Hospital could have called neighboring VA hospitals without Mr. Jablonski's consent. Records would have revealed that Mr. Jablonski had a history of homicidal ideation toward his former wife, multiple murder attempts, and a diagnosis of schizophrenia. The court emphasized the importance of, at minimum, requesting the records and leaving the burden of breaching confidentiality to the party that holds the records.

This case extends the duty to protect to a victim who had not been specifically identified by the patient. Some states (including California) have statutes that limit liability to cases involving an explicit threat.

Notably, neither the district court nor the court of appeals criticized the VA for not committing Mr. Jablonski to inpatient treatment (one clear method of satisfying a *Tarasoff* duty). One can speculate that the courts viewed Mr. Jablonski as "uncommittable" because antisocial personality disorder does not meet most statutory definitions of mental illness. For a patient to be committed to psychiatric treatment, most states require a person to meet statutory definitions for mental illness. Michigan's definition of *mental illness* is representative; it states, "a substantial disorder of thought or mood which significantly impairs judgment, behavior, capacity to recognize reality, or ability to cope with the ordinary demands of life" (Michigan Compiled Laws 330.1400a).

Fredericks v. Jonsson (2010)

In 2000, Mr. Wellington was a neighbor of the Fredericks family when he began stalking their two daughters, who were minors. This continued until January 2004, when Mr. Wellington was convicted of stalking and sentenced to 8 years' probation. One condition of his probation was that he "complete a mental health evaluation/counseling or treatment." At the request of the Colorado probation department, licensed psychologist Dr. Jonsson conducted the evaluation, which included a clinical interview and psychological testing. Mr. Wellington told Dr. Jonsson that he "used to have frequent violent fantasies involving members of the Fredericks family, but that he no longer had violent thoughts directed" at them. Dr. Jonsson did not warn the Fredericks or the probation department. Two weeks later, Mr. Wellington became intoxicated and stole a car. He drove to the Fredericks's home where he broke a window, setting off an alarm. He fled to a neighbor's yard, where he was later found unconscious.

The Fredericks sued Dr. Jonsson for negligently failing to warn them and the probation department of the danger posed by Mr. Wellington. The U.S. District Court in the State of Colorado granted Dr. Jonsson's motion for summary judgment, ruling that Section 117 of Colorado's mental health professional liability statute (Colo. Rev. Stat. § 13-21-117) applied to and protected Dr. Jonsson from their claims.

The U.S. Court of Appeals, Tenth Circuit, affirmed the District Court's summary judgment, ruling that a "special relationship" existed between Dr. Jonsson and Mr. Wellington, and thus Dr. Jonsson was bound to Section 117. The court further ruled that the statute did not require Dr. Jonsson to warn the Fredericks because Mr. Wellington had not communicated to Dr. Jonsson "a serious threat of imminent physical violence" against the Fredericks (Maxey et al. 2011).

Lessons From *Tarasoff* and Its Progeny

What can psychiatrists learn from these landmark cases involving psychiatric assessment of risk of violence? What are the "standards of the profession" for violence risk assessment in the emergency setting? Although predicting violence has no standards, there is a standard for the assessment of dangerousness (Beck 1990). In other words, when faced with a potentially violent patient in the ED, psychiatrists can and should perform a careful, thorough assessment of the risk of danger, as outlined in the earlier section "Clinical Assessment of Risk of Violence." Notably, there are no landmark cases involving inappropriate commitment to treatment. Psychiatrists have protection from litigation in commitment issues because the probate courts screen these cases with due process.

Moreover, the court's suggestions in the *Jablonski* case can be highly illustrative: psychiatrists are expected to make a legitimate attempt to obtain previous medical records and to record information from police in the medical record. The first suggestion is difficult, given the time constraints in an emergency setting. The second suggestion may require psychiatrists to overcome their reluctance to place inflammatory material in a medical record.

Conclusion

The evaluation of dangerousness to others is a necessary and vital component of any emergency psychiatric evaluation. Although psychiatrists possess no special powers of prediction, evidence-based principles used in combination with insight gained through experience can prove invaluable in preventing acts of violence perpetrated on innocents by those with mental illness.

The task of the psychiatrist practicing in an emergency setting with regard to violence risk assessment is twofold: 1) the recognition of factors commonly attributed to an increased risk of violence and 2) appropriate intervention once that determination of risk has been made. A responsible psychiatrist should employ evidence-based practices when evaluating patients for dangerousness to others and risk of violence; "shoot-from-the-hip" assessments based purely on hunches or gut feelings are dangerous and potentially destructive, and serve only to fan the flames of stigma. Likewise, although it is inadvisable and foolhardy to practice psychiatry based on unstructured assessments alone, past experience can certainly add color commentary to the play-by-play provided by evidence-based practices.

All mental health practitioners concerned for the equitable treatment of their patients should pay close attention to the effect that acts of violence committed by those with mental illnesses has on the stigma associated with mental illness. To avoid contributing to stigma, a psychiatrist must treat all patients with respect while paying careful attention to the cues detailed in this chapter.

Psychiatrists can—and in fact should—intervene when they suspect that a patient is at risk of causing physical harm to another person because of factors attributed to the exacerbation or decompensation of a mental illness. Unfortunately, there is no hard-and-fast rule to ensure the foolproof prediction of the violence perpetrated on others by psychiatric patients. There are, however, evidence-based methods that, when used in combination with clinical judgment and experience, form the basis of most accepted approaches to violence risk assessment in an ED setting.

Key Clinical Points

- Patients with mental illness do commit violent acts; however, popular media and other sources may exaggerate the risk attributable to mental illness as a category.

- Specific mental illnesses (e.g., antisocial personality disorder, substance-related disorders) carry more risk than others (e.g., major depression).

- Specific symptoms (e.g., threat-control override) carry more risk than others.

- An extensive list of risk factors should be used to guide the risk assessment.

- Although there is no perfect way to predict future violence, landmark court cases have established a "duty to protect" potential victims. This obligation may apply to evaluations in the emergency department.

References

Appelbaum PS: Foreword, in Textbook of Violence Assessment and Management. Edited by Simon R, Tardiff K. Washington, DC, American Psychiatric Publishing, 2008, pp xvii–xxii

Beck JC (ed): Confidentiality and the Duty to Protect: Foreseeable Harm in the Practice of Psychiatry. Washington, DC, American Psychiatric Press, 1990

Douglas KS, Hart DH, Webster CD, et al: HCR-20V3: Assessing Risk for Violence. Burnaby, BC, Canada, Simon Fraser University, Mental Health, Law, and Policy Institute, 2013

Fredericks v Jonsson, 609 F.3d 1096, 10th Cir. (2010)

Jablonski by Pahls v United States, 712 F.2d 391, 395, 9th Cir. (1983)

Link BG, Stueve A: Psychotic symptoms and the violent/illegal behavior of mental patients compared to community controls, in Violence and Mental Disorder: Developments in Risk Assessment. Edited by J. Monahan J, Steadman HJ. Chicago, IL, University of Chicago Press, 1994, pp 137–160

Martell DA, Rosner R, Harmon RB: Base-rate estimates of criminal behavior by homeless mentally ill persons in New York City. Psychiatr Serv 46(6):596–601, 1995 7641002

Maxey JJ, Wortzel HS, Martinez R: Duty to warn or protect: Colorado's professional liability statute provides support for summary judgment in favor of a psychologist who completed an evaluation for the Colorado probation department. J Am Acad Psychiatry Law 39(3):430–432, 2011

McNiel DE, Gregory AL, Lam JN, et al: Utility of decision support tools for assessing acute risk of violence. J Consult Clin Psychol 71(5):945–953, 2003 14516243

McNiel DE, Chamberlain JR, Weaver CM, et al: Impact of clinical training on violence risk assessment. Am J Psychiatry 165(2):195–200, 2008 18245189

Mercy J, Butchart A, Farrington D, et al: Youth violence, in World Report on Violence and Health. Edited by Krug E, Dahlberg LL, Mercy JA, et al. Geneva, Switzerland, World Health Organization, 2002, pp 25–56. Available at: http://www.who.int/violence_injury_prevention/violence/global_campaign/en/chap2.pdf. Accessed April 29, 2015.

Michigan Compiled Laws 330.1400a. Available at: http://www.legislature.michigan.gov. Accessed December 19, 2014.

Monahan J: Violence prediction: the last 20 and the next 20 years. Crim Justice Behav 23:107–120, 1996

Monahan J, Skeem JL: The evolution of violence risk assessment. CNS Spectr 19(5):419–424, 2014 24679593

Office of the Surgeon General; National Center for Injury Prevention and Control; National Institute of Mental Health; Center for Mental Health Services: Youth Violence: A Report of the Surgeon General. Rockville, MD, Office of the Surgeon General, 2001. Available at: http://www.ncbi.nlm.nih.gov/books/NBK44294/. Accessed April 29, 2015.

Resnick P: Risk Assessment for Violence: Course Outline (Forensic Psychiatry Review Course). Chicago, IL, American Academy of Psychiatry and the Law, 2009, pp 112–114

Satcher D: Mental Health: A Report of the Surgeon General. 1999. Available at: http://www.surgeongeneral.gov/library/mentalhealth/home.html. Accessed December 19, 2014.

Tarasoff v Regents of the University of California, 118 Cal Rptr 129, 529 P2d 553 (1974)

Tarasoff v Regents of the University of California, 17 Cal. 3d 425, 131 Cal Rptr 14, 551 P2d 334 (1976)

U.S. Department of Justice, Federal Bureau of Investigation: Crime in the United States, 2013. Released Fall 2014. Available at: http://www.fbi.gov/about-us/cjis/ucr/crime-in-the-u.s/2013/crime-in-the-u.s. 2013/violent-crime/violent-crime-topic-page/violentcrimemain_final. Accessed April 28, 2015.

Wong L, Morgan A, Wilkie T, et al: Quality of resident violence risk assessments in psychiatric emergency settings. Can J Psychiatry 57(6):375–380, 2012 22682575

Suggested Readings

Appelbaum PS: Legal issues in emergency psychiatry, in Clinical Handbook of Psychiatry and the Law, 4th Edition. Edited by Appelbaum PS, Gutheil T. Philadelphia, PA, Lippincott Williams & Wilkins, 2007, pp 42–79

Felthous A: Personal violence, in American Psychiatric Publishing Textbook of Forensic Psychiatry: The Clinician's Guide. Edited by Simon P, Gold L. Washington, DC, American Psychiatric Publishing, 2004, pp 471–496

Tardiff K: Clinical risk assessment of violence, in Textbook of Violence Assessment and Management. Edited by Simon R, Tardiff K. Washington, DC, American Psychiatric Publishing, 2008, pp 3–14

4

Depression, Euphoria, and Anger in the Emergency Department

Philippe-Edouard Boursiquot, M.D.

Jennifer S. Brasch, M.D.

General Approach to Mood States

Mood disturbance is a common presenting symptom or complaint for patients in a psychiatric emergency service (PES). When patients are cooperative, the assessment can be straightforward. However, angry, irritable, and euphoric patients may be agitated or potentially violent and unable to tolerate a lengthy interview. Patients with labile affect can be unpredictable and perplexing to an inexperienced interviewer. Patients who are profoundly depressed may be withdrawn and slow to reply, making it difficult to obtain full information within a busy PES. Accurate assessment of patients with abnormal mood is critical because they are at increased risk of suicide, violence, and significant morbidity (Angst et al. 2002). In this chapter, we focus on the

challenges of assessing and managing patients with extreme mood disturbances, specifically depression, mania, and anger.

When a depressed, euphoric, or angry patient arrives in the PES, safety
must be the first concern. Although it may be obvious within moments that
a patient is probably manic, attention must be directed to assessing the patient's level of agitation and need for a safe, low-stimulus environment. A safe
environment and close observation are also necessary for profoundly depressed patients, especially those who may try to die by suicide within the PES
setting. Careful assessment of risk of harm to self or others is critical because
risk issues are central in determining disposition. (For more details, see Chapter 2, "Suicide Risk Assessment and Management," and Chapter 3, "Violence
Risk Assessment.")

The assessment of and emergency interventions for a patient with extreme mood disturbance initially occur simultaneously: mood is observed and
monitored, while efforts are made to control the situation. Once immediate
safety concerns have been addressed, the assessment can proceed. Assessments
in the PES need to focus on the current presentation, including the mood disturbance, neurovegetative symptoms, and recent stressors. It is also important
to explore past episodes of abnormal mood, medical illnesses, medications,
and functional status. All patients with extreme mood states need to be
screened for comorbid psychiatric illnesses, including symptoms of psychosis,
personality disorders, and anxiety disorders. Substance use disorders are very
common among patients in the PES, and it can be a challenge to determine
whether a patient's mood disturbance is due to intoxication, withdrawal, or
drug seeking, or if the substance use is an attempt to self-treat. Previous medical notes often can be used to trace the longitudinal pattern of a mood disorder. Collateral information is often essential, especially in evaluating risk of
harm to self or others.

Depressed Mood States

Case Example 1

Ms. S, a 61-year-old woman, was brought to the PES for suicidal ideation and
nihilistic thoughts. She had a history of major depressive disorder and had
previously been treated with electroconvulsive therapy. During the interview,

she did not make eye contact. Her clothes and hair were unkempt. She appeared fatigued. Her affect was restricted. In a flat voice, she stated, "I am so sad I cannot cry." She had no plan to end her life, but she saw no possibility of recovery. She wanted to end her inner pain. She had been feeling increasingly depressed since she ran out of her medications 3 months earlier.

Depression is the third most common presenting symptom of patients in the PES, after substance use and psychotic disorders (Currier and Allen 2003). Patients who are seen in a PES or general medical emergency department following a suicide attempt should be carefully screened for depression and other mood disorders. In turn, suicide risk should be evaluated in all patients presenting with depressed mood.

Assessment

Many patients with depressed mood will readily describe their distress. Thus, open-ended questions can better elicit accurate information, in contrast to closed-ended questions, which may be more effective when interviewing a patient with thought disorganization and elevated mood (see "Elevated Mood States" section of this chapter). For example, instead of asking a yes-no question (e.g., "Would you say you have been sad and tearful more often than not for the past 2 weeks?"), the clinician could ask, "How has your mood been lately?" As part of obtaining the history of the presenting illness, the clinician should ask about major stressors and significant losses (Table 4–1) because these may trigger a major depressive episode.

Symptoms of predominant sadness or anhedonia are essential for the diagnosis of a major depressive episode. Other symptoms associated with depressive episodes include sleep disturbance, diminished energy, appetite changes, significant guilt or self-blame, impaired concentration, psychomotor retardation, and preoccupation with death or suicide. Additionally, a depressive episode can be diagnosed only if the period of depression includes a significant change in the patient's prior level of functioning.

Patients with psychomotor retardation can be slowed in their responses and provide only limited information. An inexperienced interviewer may empathize with the patient and slow down the questions until the interview almost grinds to a halt. The clinician needs to maintain the flow of the interview and persist in asking questions while demonstrating patience and con-

Table 4–1.   Categories of stressors to explore in patients with abnormal mood

Financial	Income, debt, gambling losses, theft
Employment	Instability, unemployment, dissatisfaction, retirement
Shelter	Insecurity, homelessness
Relationship	Loss (bereavement), violence, infidelity, sexual orientation, bullying, conflict, abuse, lack of support
Health	New, severe, or chronic medical illness; pregnancy; disability; chronic pain
Other	Cultural, developmental, or life transition; spiritual or environmental crisis; maladaptive coping (e.g., anxiety disorder, substance use disorder)

cern. Some patients may minimize their symptoms of depression for cultural reasons or fears of stigma and discrimination. Others may have decided to die by suicide and may deny depressed mood in order to carry out their plans. The clinician should obtain collateral information to minimize the risk of determining disposition based on insufficient or inaccurate information.

An interviewer may feel uncomfortable when a depressed patient begins to cry. The clinician should acknowledge the depth and intensity of the patient's distress, and allow some time and silence before continuing the interview. Offering a tissue demonstrates care and concern. Recognizing and addressing these manifestations of suffering can put the patient at greater ease, and empathic listening can relieve the patient's sense of emotional burden.

Asking about past episodes of mood disturbances is important. Information pertaining to past diagnoses, treatments, and compliance helps put the current presentation in context. The clinician should always inquire about a history of hypomania or mania to minimize the risk of precipitating such an episode with an antidepressant. It is important to identify mixed features because these are associated with a greater likelihood of developing bipolar disorder (American Psychiatric Association 2013).

The clinician should obtain a substance abuse history, particularly for alcohol, benzodiazepines, cocaine, opioids, and stimulants, which can be longitudinally associated with depressed mood. It can be very difficult to determine, for example, whether a patient is depressed because he or she drinks alcohol or whether the patient drinks because he or she is depressed. Some patients may use cocaine or other substances in an effort to self-treat a depressed mood. A substance-induced mood disorder must be considered if substance use has occurred within a month of the patient's depressive symptoms. (See Chapter 9, "Substance-Related Psychiatric Emergencies," for further information.)

The mental status examination of a patient with depression will often reflect the depth of his or her distress. The clinician needs to assess the patient's hygiene, eye contact, speech, and thought content. Mood-congruent themes of worthlessness, poverty, nihilism, or sickness signal severe depression and may at times reach delusional intensity. Psychotic symptoms are present in 15% of all depressed patients (Glick 2002). In adolescents, severe depression may be the first sign of bipolar disorder (DeFilippis and Wagner 2013). Depression with anxious distress can be difficult to differentiate from a mixed state; the main distinguishing feature is the absence of grandiosity and pleasure-seeking behavior in the former (Glick 2002). Because depression can be the first sign of a neurocognitive disorder in elderly patients, a brief cognitive evaluation, such as the Mini-Mental State Examination (Folstein et al. 1975) or the Montreal Cognitive Assessment (Nasreddine et al. 2005), can be useful. Alternatively, the depressed state can impair cognitive function.

The assessment also should include consideration of medical conditions that may be associated with depressed mood. This includes physical examination (Table 4–2) and investigations (Table 4–3). Pregnancy should be ruled out in women of childbearing age because it may influence choice of treatment.

Diagnosis

Depressed mood can be part of many psychiatric disorders, most commonly a major depressive episode. The clinician should be careful to consider whether the severity, duration, and impairment criteria from DSM-5 (American Psychiatric Association 2013) are met. If the patient's symptoms do not meet full criteria for major depressive episode, and a precipitating stressor exists, the clinician should consider the possible diagnosis of adjustment disorder or bereavement. If the patient is psychotic and depressed, the diagnosis is likely major depressive episode, severe, with psychotic features. Depressive episodes, with or without psychosis, can also occur in patients with bipolar disorder,

Table 4–2.   Common and noteworthy medical and substance-related disorders associated with depressed mood

Vascular: Cerebrovascular infarct, post–acute myocardial infarction, heart failure

Metabolic/endocrine: Diabetes mellitus, anemia (can also present with manic symptoms), hypothyroidism, menopausal transition, low testosterone, spontaneous abortion, vitamin B_{12} deficiency

Degenerative: Alzheimer's disease, hearing impairment

Traumatic: Head injury

Substance-related: Alcohol use disorder (current or past), cannabis use disorder, tobacco withdrawal, opioid withdrawal

Other: Sleep apnea, chronic pain, sleep deprivation

Source.   Adapted from DynaMed 1995a and Joska and Stein 2008.

Table 4–3.   Suggested investigations for patients presenting with abnormal mood

Complete blood count (CBC)

Serum glucose

Thyroid-stimulating hormone (TSH)

Urea, creatinine, electrolytes

Alanine transaminase (ALT), aspartate transaminase (AST), γ-glutamyltransferase (GGT), bilirubin

β-Human chorionic gonadotropin (β-HCG) in women of childbearing age; consider testosterone level in men

Serum alcohol level (if patient appears intoxicated)

Urine toxicology screen

Urinalysis (especially in elderly)

schizophrenia, schizoaffective disorder, or other psychotic disorders. Substance-induced mood disorder, particularly from alcohol, opioids, and cocaine, should be considered. Many patients may have more than one diagnosis. For example, high comorbidity exists between anxiety disorders and depressive symptoms. Patients with borderline personality disorder may complain of depressed or rapidly changing mood, in addition to unstable interpersonal relationships and self-image. Major depressive episode is also common in patients with eating disorders.

Table 4–4.   Criteria for hospital admission of patients with abnormal mood

Danger to self or others (risk of suicide, violence, or homicide)

Inability to care for self

Strong possibility of an acute or disabling medical condition contributing to the abnormal mood state

Symptoms that cannot be safely evaluated or treated on an outpatient basis

Lack of community follow-up care

Social isolation

Hostile home environment

Note.   Local criteria for involuntary admission also apply.

Management and Disposition

Disposition of patients is determined primarily by the risk assessment. Patients with depressed mood and significant suicidal ideation and/or psychosis generally require hospital admission (Table 4–4). Over half of all patients seen in the PES with depressive symptoms may require admission (Harman et al. 2004).

Patients with a major depressive episode who will not be admitted to a hospital can be started on an antidepressant in the emergency department. This practice is somewhat controversial, however, because of concerns regarding compliance, follow-up, and potential drug overdose (Glick 2004), but current first-line treatments for depression are generally safe in this regard. The conditions in which an antidepressant can be initiated in the PES with outpatient follow-up for monitoring are listed in Table 4–5. When prescribing an antidepressant, the clinician needs to carefully explain the purpose of the medication, describe common adverse reactions, and discuss the expected time course for symptom improvement. Patients must have follow-up with a health care provider who can monitor their response to the antidepressant and represcribe the medication (Glick 2004; Shea 1998). When available, medication samples may be offered to patients who cannot obtain or afford the medication. If possible, the patient's family or support person should be included in the discussion. Encourage patients to call a crisis line or return to the emergency department if they struggle with the treatment plan. The clinician should always document that this information was transmitted (Glick 2004).

Table 4–5.   Conditions supporting emergency department initiation of antidepressant medication with outpatient follow-up and treatment

Clear diagnosis

No substance misuse

Low suicide risk

No psychosis, agitation, or impulsivity

No acute medical problems

Clear follow-up plan

Desire to begin treatment

Ability to pay for (or having health insurance for) medications

First-line pharmacotherapy options for depression include the selective serotonin reuptake inhibitors (SSRIs; e.g., escitalopram, sertraline), serotonin–norepinephrine reuptake inhibitors (SNRIs; e.g., venlafaxine, duloxetine), norepinephrine and dopamine reuptake inhibitors (e.g., bupropion), and combined noradrenergic agonists and selective serotonin antagonists (e.g., mirtazapine) (Lam et al. 2009). The selection of a specific agent depends on known contraindications (e.g., risk of serotonin syndrome), past response (of the patient and/or a family member), adverse-effect profile, concurrent medical problems, and potential drug interactions. Mood improvement typically occurs after 4–6 weeks of therapy, although symptoms related to concentration, sleep, and energy may begin to improve in as little as 1–2 weeks. Common side effects of SSRIs and SNRIs include gastric discomfort, insomnia, jitteriness (in up to 25% of patients), and sexual disturbance (in 50%–80% of patients) (Lam et al. 2009). The starting dose should be reduced in patients with liver disease, as well as the elderly. SSRIs are generally considered safe in pregnancy, although evidence is limited (Lam et al. 2009).

For patients who present to the PES with depression and are already taking an antidepressant, consideration can be given to adding an atypical antipsychotic to accelerate or augment the antidepressant response and/or to treat insomnia or anxiety symptoms (Spielmans et al. 2013). These agents have modest efficacy but are associated with adverse effects such as weight gain, insulin resistance, and hyperlipidemia (Lam et al. 2009).

For patients with mild to moderate depression, a course of brief, structured psychotherapy can be effective. Combination of psychotherapy with pharmacotherapy may be superior to either treatment alone (Parikh et al. 2009), but access to cognitive-behavioral, interpersonal, behavioral activation, psychodynamic, or other therapies may be limited by availability or cost. Patients with bereavement or adjustment disorder may benefit from a referral to supportive counseling.

For a patient with a history of bipolar disorder, monotherapy with an antidepressant is not recommended. A mood stabilizer, such as lithium or lamotrigine, should be started before or concurrently with the antidepressant (Yatham et al. 2013). Patients presenting with psychotic features need to be treated with typical or atypical antipsychotics in conjunction with antidepressants (Glick 2002). Discussion about these treatment options can be initiated in the PES, although the decision is more likely to occur in the inpatient or outpatient setting. In cases of severe depression with suicidal ideation and no food or fluid intake, electroconvulsive therapy can be considered.

Patients with both depressive symptoms and substance use disorders do best when referred to a concurrent disorders program, but access to these services is often limited. Patients should be offered antidepressant therapy because it is safe and efficacious, may improve compliance with substance abuse treatment, and may reduce the patient's substance use (Minkoff 2005).

Case Example 1 *(continued)*

Given the high risk of self-harm and her inability to care for herself, Ms. S was certified as an involuntary patient and observed closely in the PES until an inpatient bed became available. Her diagnosis was major depressive disorder, current episode severe.

Elevated Mood States

Case Example 2

"Come in, come in!" Mr. M beckoned. "I am so glad to see you! I need to tell you what is going on. You see, today is not April the first. It is April the truth!" he exclaimed in delight. "I am a security guard for Big Town Mall. Today, I am to be promoted to field commander. You have the power to release me, doctor, so I can meet my boss. It is up to you! Up to now I have kept people's bodies safe. Now, now I know how to keep their souls safe." Mr. M smiled with satisfaction and a sense of purpose. His brother had brought Mr. M, age 28, to the PES. Mr. M had slept only 1 or 2 hours per night for the past week and did not abuse substances.

Mania is defined as a state of grandeur, often associated with an elevated, euphoric mood, although manic patients can also present with irritability. Bipolar disorder has a lifetime prevalence of 4% and is associated with a high suicide rate and significant morbidity (Ketter and Chang 2014). Interviewing a euphoric patient can be an interesting and challenging experience at times.

Assessment

Assessing a patient with elevated mood draws on an interviewer's flexibility, creativity, and patience. As in interviews with depressed patients, safety concerns are a priority. The clinician should consider having security staff present because a euphoric and elated patient may quickly become irritable, uncooperative, and threatening. Considerable interviewing skill is necessary to interject questions about symptoms consistent with mania that lead to useful information yet avoid causing irritability or excessively lengthy responses (Levinson and Young 2006). Asking questions that are short, closed-ended, and focused may increase the amount of useful information from patients who are very talkative, circumstantial, or disorganized. To obtain the history of presenting illness, the clinician should try to elicit a clear timeline of recent events and explore possible stressors. The interview should end before the patient escalates, regardless of how little factual information has been obtained. Even a short encounter provides plenty of data for the mental status examination. Information about the longitudinal pattern of mood disturbance is necessary to determine the diagnosis. Often, this information is easier to obtain from collateral sources and previous notes.

Symptoms particular to mania that often emerge spontaneously in the interview include grandiosity, increased talkativeness, flight of ideas, and distractibility. It is important to explore suicidal and homicidal ideation because manic patients often feel invincible and may lose all sense of mortality or morals. Also, the clinician should assess high-risk behaviors because manic patients often engage in actions that inadvertently result in accidents or trauma (Swann 2008). Obtaining a patient's medication and substance use

Table 4–6. Common and noteworthy medical disorders and substances associated with elevated mood

Vascular: Cerebrovascular infarct

Infectious: HIV, encephalitis, meningitis, rabies, neurosyphilis

Autoimmune: Systemic lupus erythematosus

Metabolic/endocrine: Hyperglycemia, hypoglycemia, hyperthyroidism, vitamin B_{12} deficiency

Degenerative: Alzheimer's disease

Traumatic: Head injury

Substance/medication use: Nicotine, caffeine, alcohol, cocaine, amphetamines, phencyclidine (PCP), amphetamine-like drugs, anabolic steroids, antidepressants, corticosteroids, benzodiazepine withdrawal

Other: Normal-pressure hydrocephalus, epilepsy, sleep deprivation

Source. Adapted from DynaMed 1995b and Joska and Stein 2008.

history is essential. Recent antidepressant use may be the precipitant of a manic episode. Poor compliance with prescribed mood-stabilizing medications can also contribute to a patient's presentation. Exploring the recent use of substances is important because substance misuse can mimic or mask a manic episode.

Many patients with mania have excessive motor activity and may be unable to stay seated for more than a few seconds. The mental status examination may also reveal hypervigilance, labile affect, flight of ideas, pressured speech, lack of insight, and impaired judgment.

Although patients may not cooperate with a physical examination, one should be attempted because a number of medical diagnoses are associated with euphoric or elevated mood (Table 4–6). Brief observation of the patient can suggest substance intoxication or withdrawal. Basic investigations are recommended (see Table 4–3). Because many mood stabilizers are teratogenic, pregnancy testing is recommended in women of childbearing age (James et al. 2007).

Diagnosis

The key feature of bipolar I disorder is one or more manic episodes (possibly in addition to depressive episodes), whereas bipolar II disorder is associated with hypomanic states. In hypomania, the patient has an elevated, euphoric, or irritable mood but has no psychotic features and does not require hospitalization. A patient with mania has significant impairment in social or occupational functioning, whereas a patient with hypomania can still continue to function in the community. If symptoms of both depression and mania are present, the "with mixed features" specifier should be noted in addition to the manic or hypomanic episode (American Psychiatric Association 2013), often demonstrate mood lability and severe agitation, which can make them unpredictable and difficult to manage (Swann 2008).

Manic episodes occur in a smaller number of disorders than depressive episodes. Although most commonly associated with bipolar I disorder, periods of elevated mood may also occur in schizoaffective disorder and substance-related disorders. Schizoaffective disorder requires the longitudinal predominance of mood symptoms, as well as a 2-week period of psychotic symptoms in the absence of mood symptoms. Substances associated with a euphoric mood include alcohol, amphetamines, cocaine, hallucinogens, and opioids. The state of mania is associated with disinhibition, which increases the risk of substance use. Mania is also associated with medical conditions (see Table 4–6) and can be induced by an antidepressant.

Management and Disposition

Patients in a manic state usually have little or no insight into their potentially harmful ideas and plans. In these circumstances, they need to be involuntarily admitted to the hospital (see Table 4–4). Patients with more insight and less severe mood disturbance (e.g., hypomania) may be managed in the community with medication adjustment and close follow-up.

In the emergency setting, patients in a manic state are often irritable, agitated, and intrusive (e.g., approaching others without invitation or welcome). Staff should try to decrease environmental noise and stimulation, and should offer consistent low-key interpersonal interactions (Swann 2008). Seclusion or restraints may be necessary to contain an agitated patient or prevent harm to others (see Chapter 11, "Seclusion and Restraint in Emergency Settings"). If a patient will remain in the PES for an extended period, medications should be offered proactively to prevent a re-escalation of the manic behaviors. The manic state can be alarming for patients' friends and families. Psychoeducation, including a description of the symptoms and clarification of evidence-based treatment alternatives, can provide a certain degree of reassurance (Yatham et al. 2013).

Mood stabilizers and atypical antipsychotics (e.g., risperidone, olanzapine), as monotherapy or combination therapy, are first-line agents for patients willing to take oral medication (Yatham et al. 2013). If patients refuse oral medications, then intramuscular olanzapine, ziprasidone, aripiprazole, or a combination of haloperidol and a benzodiazepine is recommended (Yatham et al. 2013). Caution is needed when using benzodiazepines in elderly patients due to the increased risk of falls. Antipsychotics are preferable to mood stabilizers if there are concerns about teratogenicity, although the risks, such as extrapyramidal symptoms, must be carefully weighed against the benefits (Yatham et al. 2013).

The clinician should keep in mind that the patient may be too agitated to consent to treatment and/or incapable of consenting, in which case administration of medications constitutes chemical restraint. Involvement of a substitute decision maker may become necessary. If hospitalization is not required, close follow-up is needed to determine the efficacy of treatment and to adjust the medication dose or type as needed.

Case Example 2 *(continued)*

Mr. M did not see the need for hospitalization. Before transfer to the ward, he became irritable and demanded to be released, but with his brother's support and encouragement, he took soluble olanzapine 10 mg orally and calmed down. He remained calm until transfer to the ward could be arranged.

Angry and Irritable Mood States

Case Example 3

Mr. W, a 17-year-old male, was brought to the emergency department by police for causing a disturbance downtown. He was resistant to the assessment, angry, and verbally abusive with staff. He refused oral sedatives, was uncooperative, and did not interact with his parents. He had a 1-year history of daily cannabis use, corresponding to an escalation of his anger reactions. His parents were unwilling to have him in their home. He was taking bupropion for attention-deficit/hyperactivity disorder (ADHD).

Anger and irritability are the most trying of the extreme moods presented in this chapter. Interviews with angry and irritable patients can be difficult because of pressures on clinicians to accurately predict risk of violence and because nobody likes to deliberately expose themselves to verbal tirades or worse. The threat of aggression is unsettling. Determining the most appropriate diagnosis can be a challenge because angry and irritable behavior can be the presenting problem for many different diagnoses. In addition, many crisis situations may develop from nonpathological angry behavior. In those situations, it is necessary for the clinician to identify the absence of a diagnosis and the limited role of the emergency department.

Assessment

For all patients, and especially for angry or irritable patients, the person's belongings and garments must be searched for weapons by security staff or trained personnel. Interviews in the PES to assess angry and irritable patients usually fall into one of two categories: 1) the assessment of a reasonably calm person who was brought in because of angry and irritable behavior in the community and 2) the assessment of a person who is angry at the time of the interview.

As with assessments of all patients in the PES, the assessment begins with ensuring everyone's safety and depends in large part on the patient's ability to cooperate. With patients who are reasonably calm and can describe their episode(s) of anger and irritability, the interviewer can gather specific details about the incident that precipitated the visit as well as about previous episodes of anger. The interviewer should ask open-ended and unbiased questions. For example, asking "How many times did you hit John?" is preferable to "Did you hit him a lot of times?" because the latter question allows the patient to minimize his or her aggressive behavior, especially if facing arrest for the actions. Once the history of the presenting illness has been explored, the interviewer can direct questions to ruling in or out specific diagnoses (Table 4–7).

Assessment of patients who are angry and irritable during the interview presents special challenges. Clinicians need to be aware of their own discomfort with angry patients and avoid revealing any irritability of their own. Setting firm limits may be necessary. It is far better for a clinician to leave the interview room to end a patient's verbal tirade than to become confrontational and thereby escalate the situation. If a patient is not psychotic or delir-

Table 4–7.   Conditions that may present with angry or irritable mood

Major depressive episode, manic episode, mixed episode

Generalized anxiety disorder, posttraumatic stress disorder

Psychotic disorders

Substance intoxication or withdrawal (alcohol, stimulants [amphetamines, cocaine], hallucinogens, phencyclidine)

Drug-seeking behavior (especially for alcohol, opioids, sedatives/hypnotics/anxiolytics)

Impulse-control disorders (especially intermittent explosive disorder)

Personality disorders (especially antisocial and borderline)

Conduct disorder, oppositional defiant disorder, disruptive mood dysregulation disorder

Attention-deficit/hyperactivity disorder, Tourette's disorder, pervasive developmental disorders

Relationship distress with spouse or intimate partner, other relational problem, adjustment disorder (with disturbance of conduct)

Mild or major neurocognitive disorder, delirium, head injury, seizure disorder

Source.   American Psychiatric Association 2013.

ious and cannot settle quickly, it may be safest to terminate the interview until the patient is calmer and more cooperative.

Certain considerations may be needed with specific populations. Youth may be more irreverent than expected, and deference to seniors may be difficult in such situations. To defuse what may quickly become a confrontational interview, it may be preferable to include a third party, such as security staff, a nurse or social worker, or even a relative.

Trying to empathize with the patient can help to establish an alliance and enable the patient to feel understood. This does not mean that the clinician must agree with the patient's ideas or beliefs, but initially debating with a patient who is angry is unlikely to be helpful. The clinician should allow the angry patient to feel heard, to be supported, and to have his or her feelings validated. Validation can lead to a joining and partnering that can support later problem solving (Shea 1998). It is important to keep in mind that patients can be angry because of long waits in the PES or from having been brought to the emergency department against their will. There is benefit for the clinician, when assessing an angry patient, to debrief with a colleague and/ or superior and to not take the anger personally.

Diagnosis

Angry and irritable behaviors are associated with many diagnoses (see Table 4–7), including mood disorders as described in DSM-5. People experiencing a depressive episode may present with irritability. This may be more common in males because certain cultural norms possibly discourage men from admitting to depression. Some authors have described a "male depressive syndrome," characterized by low impulse control, episodes of anger, and high irritability (Winkler et al. 2005). Patients experiencing a manic episode can often be angry and irritable, rather than euphoric. Table 4–8 can assist in determining whether irritability is due to depression or mania.

Patients with paranoid ideation and other psychotic symptoms can become very angry because they perceive that nobody understands their beliefs and experiences. Also, because of the high prevalence of substance use disorders in the PES, it is important to consider that patients may be intoxicated with alcohol, stimulants, phencyclidine, or other substances. Patients who are in withdrawal may become very irritable and may present to the PES seeking benzodiazepines, opioids, or other prescription medications.

Many other diagnostic categories can also be associated with anger and irritability. The family and friends of patients with borderline or antisocial personality disorders may be more concerned with the patients' outbursts of extreme and inappropriate anger than are the patients themselves. Borderline personality disorder should be suspected in patients with a longitudinal pattern of instability in interpersonal relationships and self-image, pronounced fear of abandonment, rapidly fluctuating moods, impulsivity, and self-harm behaviors. Core features in conduct disorder and antisocial personality disorder are verbal and physical aggression, destruction of property, deceitfulness, disregard for the rights of others, and the absence of remorse.

In children and adolescents, oppositional defiant disorder is associated with hostile, disobedient, and defiant behavior but not with a disregard for the rights of others, in contrast with conduct disorder, which may later progress to antisocial personality disorder. Poor impulse control can be a core

Table 4–8. Irritability in depression and mania

	Depression	Mania
To whom the irritability is directed	Irritability is much more likely to be expressed toward loved ones and people who live in close proximity.	Expressed with less selectivity. Therefore, coworkers, strangers, other drivers, etc. receive the wrath of the irritability, although simply as a virtue of time spent together, family is more likely to receive the brunt.
Triggered or not	There is often a "hook to hang the hat" of irritability on. The "infraction" may be small or insignificant, but there is usually a trigger for the irritable outburst.	The irritability is expressed virtually spontaneously. Some patients talk about walking on their own and feeling rage, and yelling, when there is no particular precipitant.
Remorseful?	People with depression most often feel awful about how they are acting and hate the fact that they are irritable.	People experiencing mania are usually remorseful only once the episode is over. During the episode, they do not recognize their behavior as irritable or feel justified in behaving that way.
Associated behavior	The irritability of depression is often associated with distress and expression of other negative emotions such as tearfulness and anguish.	The irritability of mania is often associated with rage and aggression, either verbal or physical.

Source. Reprinted from Goldstein BI, Levitt AJ: "Assessment of Patients With Depression," in *Psychiatric Clinical Skills.* Edited by Goldbloom DS. Philadelphia, PA, Elsevier Mosby, 2006, p. 350. Copyright 2006, Elsevier. Used with permission.

symptom in ADHD. ADHD is frequently comorbid with Tourette's disorder, a condition characterized by motor and vocal tics and frequently presenting with rage attacks. Intermittent explosive disorder is diagnosed in the absence of other disorders. It is more common in men. Key features include extreme expressions of anger, often to the point of uncontrollable rage, that are disproportionate to the situation at hand. The patient also exhibits genuine remorse afterward and a pleasant demeanor between outbursts.

In an effort to limit undue and excessive diagnosing of irritable youth as having bipolar disorder, the DSM-5 Task Force added disruptive mood dysregulation disorder (DMDD) as a new diagnosis (American Psychiatric Association 2013). Patients with this disorder have constant anger, superimposed on exacerbations that are disproportionate to the precipitant event and inconsistent with the developmental stage. Children or adolescents with DMDD cannot be concurrently diagnosed with bipolar disorder, oppositional defiant disorder, or intermittent explosive disorder.

Medical causes for angry outbursts should also be considered. These include dementia, delirium, a history of head injury, and seizure disorders. Any concerns about cognitive impairment should be thoroughly assessed with a standardized instrument such as the Mini-Mental State Examination (Folstein et al. 1975) or the Montreal Cognitive Assessment Test (Nasreddine et al. 2005).

It is important to remember that anger is a normal reaction to many circumstances. Anger is common in sudden losses, unexpected death of a loved one, theft, devastating medical diagnosis, discovery of betrayal, or other crisis. Anger can also be experienced during a disaster. If the anger is situational, interviewing family members may quickly reveal their role in contributing to a patient's angry outbursts.

Management and Disposition

Management of angry patients depends on their diagnoses. The clinician must carefully document the risk assessments of nonpsychotic angry patients and remind patients that they are responsible for their actions as well as the consequences of their actions when angry. Some patients may benefit from anger management sessions, which are usually delivered in a group setting and help patients learn strategies to modulate their angry outbursts, appropriately assert their needs, and develop constructive conflict resolution strategies.

Medication may have a role in the management of angry outbursts if a psychiatric disorder is present. However, if medication is prescribed, the clinician needs a clear plan for follow-up to ensure careful evaluation of any benefit. Patients with a psychiatric disorder whose anger presents a risk of injury to themselves or others usually require hospitalization.

Hospitalization or other psychiatric treatment for anger in the absence of a psychiatric disorder is generally not indicated. The most appropriate action may be to release such patients to the custody of law enforcement. Careful documentation of the decision-making process in determining disposition for an angry patient is important for medicolegal purposes.

Case Example 3 *(continued)*

An interview with Mr. W and his family revealed a 6-year history of tantrums and disputes. His mother admitted that she had insulted him about his cannabis use, social isolation, and poor academic performance. Mr. W refused to apologize for his angry outbursts. His parents wanted him to remain in the hospital. However, Mr. W did not carry psychiatric diagnoses other than his ADHD and cannabis abuse. Moreover, the ADHD appeared well controlled with his bupropion. Hospitalization was not warranted because Mr. W's anger appeared to be independent of his preexisting psychiatric diagnoses, and it would not have been appropriate to use these diagnoses to excuse his behavior. Instead, the diagnosis of parent-child relational problem was given. Reluctantly, his parents took him home. A referral for family counseling was completed.

Key Clinical Points

- In assessing patients with extreme moods, the interviewer should always address safety and risk issues first.

- Angry and depressed mood states occur in a wide range of psychiatric disorders.

- Obtaining a longitudinal history of mood states is important in establishing a mood disorder diagnosis. The clinician should screen the patient for a history of hypomania or mania before initiating treatment with an antidepressant.

- Depression and mania can each present with irritability.

- For patients with depression who do not require admission, the clinician should initiate treatment in the psychiatric emergency service and focus on maximizing adherence and follow-up.

- For patients with angry or irritable mood, the clinician should determine whether a psychiatric disorder is present and be firm about the limited role of the psychiatric emergency service in treatment of anger not due to a psychiatric or medical condition.

References

American Psychiatric Association: Diagnostic and Statistical Manual of Mental Disorders, 5th Edition. Arlington, VA, American Psychiatric Association, 2013

Angst F, Stassen HH, Clayton PJ, et al: Mortality of patients with mood disorders: follow-up over 34–38 years. J Affect Disord 68(2–3):167–181, 2002 12063145

Currier GW, Allen M: Organization and function of academic psychiatric emergency services. Gen Hosp Psychiatry 25(2):124–129, 2003 12676426

DeFilippis MS, Wagner KD: Bipolar depression in children and adolescents. CNS Spectr 18(4):209–213, 2013 23570693

DynaMed [Internet] Ipswich (MA): EBSCO Information Services. Record No 361151. Depression—differential diagnosis. 1995a. Available at: http://search.ebscohost. com.libaccess.lib.mcmaster.ca/login.aspx?direct=trueanddb=dmeandAN=361151 andsite=dynamed-liveandscope=site. Accessed December 20, 2014.

DynaMed [Internet] Ipswich (MA): EBSCO Information Services. Record No 361149. Mania—differential diagnosis. 1995b. Available at: http://search.ebscohost. com.libaccess.lib.mcmaster.ca/login.aspx?direct=trueanddb=dmeandAN=361149 andsite=dynamed-liveandscope=site. Accessed December 20, 2014.

Folstein MF, Folstein SE, McHugh PR: "Mini-mental state": a practical method for grading the cognitive state of patients for the clinician. J Psychiatr Res 12(3):189–198, 1975 1202204

Glick RL: Emergency management of depression and depression complicated by agitation or psychosis. Psychiatric Issues in Emergency Care Settings 1 (winter):11–16, 2002

Glick RL: Starting antidepressant treatment in the emergency setting. Psychiatric Issues in Emergency Care Settings 3:6–10, 2004

Harman JS, Scholle SH, Edlund MJ: Emergency department visits for depression in the United States. Psychiatr Serv 55(8):937–939, 2004 15292546

James L, Barnes TR, Lelliott P, et al: Informing patients of the teratogenic potential of mood stabilizing drugs: a case note review of the practice of psychiatrists. J Psychopharmacol 21(8):815–819, 2007 17881432

Joska JA, Stein DJ: Mood disorders, in The American Psychiatric Publishing Textbook of Psychiatry, 5th Edition. Edited by Hales RE, Yudofsky SC, Gabbard GO. Washington, DC, American Psychiatric Publishing, 2008, pp 457–504

Ketter T, Chang K: Bipolar and related disorders, in The American Psychiatric Publishing Textbook of Psychiatry, 6th Edition. Edited by Hales RE, Yudofsky SC, Roberts LW. Washington, DC, American Psychiatric Publishing, 2014, pp 311–352

Lam RW, Kennedy SH, Grigoriadis S, et al; Canadian Network for Mood and Anxiety Treatments (CANMAT): Canadian Network for Mood and Anxiety Treatments (CANMAT) clinical guidelines for the management of major depressive disorder in adults. III. Pharmacotherapy. J Affect Disord 117 (suppl 1):S26–S43, 2009 19674794

Levinson AJ, Young LT: Assessment of patients with bipolar disorder, in Psychiatric Clinical Skills. Edited by Goldbloom DS. Philadelphia, Elsevier Mosby, 2006, pp 51–70

Minkoff K: Comprehensive Continuous Integrated System of Care (CCISC): psychopharmacology practice guidelines for individuals with co-occurring psychiatric and substance use disorders (COD). January 2005. Available at: http://www.kenminkoff.com/article1.doc. Accessed December 14, 2014.

Nasreddine ZS, Phillips NA, Bédirian V, et al: The Montreal Cognitive Assessment, MoCA: a brief screening tool for mild cognitive impairment. J Am Geriatr Soc 53(4):695–699, 2005 15817019

Parikh SV, Segal ZV, Grigoriadis S, et al; Canadian Network for Mood and Anxiety Treatments (CANMAT): Canadian Network for Mood and Anxiety Treatments (CANMAT) clinical guidelines for the management of major depressive disorder in adults. II. Psychotherapy alone or in combination with antidepressant medication. J Affect Disord 117 (suppl 1):S15–S25, 2009 19682749

Shea SC: Psychiatric Interviewing: The Art of Understanding, 2nd Edition. Philadelphia, PA, WB Saunders, 1998, pp 575–621

Spielmans GI, Berman MI, Linardatos E, et al: Adjunctive atypical antipsychotic treatment for major depressive disorder: a meta-analysis of depression, quality of life, and safety outcomes. PLoS Med 10(3):e1001403, 2013 23554581

Swann AC: Mania and mixed states, in Emergency Psychiatry: Principles and Practice. Edited by Glick RL, Berlin JS, Fishkind A, et al. Philadelphia, PA, Lippincott Williams & Wilkins, 2008, pp 189–200

Winkler D, Pjrek E, Kasper S: Anger attacks in depression—evidence for a male depressive syndrome. Psychother Psychosom 74(5):303–307, 2005 16088268

Yatham LN, Kennedy SH, Parikh SV, et al: Canadian Network for Mood and Anxiety Treatments (CANMAT) and International Society for Bipolar Disorders (ISBD) collaborative update of CANMAT guidelines for the management of patients with bipolar disorder: update 2013. Bipolar Disord 15(1):1–44, 2013 23237061

Suggested Readings

Edwards CD, Glick RL: Depression, in Emergency Psychiatry: Principles and Practice. Edited by Glick RL, Berlin JS, Fishkind A, et al. Philadelphia, PA, Lippincott Williams & Wilkins, 2008, pp 175–188

Swann AC: Mania and mixed states, in Emergency Psychiatry: Principles and Practice. Edited by Glick RL, Berlin JS, Fishkind A, et al. Philadelphia, PA, Lippincott Williams & Wilkins, 2008, pp 189–200

5

The Psychotic Patient

Patricia Schwartz, M.D.
Mary Weathers Case, M.D.
Joshua Berezin, M.S., M.D.

Case Example

Mr. L is a 57-year-old undomiciled black veteran with unknown past psychiatric history, who arrived by ambulance after he was found naked under the highway in the rain, stating that he needed to take a shower. He used military language, asking for a "debriefing" and demanding to see a "medic." He reported that he was a "three-star general" and demanded that staff call the Pentagon.

Definitions

Psychosis is characterized by "delusions, hallucinations, disorganized thinking (speech), grossly disorganized or abnormal motor behavior (including catatonia), and negative symptoms" (American Psychiatric Association 2013, p. 87) and is a common reason for patients to present to the psychiatric emergency room. *Delusions* are "fixed beliefs that are not amenable to change in light of conflicting evidence" (American Psychiatric Association 2013, p. 87). *Hallucinations* are "perception-like experiences that occur without an external stimulus" (American Psychiatric Association 2013, p. 87) and can be olfactory, visual, tactile, gustatory, and auditory; the latter are the most common in schizophrenia and related psychotic disorders. *Disorganized speech* occurs when the patient no longer expresses himself or herself coherently, switching from topic to topic, giving unrelated answers to questions, or, in its most severe presentation, being unable to maintain sentence structure ("word salad"). *Disorganized behaviors* can include sudden, unprovoked acts of violence, sexually inappropriate behavior, or even the inability to perform activities of daily living such as putting on clothing correctly. *Catatonic behaviors* include negativism (a resistance to instructions), immobility, posturing, and mutism. *Negative symptoms* include diminished emotional expression, avolition (decreased motivation to engage in purposeful activities), alogia (decreased speech output), anhedonia (decreased ability to experience pleasure from positive experiences), and asociality (decreased interest in social interactions).

Initial Survey of the Patient

The evaluation of the patient with psychotic symptoms in the emergency setting begins the moment the patient arrives at the hospital, if not before. The clinician should carefully note the circumstances of the patient's arrival and his or her initial appearance to determine how to safely proceed with the assessment.

Mode of Presentation

Psychotic patients present by a number of means and under a variety of circumstances, all of which are relevant to evaluation and treatment. An individual can be taken to the emergency room by ambulance; arrive under his or her own volition; or be brought by family, friends, strangers, or law enforcement personnel (Dhossche and Ghani 1998). Individuals who self-present to the emergency room for psychosis generally fall into one of three major categories:

1) those who present with medical and somatic complaints, 2) those who present with social complaints, and 3) those who present with psychiatric complaints. Of psychotic patients with psychiatric complaints, the chief subjective complaint is often unrelated to psychosis. Common reasons for such patients to request help are mood symptoms or social stressors, and when they present with more overtly psychotic complaints, such as hallucinations, feelings of persecution, or paranoid ideation, they often lack insight into the psychotic nature of their complaints. Persons who present complaining of homelessness, financial difficulties, or other social issues often reveal themselves to be flagrantly psychotic as well. An individual who requests a social intervention or who appears to have secondary motives for presenting to the emergency room requires a full evaluation.

Psychotic patients are often referred to the emergency room by someone else. Behavior intolerable to the community, such as violence, aggression, agitation, and disorganized or inappropriate behavior, will commonly result in the involvement of either law enforcement or emergency medical services. Patients with persecutory delusions may make frequent complaints about others to law enforcement agencies and end up being referred for evaluation, thanks usually to a concerned law enforcement officer. Families of psychotic individuals may bring their loved ones to emergency services for aggressive behaviors, or they may report that the patients have stopped eating, are not sleeping, are behaving oddly, or are otherwise unable to care for themselves. After some change in their baseline behavior occurs, patients already connected to the mental health system may be referred for evaluation by health care providers, case managers, counselors, social workers, staff in shelters or prison systems, or other public agencies.

Choosing a Setting for the Initial Patient Evaluation

Having considered the psychotic patient's mode of presentation, a clinician needs to determine the appropriate setting for the evaluation. In many hospitals, patients are seen in the medical emergency department, and psychiatric consultation is available at the request of emergency department staff. Larger tertiary care centers may have a designated psychiatric emergency room that is separate from the medical emergency room. In such cases, staff must decide whether to evaluate a patient in the psychiatric or medical emergency room.

The initial patient contact is often a triage nurse, who briefly interviews the patient, obtains a set of vital signs, and determines whether the chief complaint is primarily medical or psychiatric. Vital sign abnormalities, somatic complaints, physical signs, marked intoxication, disorientation, rapid onset of psychotic symptoms, or a waxing and waning mental status are all strong indications for evaluation in the medical emergency department, even when a designated psychiatric emergency room is available, at least until the patient is determined to be medically stable. Other patients who warrant a thorough workup in a medical emergency department include patients who are experiencing psychotic symptoms for the first time, elderly patients, and patients with a history of trauma, falls, or significant medical comorbidities (Marco and Vaughan 2005). Regardless of the setting, the psychiatrist plays a critical role in the medical management of psychiatric patients by generating a differential diagnosis that takes into account possible medical etiologies for psychosis (see later section "Differential Diagnosis") and by effectively communicating specific concerns about a patient's presentation to other physicians, nurses, and hospital staff. Under no circumstances should a potentially medically ill patient with psychosis be simply referred to the emergency room for "medical clearance" without a conversation between the psychiatrist and the emergency room physician that addresses the exact nature of the concern.

Initial Assessment and Management

After the setting is determined, the next decision is whether the patient can wait to be fully evaluated or must be seen immediately. If the patient is being evaluated in a medical emergency department, either because the patient is medically unstable or because the facility does not have a designated psychiatric emergency room, the patient should be seen as quickly as possible.

The initial psychiatric assessment, which is separate from the full interview that will follow, has one primary purpose: to assess danger and maintain a safe environment for both patients and providers. Any patient who is physically violent on arrival requires immediate assessment and may require urgent behavioral and/or pharmacological intervention. Conversely, a patient who arrives in some form of restraint may no longer need it. Patients brought in by emergency medical services, for example, may have been agitated and dangerous at the time of their initial point of contact but may have calmed sufficiently in transit. For this reason, any patient arriving in physical restraints should be assessed immediately, and a decision needs to be made as to whether physical restraint is absolutely necessary to avoid imminent danger; almost always a less restrictive intervention is available. Other patients who require immediate assessment include those who appear frightened or paranoid, are verbally responding to internal stimuli, are verbally aggressive or threatening, have psychomotor agitation (e.g., pacing or shadowboxing), or are attempting to leave the area without being evaluated. In general, special care must be taken in the initial assessment of psychotic patients who present involuntarily to the emergency room setting.

A safe and well-run psychiatric emergency department will have adequate staff available to rapidly and effectively deal with any sudden violent outburst with a certain amount of sensitivity to the special needs of this patient population. The psychiatrist should not approach an agitated patient to perform an initial assessment without support staff in the room. On the other hand, the psychiatrist should not leave the initial assessment to the support staff; a team approach works best, and an adequate "show of force" will often be enough to defuse a potentially dangerous situation. The psychiatrist should approach the patient and introduce himself or herself as the doctor who will be performing the evaluation. Patients should be given information about what to expect in language they can understand. It may be appropriate to explain the emergency room procedures, such as performing a search, holding personal valuables in a safe place, or changing into hospital clothes, with emphasis on the fact that these are standard procedures. Any reasonable wants or needs of the patient, such as hunger or thirst or the need for a bathroom, should be addressed. Often, offering food or drink even when the patient has not asked for it may have a calming effect. Patients who want to contact their family or legal services should be given the opportunity to do so.

Unfortunately, some patients with acute psychosis will remain too agitated to be initially assessed, or will become agitated during their evaluation or disposition to the point where they become potentially dangerous to themselves, staff, or other patients. In such cases, when verbal de-escalation techniques have been exhausted, the next step generally involves the use of pharmacological interventions, physical restraints, or both. The subject of seclusion and restraint is covered more fully in Chapter 11, "Seclusion and Restraint in Emergency Settings."

The treating physician has several choices to make in determining which medications to use, by which route, and in what doses (Wilson et al. 2012).

Although time is of the essence and information is often lacking, the first step in managing agitated patients is to establish a working diagnosis, which will guide the choice of medication. For these purposes, diagnostic categories can be broad and include alcohol intoxication, alcohol withdrawal, stimulant intoxication, delirium, and primary psychotic illnesses. Acute alcohol intoxication raises concerns for oversedation, so when medications are absolutely necessary, monotherapy with haloperidol is likely the safest choice. Alcohol withdrawal and stimulant intoxication should be managed with benzodiazepines. Delirium should be managed first and foremost with correction of the underlying abnormality, with low-dose antipsychotics as adjunctive treatments. Traditionally, agitation secondary to underlying psychotic illnesses has been managed with haloperidol, often in combination with lorazepam. Although this combination is widely used, guidelines now recommend atypical antipsychotics as first-line treatment given their more favorable safety profiles (Wilson et al. 2012).

The choice of drug also depends on the route of administration. In general, unless a patient is physically violent or in imminent danger of becoming so, providers should offer even the most seemingly agitated patient the option of taking medications by mouth and can similarly involve the patient in choosing a medication that has worked well for him or her in the past (Currier et al. 2004). These steps can maintain patient rapport in an otherwise coercive context, and giving the patient some power over the situation may itself aid in de-escalation. For management of agitation secondary to an underlying psychotic illness, oral risperidone (available in solution) or olanzapine is a reasonable first-line choice, with haloperidol with lorazepam as an additional option. When intramuscular medication is required, it is advisable to first have the necessary staff on hand to restrain the patient physically, if necessary, because attempting to give an injection to an unwilling agitated patient without at least temporary restraint poses a significant risk of needlestick or other injury to all involved. Among the second-generation antipsychotics, olanzapine, ziprasidone, and aripiprazole are all available in intramuscular formulations. In terms of dosing, one should keep in mind that patients who are naïve to antipsychotics are likely to be more quickly and heavily sedated and therefore may require less medication. Standard dosages do not need to be increased for obese, large, or severely agitated patients. As with all medications, dosages used in elderly patients are typically much less than the dosage for a typical younger adult. Concomitant use of intramuscular olanzapine and intramuscular benzodiazepines should be avoided.

All antipsychotic medications have the potential to cause side effects. The patient in the emergency setting is at particular risk for two reasons: patients may at times need to be medicated without sufficient knowledge of medical comorbidities or previous reactions to medications, and patients treated in the emergency department and subsequently discharged are often lost to follow-up. Patients treated with typical antipsychotics or risperidone in the emergency room should be observed for signs of acute dystonia, such as muscle spasm or stiffness. Acute dystonia is treated with intramuscular injection of anticholinergic drugs, such as diphenhydramine or benztropine. Intramuscular injection of chlorpromazine can lead to orthostasis, lowering of the seizure threshold, and anticholinergic effects. Other potential side effects of antipsychotics are akathisia (i.e., the subjective sense of being unable to sit still or stop moving) and tardive dyskinesia (i.e., abnormal choreiform movements than can often be observed in patients with a history of treatment with typical antipsychotics; these are unlikely to be caused or significantly worsened by a single antipsychotic dose in the setting of agitation).

Although the ideal intervention would control agitation without putting the patient to sleep, in practice, shortly after receiving medications, many patients will often become too sedated to answer questions. It is therefore of vital importance to gather as much information from the patient as possible prior to pharmacological intervention. If nothing else, information about medical history, substances used, allergies, current medications, any recent trauma, and emergency contacts are all important to obtain.

Case Example *(continued)*

Mr. L arrived on a stretcher to the psychiatric emergency room. A cursory examination of his property revealed a veteran's identification card. He was agitated and paranoid during the interview, refusing to answer the majority of questions. He reported that he was in a car with President Bush just 2 weeks ago but said that it would be too dangerous to say why. He asked the medical students present during the interview, "Which one of you jokers grabbed me this morning?" When asked what war he is a veteran of, Mr. L replied, "I'm at war now!" He was malodorous, disheveled, and continually scratching his skin. Mental status examination revealed that he was disoriented to place and time. Because of his agitation, he received medications as needed.

Evaluation of the Psychotic Patient

Following the initial triage and assessment of the patient with psychosis, the patient should be searched and placed in a safe environment. The full psychiatric evaluation can then begin. During the interview, the same basic safety precautions that apply to all psychiatric patients should be closely followed.

The Interview

The evaluation of the patient with psychotic symptoms should include, as much as the patient will tolerate, a complete history and mental status examination. Wording questions in a nonthreatening, validating manner is critical to establishing the therapeutic alliance. Important areas of focus in the mental status examination of the patient with psychotic symptoms include abstraction, characterization of thought process and content, and characterizing internal preoccupation.

Patients, especially those experiencing their first psychotic episode, should be asked about hallucinations in the least stigmatizing way possible. When auditory hallucinations are present, patients should be asked about the number of voices they hear, what the voices say, whether they speak *to* the patient or *about* the patient, and whether they ever command the patient to do anything. Command auditory hallucinations are particularly concerning. It is of critical importance to obtain a detailed history of the nature of the commands and to assess whether they are of a violent or suicidal nature, and whether the patient has ever acted on them.

Questions about delusions should cover the range of common delusional types: persecutory, somatic, religious, and grandiose. When inquiring about delusional thoughts, the interviewer should tread carefully, because any fragile rapport he or she has managed to build with a paranoid or frankly delusional patient may be negated if the clinician appears to doubt or challenge a patient's firmly held belief; on the other hand, it is never acceptable practice to collude with a patient's delusions. In the case of somatic delusions, a patient presenting with a somatic complaint must receive a thorough and appropriate medical workup, even if the patient has a primary psychotic disorder, and particularly if there is no documentation of such a workup having been done in the past.

During this nuanced assessment, it is crucial that patients are able to express themselves in the language with which they are most comfortable and that their responses can be clearly understood by the interviewer. For this reason, foreign language interpretation services should be used when patients and interviewers do not speak the same language, and sign language interpretation should be used for patients with hearing impairments. Although it may seem more expedient at times to make use of other assessment means (e.g., using a family member for translation, or using writing with a patient who has a hearing impairment), these methods should be avoided when possible because they often fail to capture the complexity of the symptoms being described and (in the case of family member translation) pose issues surrounding privacy rights of the patient and potential bias in translation.

Collateral Sources of Information

The importance of collateral information from other sources, such as friends, family, providers, and outside observers, cannot be overestimated. Patients presenting with psychotic symptoms may be paranoid and refuse to give correct or complete information, or may be too disorganized to give such information. Health Insurance Portability and Accountability Act (U.S. Department of Health and Human Services 2003) regulations allow a clinician to contact outside sources of information in the case of an emergency, so that the patient who lacks capacity to give consent can receive emergency care. Other potential sources of (or clues to) collateral information include the patient's own property and medical records. If the patient will permit a search, his or her cell phone, wallet, and other items might provide important information that the patient may not be able to recall. Some states have prescription drug monitoring programs and Medicaid registries that can provide helpful historical information. Use of Internet search tools and social media sites should be considered on a case-by-case basis after taking into account what the clinician's motivations are for the search, what the potential effect on treatment might be, whether or not informed consent is appropriate, whether and how results will be shared with the patient, and how results will be documented (Clinton et al. 2010).

Case Example *(continued)*

Collateral information obtained from a nearby Veterans Administration hospital revealed that Mr. L was HIV positive, his last CD4 lymphocyte count was 232, and he had been treated with atovaquone and the combination drug Atripla. When asked about his HIV status, Mr. L reported noncompliance with his medications. The hospital's records also indicated a history of a parotid mass that had not yet been fully worked up. Although the hospital's notes indicated that Mr. L had a history of alcohol dependence, there was no record of any previous psychiatric treatment. Vital signs on arrival to the hospital were within normal limits, and Mr. L was not noted to have any alcohol on his breath.

Differential Diagnosis

After completing the psychiatric evaluation, the clinician must form a differential diagnosis. For all patients presenting to the psychiatric emergency service, it is generally helpful to think about differential diagnosis in terms of several broad categories into which symptoms might fit: 1) medical conditions, 2) substance-induced conditions, 3) psychotic disorders, 4) mood disorders, 5) anxiety disorders, and 6) other miscellaneous conditions.

Medical Conditions

Medical issues are often the least frequent cause of symptoms in patients who have already been triaged to psychiatry. However, patients should be examined for medical conditions first, both because a medical issue presents a potentially quickly reversible cause of symptoms and because missing a medical condition can have dire consequences. This situation is clearly illustrated by the clinical case of Mr. L. The clinician should not rush to conclude that a patient who appears psychotic has a primary psychiatric condition.

Table 5–1 presents a list, albeit not exhaustive, of medical conditions that can present with psychosis, along with the signs and symptoms they commonly cause. These symptoms often include delirium, a syndrome characterized by waxing and waning mental status that can also be accompanied by psychotic symptoms, including disorganization, hallucinations (particularly visual hallucinations), and false beliefs that are usually not fixed.

Given all the possible medical causes of psychotic symptoms, it is difficult to determine the appropriate medical workup for the patient with psychotic symptoms, particularly given that most of these conditions are rare and tests will likely be low yield. However, a medical workup serves other purposes beyond identifying medical causes of the presenting symptoms: it establishes a

Table 5–1. Medical conditions that can present with psychosis

Condition	Signs and symptoms
Electrolyte imbalances *Causes:* primary medical conditions (e.g., renal failure) or related to psychiatric conditions (e.g., eating disorders, psychogenic polydipsia)	Delirium; physical stigmata of underlying cause of electrolyte imbalance (e.g., enlarged parotid glands, dental disease in bulimia)
Hepatic encephalopathy *Cause:* acute or chronic liver failure	Delirium; asterixis; jaundice; day-night sleep reversal
Brain tumors	Hallucinations and/or delusions accompanied by headache; disorganization not usually present if tumor is focal
Infections (both systemic and central nervous system)	Delirium; elevated temperature; elevated white blood count; focal signs of infection (e.g., nuchal rigidity)
HIV	Mania; major neurocognitive disorder (dementia) featuring prominent psychomotor retardation; opportunistic infections can cause delirium or focal symptoms
Wilson's disease	Bizarre behavior; psychosis; motor symptoms; liver and kidney function abnormalities
Huntington's disease	Personality changes; depression; psychosis; choreiform movements; family history usually present
Acute intermittent porphyria	Psychosis; abdominal pain; neuropathy; autonomic dysfunction
Tertiary syphilis	Psychosis; major neurocognitive disorder (dementia); ataxia; Argyll Robertson pupils
Hyperthyroidism or hypothyroidism	Mood and psychotic symptoms; physical symptoms of each syndrome (e.g., heat or cold intolerance, hair loss, weight loss/gain)

Table 5–1.   Medical conditions that can present with psychosis *(continued)*

Condition	Signs and symptoms
Seizures	Interictal or postictal psychosis; hyperreligiosity; "viscous" or "sticky" style of interaction; auditory hallucinations in temporal lobe epilepsy
Major neurocognitive disorder (dementia)	Visual hallucinations (particularly in DSM-5 major neurocognitive disorder with Lewy bodies); paranoid ideation (most typically that people are stealing from them)
Medications *Examples:* steroids, interferon, levetiracetam, dopamine agonists	Psychosis is usually temporally related to when the patient began taking the medication; would be classified as substance/medication-induced psychosis by DSM-5

Note.   DSM-5 = *Diagnostic and Statistical Manual of Mental Disorders*, 5th Edition (American Psychiatric Association 2013).

medical baseline for patients without previous psychiatric treatment (a useful tool in assessing for potential side effects of medication should this treatment be instituted in the future), it screens for side effects in patients already engaged in pharmacological treatment, and it screens for unrelated medical illnesses in this vulnerable population. In fact, a growing body of evidence supports the contention that people with primary psychotic disorders such as schizophrenia have a much higher rate of medical comorbidity (e.g., cancer, heart disease, diabetes) than the general population (Newcomer 2006), and when such medical conditions exist, the patients' mortality is also well above the average. Regardless of psychiatric history, every patient who presents with psychotic symptoms should at minimum have a complete blood count, a comprehensive metabolic profile, thyroid-stimulating hormone test, and syphilis screening. HIV testing should also be encouraged given the prevalence of HIV and the added benefit as a public health measure. A more extensive workup should be considered for patients with new-onset psychotic symptoms: imaging, preferably magnetic resonance imaging, should be strongly considered to rule out tumors and other intracranial lesions as the cause of psychotic symptoms, and electroencephalography can be considered to rule out seizures (particularly temporal lobe epilepsy) in patients with a suggestive clinical history. Further tests should be ordered if personal history, family history, or the results of initial testing are suspicious for a rare medical cause (Freudenreich et al. 2009). For instance, a patient with psychotic symptoms who is found to have elevated liver function tests might warrant further workup for Wilson's disease, including an ophthalmological exam looking for Kayser-Fleischer rings and serum ceruloplasmin. Similarly, a patient with a history of brief psychotic episodes associated with neuropathy and abdominal pain should have urine sent during an episode (checking for uroporphyrin, porphobilinogen, and aminolevulinic acid) to rule out acute intermittent porphyria. Treatment for psychosis secondary to a general medical condition should be directed toward addressing the underlying medical condition and is usually best accomplished on a medical unit with psychiatric consultation.

The timing of this medical workup is an issue of some debate in both the psychiatric and the emergency medicine literature, given the competing interests of 1) promptly clearing patients to receive definitive care in an appropriate psychiatric setting (thereby reducing the burden of care on the busy emergency department) and 2) not inappropriately sending medically ill patients to these psychiatric settings. In the patient with preexisting psychiatric illness who presents similarly to previous episodes, a full history, physical examination, and vital signs are often sufficient to determine medical stability for transfer from the emergency department to a psychiatric setting (presuming that setting has the capacity to conduct further laboratory screening and medical workup as deemed appropriate). In contrast, for patients with new-onset symptoms or those who are unable to provide an adequate history, some laboratory screening is indicated in the emergency department (Zun 2012).

Substance-Induced Conditions

A variety of substances can cause psychotic symptoms, during either intoxication or withdrawal. Table 5–2 lists some of the psychosis-causing substances commonly encountered in the emergency setting and their accompanying symptoms. All patients presenting with psychotic symptoms in the emergency department should be screened for substance use with urine or serum toxicology; notably, however, synthetic cannabinoids ("K2," "spice"), cathinones ("bath salts"), and an ever-expanding array of designer drugs are not picked up on commercially available screening tests. Additionally, the formulations of these drugs differ across and even within products, so even patient reports of designer drug use are often unreliable predictors of intoxication syndromes (Rosenbaum et al. 2012).

Substance use can also predispose patients to falls and other accidents with consequent head trauma, which can then present with psychiatric symptoms. It is important not to fall into the trap of incorrectly attributing these symptoms to the substance use, because missing a head injury can lead to serious consequences for the patient. Patients with substance abuse who present with new-onset psychotic symptoms should be examined for evidence of head trauma; if evidence is found, head imaging should be obtained.

Treatment for substance-induced psychosis usually involves maintaining the patient's safety in a psychiatric setting with supportive interventions until the symptoms resolve. In cases of delirium tremens, however, aggressive medical management (often in an intensive care unit) is required to prevent seizures, aspiration, and death. Despite the fact that patients with substance-induced psychosis often do not have an underlying psychotic illness, they can benefit from antipsychotics and benzodiazepines on an as-needed basis during the episode to address their symptoms, particularly if agitation is prominent.

Psychotic Disorders

The most obvious diagnoses to consider when a patient presents with psychotic symptoms in the psychiatric emergency setting are described in DSM-5 (American Psychiatric Association 2013) as schizophrenia spectrum and other psychotic disorders. These include schizophrenia, schizoaffective disorder, schizophreniform disorder, brief psychotic disorder, delusional disorder, and schizotypal personality disorder. These diagnoses are distinguished from one another by history obtained from the patient and collateral information about time course, mood symptoms, and stressors. The following is a brief review of the DSM-5 criteria for each diagnosis:

- *Schizophrenia:* At least 6 months of symptoms, and at least 1 month of meeting two of the following symptoms: delusions, hallucinations, disorganized speech, grossly disorganized or catatonic behavior, or negative symptoms.

Table 5–2.   Substances that can cause psychosis

Substance	Signs and symptoms
Alcohol	*Intoxication:* agitation may appear psychotic *Withdrawal:* hallucinations with alcoholic hallucinosis; hallucinations and delirium with delirium tremens
Amphetamines	*Intoxication:* psychosis similar to that seen with cocaine but often prolonged (3–5 days), dilated pupils; often accompanied by stigmata of chronic amphetamine use (e.g., anorexia, poor dentition)
Cannabis	*Intoxication:* paranoid ideation; if severe, drug may have been laced with other substances (e.g., PCP)
Cathinones ("bath salts," mephedrone, MDPV)	*Intoxication:* manic symptoms, paranoia, reports of bizarre and aggressive behavior; negative urine toxicology test
Cocaine	*Intoxication:* disorganization, manic symptoms, delusions, hallucinations (including tactile), dilated pupils; lasts for hours after use *Withdrawal:* depressed mood, hallucinations, somnolence, social withdrawal; beginning hours after use and lasting 24–72 hours
Hallucinogens (LSD, psilocybin mushrooms)	*Intoxication:* vivid visual hallucinations, dissociative symptoms; occasions of recurrence of symptoms of intoxication ("flashbacks") can occur months or years after use
PCP	*Intoxication:* hallucinations, delusions, unpredictable violence; symptoms wax and wane and can last 3–5 days; associated with hyperacusis and nystagmus
Synthetic cannabinoids ("K2", "spice," "potpourri," etc.)	*Intoxication:* agitation, paranoia, hallucinations, perceptual disturbances; negative urine toxicology test

Note. LSD = lysergic acid diethylamide; MDPV = 3,4-methylenedioxypyrovalerone; PCP = phencyclidine.

- *Schizoaffective disorder:* Criteria are met during an uninterrupted period of illness for both a major mood episode (major depressive or manic) and the above criterion for schizophrenia, with delusions or hallucinations present for at least 2 weeks in the absence of mood symptoms at some point during the illness.

- *Schizophreniform disorder:* At least 1 month but less than 6 months of psychotic symptoms.
- *Brief psychotic disorder:* Psychotic symptoms appear and resolve fully in less than 1 month; symptoms are often caused by the presence of an acute stressor.
- *Delusional disorder:* At least 1 month of one or more delusions without marked impairment in functioning and without other associated psychotic symptoms.
- *Schizotypal personality disorder:* A pervasive pattern of decreased capacity for close interpersonal relationships, cognitive and perceptual distortions, and eccentricities of behavior.

Treatment for these psychotic disorders varies by diagnosis but usually involves the use of antipsychotic agents combined with psychosocial treatments.

Mood Disorders

Both manic and major depressive episodes can present with psychotic features. Given that mood disorders are much more common than primary psychotic disorders, and that the treatment and prognosis are different for patients with mood disorders with psychotic features than for patients with primary psychotic disorders, all patients presenting with psychotic symptoms should be evaluated closely, both during the interview and in the gathering of collateral information, for the presence of mood symptoms. Psychotic symptoms that are present during mood episodes are usually mood congruent (e.g., the manic patient may have grandiose delusions, whereas the depressed patient may have negativistic delusions, such as that his or her organs are rotting). Treatment for mood disorders with psychotic features involves pharmacological treatment, both for the mood symptoms and for the psychotic symptoms, as well as psychotherapy.

Anxiety Disorders

Severe presentations of some anxiety disorders may appear to be psychosis, and this possibility should be considered in patients presenting to the emergency department. Some patients with obsessive-compulsive disorder can hold their obsessive thoughts so rigidly or engage in such bizarre rituals as to appear psychotic. Patients who are in the midst of reexperiencing episodes of posttraumatic stress disorder (particularly when intoxication is also involved) can also appear psychotic. This phenomenon highlights the importance of obtaining a full psychiatric review of symptoms during the interview, because the treatment for these disorders will be very different from treatment for primary psychotic disorders.

Miscellaneous Conditions

Several other conditions should be considered in the differential diagnosis for patients presenting to the emergency department with psychotic symptoms. Although DSM-5 describes schizotypal personality disorder as a primary psychotic disorder based on its apparent genetic relationship with schizophrenia (because this personality disorder is more common among first-degree relatives of individuals with schizophrenia), paranoid personality disorder (another Cluster A personality disorder) can also be considered in patients who present with a persistent pattern of distrust and suspicion of others but without frank delusions. Patients with borderline personality disorder, as well as other Cluster B personality disorders, can develop micropsychotic episodes, particularly in the context of acute stressors. Patients with dissociative disorder can appear disorganized and psychotic. Additionally, the stereotyped behavior and deficits in communication and social interaction typical of autism spectrum disorder can be difficult to distinguish from psychotic symptoms, particularly when a developmental history is not readily available (Dossetor 2007).

Although it should always be a diagnosis of exclusion, malingered psychosis is unfortunately not at all uncommon in the psychiatric emergency setting. In general, malingering should be considered in patients who have clear motives for doing so (as in patients under arrest), who exhibit inconsistencies in their history and mental status examination, or who are very vague in their descriptions of their symptoms. Also suspect are patients who report dangerous symptoms that are inconsistent with their affect, behavior, and thought process (e.g., a patient who appears cheerful in the waiting area but subsequently reports to the doctor, "I'm hearing voices telling me to kill myself and others"). The more detail the psychiatrist presses for during the interview, the more difficult it will become for a malingering patient to keep his or her story straight (Resnick 1999). When available, medical records from within the same institution should be examined; a history of malingering or a pattern of brief inpatient admissions from which the patient frequently signs out against medical advice would be added evidence of a malingering diagnosis. In practice, differentiating psychotic disorders from malingering can be complicated, because patients with genuine psychotic disorders may at times present primarily for secondary gain. In these cases, a careful risk assessment should guide disposition.

Risk Assessment: Important Risk Factors in the Psychotic Patient

The risk assessments of patients who are judged, after careful consideration of the differential diagnoses, to most likely have a disorder other than a primary psychotic disorder are addressed in the chapters appropriate to the determined underlying diagnoses. In this section, we focus on the evidence-based risk assessment of patients who are thought to have a primary psychotic disorder, although many of the risk factors for this population can be extrapolated to other populations who experience psychotic symptoms in the context of other disorders. This is certainly not an exhaustive listing of all of the risk factors for suicide and violence; this discussion is meant to highlight those factors that are most relevant to the emergency psychiatric assessment.

Risk Factors for Violence

The public perception that patients with psychosis are at elevated risk of violence has sparked a debate in the psychiatric literature that is still far from being resolved, despite the existence of several large-scale studies on the topic (Torrey et al. 2008). Although the jury is still out on this larger question, it is clear from the literature that several factors can predict violence in this population. As might be expected, *past history of violence and criminal behavior* is one of the strongest predictors of future violence and, if present, should be weighted heavily in the risk assessment of any patient. In a risk assessment, however, the clinician cannot rely exclusively on past behavior as a predictor of future violent behavior. On the one hand, if past behavior were the only factor considered, the risk assessment would fail to identify patients with no such history who go on to become first-time perpetrators of violence (Buchanan 2008). On the other hand, a history of violence is always present in patients who have engaged in that behavior, and therefore a focus on history fails to consider the patient's acute risks and current symptoms.

Comorbid substance abuse may be one of the largest contributors to violence among patients with a primary psychotic illness (Monahan et al. 2001). However, some authors have found that it is not the substance abuse itself but other factors associated with substance abuse (e.g., childhood conduct disorder and current psychotic symptoms) that are most predictive of violence (Swanson et al. 2006). *Intoxication* certainly raises the risk of violence due to its disinhibiting effects, but it is an easily modifiable risk factor in that the patient's risk can be significantly reduced just by retaining the patient until he or she is no longer intoxicated. *Akathisia* can similarly increase risk of violent acting-out behavior due to the physical discomfort that it causes, and it can be easily modified by changing the psychopharmacological regimen.

Positive psychotic symptoms, including hallucinations and delusions (particularly hallucinations of a command nature and delusions of a persecutory nature), are associated with higher rates of violence, whereas negative symptoms may actually lower the risk of serious violence (Swanson et al. 2006). Command auditory hallucinations to harm others are particularly concerning if the patient has any history of acting on command auditory hallucinations in the past. Given the important role of antipsychotics in preventing positive symptoms, *noncompliance with antipsychotics* increases the risk of violence.

Recent violent threats and behavior leading up to presentation in the psychiatric emergency setting must be given significant weight in the risk assessment, particularly if the patient has a past history of violence or arrest. *Homicidal ideation,* even if it has been communicated as violent fantasies shared only with the assessing clinician rather than as threats toward a target, will also increase the acute risk of violence. Even when violent ideation or behavior is absent from the current presentation, the risk of repeated violence if the patient has a history of violent behavior when experiencing similar symptoms can be serious enough to justify the classification of the patient as at elevated acute risk.

Risk Factors for Suicide

When assessing suicide risk, past history is strongly predictive of future behavior, and a history of *past suicide attempts* will chronically elevate a patient's risk of future suicide attempts. Approximately 5%–6% of patients with schizophrenia die from suicide (American Psychiatric Association 2013, p. 104). Suicidality risk is generally thought to be highest early in the course of the illness, highlighting the importance of engaging patients with psychosis early in the course of their symptoms (Melle et al. 2006). *Comorbidity with depressive symptoms or with substance abuse* is thought to increase the risk of suicide attempts among patients with psychotic symptoms, as is the presence of *command auditory hallucinations to harm oneself* (particularly when the patient has a history of acting on command auditory hallucinations). *Current suicidal ideation,* particularly if there is evidence of planning, should be weighted heavily in the risk assessment. However, the presence of contingency to this suicidal ideation (e.g., "If you don't admit me, I will kill myself") is less predictive than noncontingent suicidal ideation (Lambert 2002). *Social isolation* likely also contributes to suicide risk, whereas the presence of good social and treatment supports may serve as a protective factor. *Akathisia* may also worsen suicide risk and should be given particular attention because this is a modifiable risk factor. For psychotic patients, as for all psychiatric patients, *access to weapons* will elevate concern about suicide risk.

Other Risk Factors for Harm to Self

A risk assessment also must include a consideration of the potential danger to a patient from inability to care for self. Much of this assessment can be ascertained from the first contact with a patient: if the patient is disheveled, suffering from parasite infestation, or suffering from visible consequences of untreated medical illness that on evaluation appear to be related to the patient's psychotic symptoms, then the patient clearly is unable to care for himself or herself. For example, diabetes-related leg ulcers may turn out to have been caused by the patient not taking prescribed insulin, under the delusion that he or she is cured of diabetes.

If the individual's inability to care for self is not obvious, the clinician must ask questions—often subtle questions—to assess a patient's ability to care for self. For instance, a patient who is afraid to stay in her apartment due to persecutory delusions might choose instead to stay in a shelter. Does this indicate the patient's inability to care for self? The answer to that question hinges on several subsidiary questions about whether the behavior (staying in the shelter) results in adverse consequences for the patient that can lead to potential worsening of her physical or mental health. Appropriate questions might include the following: Does she have access to her psychiatric medications in the shelter? Is she still able to attend her outpatient treatment? Does she still have access to her family and social supports? Has similar behavior led to harm in the past? The availability of support services may alter decisions about whether such a patient needs inpatient psychiatric hospitalization or can be maintained in the community with greater oversight.

Making a Decision About Appropriate Treatment

Having made a thorough risk assessment, the clinician will usually have a good impression of what he or she believes is the appropriate setting for a pa tient's treatment. If the patient with psychotic symptoms is motivated to follow the clinician's recommendations, the decision about what to do at this point is easier. If the clinician believes that the patient would benefit from inpatient stabilization (either because of the degree of risk or because inpatient treatment would facilitate a more rapid workup and treatment of the patient's symptoms), then the patient can be admitted on a voluntary basis. Alternatively, if the clinician feels that the patient can be safely discharged with a higher level of outpatient care, he or she can feel reassured that the patient is likely to comply with such interventions. The degree of community services that can be accessed from the emergency setting varies in different locations, as discussed further in Chapter 1, "Approach to Psychiatric Emergencies." For patients discharged during their first psychotic episode, many states and municipalities offer special services with which emergency providers should be familiar.

If a patient with psychotic symptoms is not motivated for treatment, or if the patient actively opposes treatment, then the choice of an appropriate treatment setting is far more difficult. A lack of motivation for treatment is often associated with greater severity of symptoms, increased clinical impression of dangerousness to others, high suspiciousness, and grandiosity (Mulder et al. 2005). Often, such situations require involuntary hospitalization. The clinician faces difficulties when the patient does not meet the legal standards for involuntary commitment but is unlikely to follow up with outpatient treatment. In such cases, the clinician can try to build a therapeutic alliance and to increase the patient's motivation (possibly by using techniques such as motivational interviewing) in the emergency setting. The clinician can also attempt to mobilize the patient's social supports (including family, friends, and treatment providers such as case managers) to encourage the patient's compliance with outpatient follow-up and to monitor closely for any worsening of symptoms that might warrant the patient's return to the emergency room.

Once a decision has been made to hospitalize a patient on either a voluntary or an involuntary basis, the clinician in the emergency department is also charged with formulating and executing a plan for treatment until the patient is reassessed by the inpatient team. At that point, the medical workup should have already been initiated, and the clinician should communicate to the inpatient team what tests or medical issues need to be pursued further. The emergency clinician is also responsible for sending the patient to the inpatient unit at the appropriate level of observation and for communicating to the inpatient team the patient's level of risk for violence or suicidality. The emergency clinician should also alert the inpatient team to any other management issues that he or she believes the patient may pose (e.g., if the patient is at risk of sexual acting-out or elopement based on history or clinical presentation).

Emergency clinicians are often responsible for initiating or changing a patient's pharmacological regimen. Pharmacological modifications are often required to reduce the patient's level of risk on the inpatient unit, for instance, if he or she has already demonstrated agitation in the emergency setting. However, in this era of managed care and brief hospitalizations, it is often necessary, even in less acute situations, to make medication changes immediately rather than waiting for the inpatient team to make a decision the next day. What follows is a brief list of factors that should be considered in the choice of antipsychotic agents for the patient with psychotic symptoms:

- *Side effects:* Atypical (second-generation) antipsychotics pose a greater risk of metabolic syndrome, whereas typical (first-generation) antipsychotics pose an increased risk of extrapyramidal symptoms, tardive dyskinesia, and neuroleptic malignant syndrome. Each patient's situation should be considered individually based on the tolerability of these side effects and any personal or family history (e.g., diabetes) that might put the patient at greater risk of these side effects.

- *History:* Personal or family history of response to a particular agent may affect the selection.
- *Potential for noncompliance:* The patient considered at high risk of "cheeking" while in the hospital may require an antipsychotic available in liquid or dissolving tablet form. The patient who may require a court order for medications over objection may benefit from an antipsychotic that is also available in a short-acting injectable form. The patient who is at chronic risk of noncompliance in the outpatient setting, even after being stabilized in the inpatient setting, might be best served by being started on the oral form of an antipsychotic that is also available as a long-acting injectable preparation, onto which the patient may later be titrated.
- *Cost and access issues:* It is important to ensure that after discharge, the patient will still be able to obtain the medication started during inpatient treatment; otherwise, the patient is more likely to become noncompliant in the future. If uninsured, the patient should be started on a medication that he or she will be able to afford when discharged, or the clinician should initiate efforts to get the patient insured. If the patient is insured but the insurance plan restricts the formulary of available agents, the patient should be started on a formulary agent if possible, or a request to the insurance company for the nonformulary agent needs to be made.
- *Frequency of dosing:* Patients tend to have greater rates of compliance with medications that have once-daily dosing as opposed to more frequent dosing.

Case Example *(continued)*

Suspicion for a medical or substance-induced cause for Mr. L's psychosis was high, given the absence of a history of psychosis, the presence of a history of alcohol dependence and multiple medical problems that could present with brain involvement, and the presence of disorientation on mental status examination. Nevertheless, the decision was made that Mr. L could be treated on the psychiatric service (rather than a medical service) because his vital signs were normal and he did not otherwise appear medically unstable, and because he would benefit from being treated in a secure, locked area given his agitation. A medical workup, including blood work, urine toxicology, chest X ray, and head computed tomography (CT), was initiated promptly. Preliminary read of a head CT scan without contrast revealed a large acute right parietal subdural hematoma, extending from the vertex to the level of the body of the lateral ventricles. A second extra-axial collection along the right frontoparietal convexity, with a more heterogeneous appearance, suggested acute or chronic subdural hematomas. There was also a 1.3-cm leftward midline shift and right uncal herniation. The etiology of these injuries was presumably multiple prior falls while intoxicated.

At this time, Mr. L was transferred to the medical emergency department, and neurosurgery was called. By this point, he had become more obtunded, either from the as-needed medications or from the uncal herniation. Mannitol was administered, but the patient continued to deteriorate, so the decision was made to take him to surgery, where his subdural hematoma was successfully evacuated and a drain was left in place. Follow-up after he was transferred to a rehabilitation unit revealed that Mr. L was organized and able to give a coherent history, with no residual psychotic symptoms. Although he had some residual left-sided weakness, he was able to walk and move independently.

Role of the Emergency Psychiatrist as Psychoeducator

The emergency psychiatrist plays a vital role in providing psychoeducation to patients and their families. Often, the emergency clinician is the first mental health contact for patients with first-break psychosis who may have no knowledge about their diagnosis or the way that the mental health system works. Frequently, patients with psychosis present to the psychiatric emergency room in a paranoid state. The clinician's failure to adequately explain the reasoning behind decisions about treatment and disposition only serves to enhance this paranoia, leaving the patient to guess at the clinician's intent and often to ultimately ascribe a malevolent motive to the clinician. The same can often be true for families, who see that their loved one is ill but often overestimate the patient's ability to care for him- or herself. The family then perceives coercive measures, such as as-needed medications and involuntary admission, as victimizing rather than as caring for their loved one. Psychoeducation serves to reverse these misconceptions and helps to build an alliance in which the patient and family are active participants in the treatment plan. This alliance is well worth the time necessary to provide psychoeducation even in the busiest of emergency settings.

Key Clinical Points

- Psychosis is characterized by delusions, hallucinations, and disorganization of speech and behavior.

- Although primary psychotic disorders such as schizophrenia are the most obvious cause, patients presenting with psychosis need to be carefully evaluated for the presence of medical conditions, substance use, and other psychiatric conditions that could be causing their symptoms.

- Care must be taken in evaluating the patient with psychotic symptoms to maintain safety while obtaining a history from the patient and collateral sources.

- Examining the history for risk factors for violence and self-harm will inform the clinician's decision regarding the need for hospitalization and further treatment.

- Antipsychotic medications play a key role both in controlling agitation and in addressing psychotic symptoms, but nonpharmacological interventions such as psychoeducation also are vital in the treatment of patients with psychotic symptoms in the emergency setting.

References

American Psychiatric Association: Diagnostic and Statistical Manual of Mental Disorders, 5th Edition. Arlington, VA, American Psychiatric Association, 2013

Buchanan A: Risk of violence by psychiatric patients: beyond the "actuarial versus clinical" assessment debate. Psychiatr Serv 59(2):184–190, 2008 18245161

Clinton BK, Silverman BC, Brendel DH: Patient-targeted googling: the ethics of searching online for patient information. Harv Rev Psychiatry 18(2):103–112, 2010 20235775

Currier GW, Chou JC, Feifel D, et al: Acute treatment of psychotic agitation: a randomized comparison of oral treatment with risperidone and lorazepam versus intramuscular treatment with haloperidol and lorazepam. J Clin Psychiatry 65(3):386–394, 2004 15096079

Dhossche DM, Ghani SO: Who brings patients to the psychiatric emergency room? Psychosocial and psychiatric correlates. Gen Hosp Psychiatry 20(4):235–240, 1998 9719903

Dossetor DR: "All that glitters is not gold": misdiagnosis of psychosis in pervasive developmental disorders—a case series. Clin Child Psychol Psychiatry 12(4):537–548, 2007 18095536

Freudenreich O, Schulz SC, Goff DC: Initial medical work-up of first-episode psychosis: a conceptual review. Early Interv Psychiatry 3(1):10–18, 2009 21352170

Lambert MT: Seven-year outcomes of patients evaluated for suicidality. Psychiatr Serv 53(1):92–94, 2002 11773656

Marco CA, Vaughan J: Emergency management of agitation in schizophrenia. Am J Emerg Med 23(6):767–776, 2005 16182986

Melle I, Johannesen JO, Friis S, et al: Early detection of the first episode of schizophrenia and suicidal behavior. Am J Psychiatry 163(5):800–804, 2006 16648319

Monahan J, Steadman HJ, Silver E, et al: Rethinking Risk Assessment: The MacArthur Study of Mental Disorders and Violence. New York, Oxford University Press, 2001

Mulder CL, Koopmans GT, Hengeveld MW: Lack of motivation for treatment in emergency psychiatry patients. Soc Psychiatry Psychiatr Epidemiol 40(6):484–488, 2005 16003598

Newcomer JW: Medical risk in patients with bipolar disorder and schizophrenia. J Clin Psychiatry 67 (suppl 9):25–30, discussion 36–42, 2006 16965186

Resnick PJ: The detection of malingered psychosis. Psychiatr Clin North Am 22(1):159–172, 1999 10083952

Rosenbaum CD, Carreiro SP, Babu KM: Here today, gone tomorrow...and back again? A review of herbal marijuana alternatives (K2, Spice), synthetic cathinones (bath salts), kratom, Salvia divinorum, methoxetamine, and piperazines. J Med Toxicol 8(1):15–32, 2012 22271566

Swanson JW, Swartz MS, Van Dorn RA, et al: A national study of violent behavior in persons with schizophrenia. Arch Gen Psychiatry 63(5):490–499, 2006 16651506

Torrey EF, Stanley J, Monahan J, et al; MacArthur Study Group: The MacArthur Violence Risk Assessment Study revisited: two views ten years after its initial publication. Psychiatr Serv 59(2):147–152, 2008 18245156

U.S. Department of Health and Human Services: Summary of the HIPAA privacy rule, May 2003. Available at: http://www.hhs.gov/ocr/privacy/hipaa/understanding/summary/privacysummary.pdf. Accessed December 21, 2014.

Wilson MP, Pepper D, Currier GW, et al: The psychopharmacology of agitation: consensus statement of the American Association for Emergency Psychiatry Project Beta Psychopharmacology Workgroup. West J Emerg Med 13(1):26–34, 2012 22461918

Zun LS: Pitfalls in the care of the psychiatric patient in the emergency department. J Emerg Med 43(5):829–835, 2012 22698827

Suggested Readings

Freudenreich O, Schulz SC, Goff DC: Initial medical work-up of first-episode psychosis: a conceptual review. Early Interv Psychiatry 3(1):10–18, 2009

Monahan J, Steadman HJ, Silver E, et al: Rethinking Risk Assessment: The MacArthur Study of Mental Disorders and Violence. New York, Oxford University Press, 2001

Zun LS: Pitfalls in the care of the psychiatric patient in the emergency department. J Emerg Med 43(5):829–835, 2012

6

The Anxious Patient

Steven Storage, M.D.
Divy Ravindranath, M.D., M.S.
James Abelson, M.D., Ph.D.

Case Example

Ms. D, a 28-year-old female graduate student with no prior psychiatric history, was referred to the psychiatric emergency service from the medical emergency department for further evaluation after a negative workup for chest pain. The referring doctor's diagnosis was anxiety. Ms. D characterizes herself as having been an anxious person for the majority of her life. She states that her mind often jumps from worry to worry, leaving her distracted and keeping her up at night. Her tension tends to embody itself in her muscles. She frequently experiences abdominal distress and heartburn but has never been diagnosed with an ulcer. She also says that she cannot think about going out

The authors would like to acknowledge the thoughtful comments of Dr. Brian Martis in the preparation of this chapter.

with friends without developing a panic attack. At the suggestion of going out, she develops a sense of dread, hyperventilates, and feels as if her heart is racing. She gets preoccupied with these physical symptoms, and her panic worsens. She calms herself by slow breathing and counting, and uses alcohol if she goes out. She had a fight with her fiancé a few days ago over "something insignificant." She subsequently tried to call him, but he responded only with a one-word text message: "Later." She began to worry about the stability of the relationship, the years she had invested in it, and her future in general. She found the distress intolerable, decided she was better off without him, and went to his house to break off the engagement. He was speechless. She departed abruptly, worrying about what she had done. Since that time, the panic attacks have occurred more frequently and without clear triggers. It has become harder to talk herself out of the panic. She spoke with her ex-fiancé and thinks they will be able to reconcile, but she thinks she needs something to help herself cope better. She doesn't want to become an alcoholic.

Ms. D is a clearly anxious woman with a classic emergency room presentation featuring elements of multiple DSM-5 (American Psychiatric Association 2013) anxiety disorder diagnoses and a broad anxious predisposition. She demonstrates behavioral tendencies that amplify anxiety (e.g., focusing on physical symptoms) and some reasonable coping efforts to alleviate her anxiety (e.g., taking slow breaths). She also demonstrates one highly dysfunctional but common consequence of anxiety: a vulnerability to impulsive action.

Everyone experiences anxiety. Its complete absence is probably extremely rare, highly pathological, and perhaps incompatible with a long life. Anyone under acute threat should experience some elements of anxiety, both psychologically/emotionally and physically. Activation of the sympathetic nervous system is a normal aspect of the response to threat and is a normal component of physical preparations needed to cope with threat. However, anxiety can also occur in the absence of genuine threat or in gross excess relative to the magnitude of the threat. When it occurs inappropriately, excessively, or uncontrollably and produces impairment in critical life functions, as seen in the case of Ms. D, anxiety is considered pathological and an anxiety disorder or related condition is likely present.

The first challenge in assessing patients who present to the emergency department is differentiating true medical emergencies from acute situations that entail less immediate risks. The presence of extreme anxiety does not by itself mean that the risk of a medical emergency is low, because serious medical threats, such as chest pain from an impending myocardial infarction, can generate very intense fear. Therefore, the first rule in managing anxiety in the emergency department is to not let its presence hinder a clinician from performing a careful assessment for medical emergencies requiring immediate intervention.

Once immediate medical risks are ruled out and a psychosocial problem is identified, safety is still not assured. The next step is to perform a careful assessment of psychiatric risk. The primary concerns at this point are risk of suicide or self-harm behaviors and risk of violence against others. Patients with only anxiety disorders are rarely violent, but anxiety does increase the risk of suicide, and highly anxious patients may well have other disorders (e.g., paranoid psychosis, borderline personality disorder) in which risk of injurious behavior toward self or others is elevated. (For guidance in assessing these types of risks, see Chapter 2, "Suicide Risk Assessment and Management," and Chapter 3, "Violence Risk Assessment.")

Anxiety disorders are very common; as many as one in four people may be affected by at least one of the anxiety disorders defined in DSM-IV-TR (American Psychiatric Association 2000). These disorders occur more frequently in women than men (at a ratio of approximately 2:1) and are more common in people at lower socioeconomic levels. Panic disorder has a lifetime prevalence of 1.5%–5.0% and is highly comorbid with other disorders (Sadock and Sadock 2003).

Clearly, many people have anxiety disorders, and anxious people use health care systems much more frequently than do other people, increasing their likelihood of presenting to emergency departments and adding to health care costs. Of 171 consecutive patients referred to an anxiety disorders specialty clinic, those with anxiety had visited nonpsychiatric medical providers six times, on average, in the prior year. Patients with panic disorder were the most frequent medical care users, followed by patients with phobias, generalized anxiety disorder, and social anxiety disorder. The majority of these visits were to the emergency room, cardiology clinic, and primary care clinic (Deacon et al. 2008).

Given the high rates at which anxious patients present to emergency rooms, it is important for emergency department staff to be well acquainted with their presentations and management. In this chapter, we present material related to the chief complaint of "anxiety" in the emergency department.

Given that panic attacks are a primary manifestation of this chief complaint and represent a paradigm for understanding acute exacerbation in any anxiety (or other psychiatric) disorder, we focus in the first two sections of this chapter on panic attacks and panic disorder. In the third section, we examine somatic symptom disorder and other disorders with prominent somatic symptoms. Somatic symptom and related disorders involve intense anxiety about physical symptoms, and even though they are not technically classified as anxiety disorders, they will bring highly anxious patients into the emergency department. In the final section, we briefly discuss other anxiety and anxiety-related conditions.

Panic Attacks

Panic Attacks and Associated Conditions

Anxiety can be a chronic or subchronic condition, but it is also experienced acutely. A sudden rise in fear may well be an appropriate response to a real threat, but it can also occur in the absence of true threat in the form of a panic attack. A panic attack is characterized by an abrupt surge of intense fear or intense discomfort that reaches a peak within minutes. Panic attacks may be *expected* (with an obvious trigger or cue) or *unexpected* (without an obvious trigger or cue). The sudden onset of fear is often accompanied by activation of the sympathetic nervous system, which may lead to increased heart rate, dilated pupils, and other physiological changes that prepare the organism to respond to threat. It triggers a heightened vigilance to both external cues and internal (bodily) states as the organism scans for sources of risk that may require immediate responses. This vigilance is associated with heightened awareness of physical sensations. In a panic attack, especially when real environmental threats are not present, these physical sensations are interpreted as a source of threat themselves, causing attention to be focused on them and leading to escalating sensations that might include palpitations, shortness of breath, lightheadedness, derealization, paresthesias, and/or nausea. These sensations in turn further heighten vigilance and the sense of threat and generate catastrophic cognitions (e.g., "I am having a heart attack" or "I am going to die"), thereby creating an escalating "fear-of-fear" cycle that culminates in a full-blown attack. The subjective sensation of altered bodily states usually far exceeds any real changes in physiological parameters.

Although a panic attack may reflect an abnormal activation of fear systems, having a panic attack does not necessarily mean that a person has panic disorder. Over one-third of the population will have a panic attack sometime in their life, but less than 5% will develop panic disorder (Sadock and Sadock 2003). All humans carry the capacity to panic in response to perceived threat. A single attack, whether in response to an identified cue or not, does not constitute a disorder. Some people even have recurrent attacks but manage them effectively and suffer no impairment, and therefore do not qualify for a diagnosis. However, if at least one attack has been spontaneous, fear of further attacks develops, and functioning is impaired, then panic disorder is likely present. Many patients with panic also develop agoraphobia, a separate DSM-5 diagnosis, which involves fear and avoidance of places from which escape might be difficult, with particular fear of having a panic attack and being unable to flee. Panic attacks can occur in the context of any psychiatric disorder, and DSM-5 now lists panic attack as a descriptive specifier that can function as a marker and prognostic factor. For example, when attacks never occur spontaneously but are consistently triggered by specific, feared cues, specific phobia with panic attacks may be a more appropriate diagnosis. Typical phobic cues can range from animals (e.g., spiders, snakes, dogs) to particular situational cues (e.g., heights, closed places, airplanes, storms). If the triggers focus on social scrutiny and fear of public embarrassment, the diagnosis might be social anxiety disorder with panic attacks. Some patients only experience abrupt surges of intense fear in response to reminders of traumatic events and might carry a diagnosis of posttraumatic stress disorder (PTSD) with panic attacks.

People with panic attacks that are always triggered by specific cues can often successfully manage the attacks through careful avoidance of their triggers, although the ability to do this depends on how readily avoidable the triggers are and the "costs" incurred by avoidance behavior. For example, avoiding spiders is much easier than avoiding social situations or all forms of public transportation. When attacks occur spontaneously, as they do in panic disorder, use of avoidance as a coping technique is more challenging and less effective; because the triggers are not circumscribed, the avoidance can become pervasive and disabling. Patients can become housebound.

The differences in diagnoses have bearing on treatment decisions. Panic and avoidance linked to specific, circumscribed triggers can be treated nonpharmacologically with exposure and desensitization-based cognitive-behavioral therapy (CBT). This treatment is based on the simple principle that fear-based avoidance usually involves automatic, cued triggering of alarm signals in the brain, and the best way to decouple the triggering cues from the automatic responses is through systematic, graded exposure to the cues in a controlled setting. Although patients with panic attacks may have avoidance behaviors for which this type of exposure therapy may be useful, patients with panic disorder are much more likely to also require pharmacological intervention. The differential thus becomes important even in the emergency department, because initiation of pharmacological treatment for well-diagnosed panic disorder might be appropriate, but evaluation by an anxiety specialist might be important before medication is started for a phobia or social anxiety, for which CBT might be the first-line treatment.

Management of a Panic Attack

Panic attacks are obviously frightening and uncomfortable. Patients with panic attacks will present to the emergency department with intense anxious distress, and the anxiety can be "contagious," especially when a threat eliciting this strong response cannot be located. When interacting with a panicking patient, a clinician needs to avoid being pulled into the whirlwind of anxiety. False assurance, such as insisting that nothing threatening is happening even before any data that can support that impression have been collected, is not likely to be helpful. However, the patient may be calmed by assurance that appropriate steps will be taken to identify and address any threats, and that the expressed distress will be taken seriously and reduced. This calm approach will be critical in building the rapport needed to fully evaluate the presenting symptom, to obtain the history and testing needed to ensure that the patient does not have a more emergent medical condition, and to build a foundation for productively addressing the acute anxiety.

In addition to maintaining a calm and confident demeanor, but without false or condescending reassurance, the clinician can take additional steps to help calm the patient. Panic attacks are sometimes associated with hyperventilation, which can trigger and intensify physical symptoms. Helping the patient to slow his or her breathing through attention and control can be helpful, emphasizing that the key is slow breathing, not deep breathing, with enough tidal volume for adequate oxygenation but not with huge breaths that will keep partial pressure of carbon dioxide (pCO_2) low. Progressive muscle relaxation, with systematic tensing and then relaxing of the various muscle groups of the body, is useful for some patients. Reassurance, as data are obtained, that the patient does not appear to be in acute medical danger can also help. Initiation of education—informing the patient that he or she might be experiencing a panic attack; that panic attacks are overwhelming and frightening but not truly threatening; and that it will pass quickly if the patient lets it run its course— can both calm and lay groundwork for subsequent treatment efforts. This education provides foundation for the cognitive component of CBT. The behavioral component involves exposure and desensitization to cues that trigger fear, but the acute setting is not likely to be an appropriate context for initiation of this part of the treatment.

Another cognitive tool used in CBT for panic might also be useful for some patients in the emergency department. This involves directly addressing the catastrophic interpretations that patients with panic often attach to their symptoms with an exploration of past evidence relevant to their interpretations. For example, a patient who interprets chest pain as evidence that he or she is having a heart attack can be asked to review cardiac risk factors with the doctor and can usually be helped to see that he or she has many factors that make a heart attack unlikely; the patient may be young, lack a family history of cardiac disease, have favorable metabolic profiles, be normotensive, and so on. If the patient has had previous episodes like this one that did not prove to be a heart attack, this can be discussed. The provider can also share his or her own experience with other patients with identical symptoms who have come to the emergency room and were proved not to be having heart attacks.

If the patient is preoccupied with fearful beliefs that can be directly addressed with behavioral tests, this can have a strong, beneficial impact. For example, some patients may be convinced that if they stand up, their blood pressure will drop and they will faint. With appropriate support, they may be willing to test this belief, by trying to stand with an automatic blood pressure monitor in place and seeing exactly what happens to their heart rate and blood pressure, with education provided so they understand the changes. Activating these kinds of cognitive processes can help reduce the emotional focus and intensity.

If the patient's attack cannot be managed with reassurance and the types of techniques described above, use of a benzodiazepine can be considered. A relatively short-acting agent, such as lorazepam 0.5–1.0 mg orally, is usually sufficient in a benzodiazepine-naïve individual. Lorazepam can also be administered intramuscularly if the patient is unable to take an oral medication.

Use of medication is presented as a secondary technique because benzodiazepines, even fast-acting ones like alprazolam (peak effect in 1–2 hours), take time to enter the bloodstream and exert their effect on the brain. Panic attacks often abate naturally before the medication takes effect, but patients will falsely attribute their recovery to the drug and can rapidly develop psychological reliance on access to it. Even when a benzodiazepine does provide relief, its use can suggest to the patient that the anxiety symptoms cannot be controlled or endured without external assistance, diminishing the patient's self-efficacy and undermining the kind of cognitive and psychological work that is important in optimizing long-term recovery.

Differential Diagnosis and Further Evaluation

As discussed in the previous section, panic attacks can be associated with a number of anxiety disorders as well as non-anxiety-related psychiatric conditions and medical conditions. Table 6–1 presents a differential of psychiatric and nonpsychiatric conditions that may produce anxiety, panic attacks, or panic-like attacks.

Once the patient is sufficiently calm to participate in his or her care, then evaluation for the etiology of the panic attack should proceed. As with all psychiatric emergencies, the patient should be "cleared" of any medical conditions that may present with psychiatric symptoms forming the chief complaint. A complete discussion of the evaluation for and management of these medical conditions is beyond the scope of this chapter.

For the associated psychiatric conditions, indications for hospitalization (e.g., acute suicidal or homicidal ideation) should be assessed. If there are no indications for hospitalization, then the patient should be discharged with reassurance that the panic attack, though frightening, is not life threatening and with advice that outpatient psychiatric treatment could reduce the patient's chances for experiencing future panic attacks. (For a brief discussion of outpatient follow-up, see Chapter 1.)

One psychiatric condition, panic disorder, merits additional discussion because the anxiety in panic disorder influences emergency room utilization

Table 6–1.   Disorders associated with anxiety syndromes

Psychiatric

Cognitive disorders

Depressive episodes with anxiety

Generalized anxiety disorder

Obsessive-compulsive disorder

Panic disorder

Personality disorders
(especially Clusters B and C)

Posttraumatic stress disorder

Psychotic disorders

Social anxiety disorder

Specific phobia

Cardiovascular

Angina pectoris

Arrhythmias

Congestive heart failure

Hypertension

Hyperventilation

Hypovolemia

Myocardial infarction

Shock

Syncope

Valvular disease

Endocrine

Cushing's syndrome

Hyperkalemia

Hyperthermia

Hyperthyroidism

Hypocalcemia

Hypoglycemia

Hyponatremia

Hypoparathyroidism

Hypothyroidism

Menopause

Neurological

Cerebral syphilis

Cerebrovascular insufficiency

Encephalopathies (infectious,
metabolic, and toxic)

Essential tremor

Huntington's chorea

Intracranial mass lesions

Migraine headaches

Multiple sclerosis

Postconcussive syndrome

Posterolateral sclerosis

Polyneuritis

Seizure disorders (especially temporal
lobe seizures)

Vasculitis

Vertigo

Wilson's disease

Respiratory

Asthma

Chronic obstructive pulmonary disease

Pneumonia

Pneumothorax

Pulmonary edema

Pulmonary embolus

Drug related

Stimulant, marijuana, or hallucinogen
abuse

Alcohol or sedative-hypnotic
withdrawal

Akathisia (secondary to antipsychotic
medications or SSRIs)

Anticholinergic, digitalis, or
theophylline toxicity

Abuse of over-the-counter diet pills

Table 6–1.   Disorders associated with anxiety
syndromes *(continued)*

Dietary	Neoplastic
Caffeinism	Carcinoid tumor
Monosodium glutamate	Insulinoma
Tyramine-containing foods in those	Pheochromocytoma
taking MAOIs	**Infectious/inflammatory**
Vitamin deficiency	Acute or chronic infection
Hematological	Anaphylaxis
Acute intermittent porphyria	Systemic lupus erythematosus
Anemias	

Note.   MAOIs = monoamine oxidase inhibitors; SSRIs = selective serotonin reuptake inhibitors.
Source.   Milner et al. 1999.

and increases the chances that the patient presents to the emergency department with "physical" complaints. The next section focuses on panic disorder.

Panic Disorder

Why Focus on Panic Disorder?

Panic disorder is a particularly important anxiety disorder for emergency department personnel to understand. The patient's heightened sensitivity to bodily sensations and catastrophic misinterpretation of them as serious medical threats that is typical of panic lead to frequent emergency room visits and hospital admissions to rule out myocardial infarctions, manage dyspnea, and evaluate presyncope. Repeated emergency department visits from patients with panic disorder cost the medical system a substantial amount of money; these costs could be significantly reduced with early recognition and effective management of the panic disorder (Coley et al. 2009).

One characteristic of panic disorder that can help differentiate it from other types of anxiety problems is an extreme sensitivity to bodily sensations. Patients with panic disorder pay considerable attention to the normal "sounds of the bodily machinery" and are quite frightened by them, whereas most people have habituated and learned to screen out these "sounds" unless something clearly changes or goes awry. Panic attacks are often triggered in patients with panic disorder when what should be a "silent" event is attended to and interpreted as a danger signal (Austin and Richards 2001). Instead of thinking about a perceived palpitation as a normal sensation, a patient with panic disorder is prone to catastrophic interpretation (i.e., jumping to the conclusion that a heart attack might be imminent). This reactivity to bodily sensations has been labeled *anxiety sensitivity*. It can be measured using the Anxiety Sensitivity Index (Reiss et al. 1986) and can be helpful in predicting the appearance of spontaneous panic attacks as are seen in panic disorder (Schmidt et al. 2006). This trait also contributes to the frequent appearance of panic disorder patients in emergency departments.

Numerous studies have examined presentation of patients with panic disorder to the medical emergency room, and multiple factors that make symptoms such as chest pain more likely to be due to panic disorder have been distilled. If a patient is younger, female, without known coronary artery disease, presenting with atypical chest pain, and reporting high levels of anxiety, the probability of panic disorder is higher than in the absence of these factors (Huffman and Pollack 2003). All of these factors should be readily identified in the initial evaluation of the chest pain complaint. In patients with low risk of cardiac-related chest pain, a simple set of screening questions can provide data that correlates well with gold-standard techniques for diagnosing panic disorder. Wulsin et al. (2002) have shown that emergency department physicians with no additional training in psychiatric assessment can diagnose panic disorder in patients with low to moderate risk of acute coronary syndrome, with fairly good agreement with psychiatric experts ($\kappa = 0.53$; 95% confidence interval, 0.26–0.80), by asking 1) whether a sudden attack of fear or anxiety has occurred in the 4 weeks prior to the emergency department presentation; 2) whether similar attacks have occurred previously; and 3) whether these attacks come out of the blue, cause worry about having another attack, and feature any cardinal symptoms of panic attacks (shortness of breath, chest pain, heart racing or pounding, sweating, chills or flushing, dizziness, nausea, choking sensation, or tingling or numbness). In this study, diagnosis and initiation of selective serotonin reuptake inhibitor (SSRI) treatment in the emergency department correlated with a significant enhancement of continued treatment at 1-month and 3-month follow-ups.

It can be critically important to screen for and make the diagnosis of panic disorder in the emergency department. Patients come to the emergency room disturbed or distressed by their symptoms and wanting to know what is wrong with them. Simple reassurance that nothing serious can be identified and that tests have "ruled out" the heart attack or other "catastrophic" diagnosis that patients feared often falls on unhearing ears. The fear associated with a panic attack amplifies the personal importance of the symptoms being experienced, so a provider's assertion that "nothing is wrong" does not match the patient's experience.

Receiving a clear diagnosis of a fairly easily treatable brain-based pathology, based on a carefully done screening approach with proven efficacy, may be far more satisfying to the patient. This diagnosis, however, must be delivered with an appropriate amount of compassion and recognition of the potential need to reduce the stigma attached to psychiatric disorders. It may also help to assure the patient that he or she is not being told that the symptoms are "all in the head," even if those symptoms are generated by misfiring neurons in the brain. Simply ruling out a heart attack, for example, leaves open the possibility of innumerable other interpretations of the symptoms. A panic-prone patient may well go home, do some online research, and become convinced the problem was an arrhythmia or something wrong with the lungs. The patient will return to the emergency room for further rule-outs each time symptoms recur, inconveniencing the patient and increasing medical costs. When a careful diagnosis of panic disorder is made during an emergency department visit, it usually proves to be stable 2 years later; in contrast, patients with panic disorder who do not receive a panic diagnosis and appropriate panic treatment do worse over that 2-year period, both psychiatrically and medically (Fleet et al. 2003).

Initial Treatment of Panic Disorder

If panic is accurately diagnosed, appropriate treatment can be initiated in the emergency department, using both medications and nonpharmacological treatments. SSRI antidepressants are the drugs of choice; they can reduce both the frequency and intensity of panic attacks, and can be initiated in the emergency department (Wulsin et al. 2002). SSRIs have the advantage of also being useful for treating many of the comorbidities that are common in patients with panic disorder, including social anxiety, generalized anxiety disorder, PTSD, and depression.

When prescribing SSRIs, the clinician should keep in mind that these patients have a heightened propensity for catastrophic thinking around bodily sensations. Because SSRIs can cause bodily sensations in the first days to weeks of treatment, the risk of having a panic attack and abruptly discontinuing the medication in the titration phase is high. If started at too high a dose or without adequate preparation, this early activation effect can lead some patients with panic disorder to refuse all future efforts to prescribe an SSRI for them. This early risk should be managed with clear instructions to the patient about what to anticipate and very gradual titration of the medication from the lowest initiation dose. Sertraline or citalopram are good first-choice drugs for patients with panic disorder. Sertraline has a very broad dosing range, so it can be started at very low levels (25 mg/day) and titrated slowly to a target dosage of 100 mg/day. Citalopram is a good alternative, because it tends to be minimally activating, with fewer bodily sensations for the patient to misinterpret during titration. It can be started at 5 mg/day and titrated to a target dosage of 20 mg/day. With either drug, the titration pace can be adjusted to individual sensitivities and should be done under supervision, so close follow-up is important. Long-acting benzodiazepines, such as clonazepam, can be prescribed in a scheduled fashion to reduce the patient's sensitivity to side effects during the titration of an SSRI antidepressant, although this approach must be taken judiciously and is not appropriate for all patients. Rapid follow-up and active management of the medication titration is key to successful treatment.

Cognitive management of panic attacks is a cornerstone of treatment for panic disorder. Although the emergency room will not likely lend itself to performing intensive CBT, the emergency physician should at least inform the patient that a nonpharmacological treatment for panic disorder exists. Knowing that treatment other than medication is available can help alleviate some of the patient's anxiety about treatment side effects and may make him or her more willing to pursue outpatient follow-up. Relaxation techniques—slow breathing and progressive muscle relaxation—were discussed earlier in the chapter (see "Management of a Panic Attack") as useful approaches to managing acute anxiety within the emergency room. Evidence is mixed as to whether these techniques add meaningfully to the standard CBT package used to treat panic, but they definitely will have some value to some patients during initial efforts to manage overwhelming anxiety and initiate a fuller treatment.

As discussed in the earlier section on managing panic attacks, full treatment of anxiety disorders often includes an exposure-based component in the CBT package. However, the patient in an acute crisis may be too unstable to begin this form of treatment, and the emergency room is not the place to initiate it. Instead. rapid follow-up should be arranged with a skilled clinician experienced with these techniques to produce the greatest impact and enhance outcomes.

Somatic Symptom and Related Disorders in the Medical Setting

DSM-5 includes a new category of psychiatric diagnoses known as the somatic symptom and related disorders, which includes the diagnoses of somatic symptom disorder, illness anxiety disorder, and conversion disorder (functional neurological symptom disorder), along with others. These diagnoses represent a reorganization of related DSM-IV-TR diagnoses, such as somatoform disorder and hypochondriasis, and now emphasize the presence of distress associated with perceived somatic symptoms rather that the absence of a medical explanation for these symptoms. Although somatic symptom and related disorders are not classified as anxiety disorders, they all share a common feature: pronounced somatic symptoms associated with significant distress and impairment, which will cause highly anxious patients to seek medical care. These somatizing patients have disproportionately high rates of medical care utilization. Barsky et al. (2005) found that compared with non-somatizing patients, the somatizing patients had approximately twice the number of outpatient, inpatient, and emergency department visits over a 12-month period. In fact, due to the nature of their condition, patients with somatic symptom and related disorders are much more likely to present to the emergency department or other medical setting than they are to seek help from a mental health professional.

A diagnosis of somatic symptom disorder may be appropriate for an individual who has one or more somatic symptoms that are distressing or causing a significant disruption in daily life. Although the prevalence of somatic symptom disorder is not known, the disorder is thought to occur in 5%–7% of the adult population, likely more commonly in females (American Psychiatric Association 2013). An individual diagnosed with this disorder may devote a disproportionate amount of time to thinking about the perceived seriousness of his or her symptoms; may demonstrate high levels of anxiety associated with the symptoms; and may expend a great deal of time, energy, and resources on these health concerns. In severe cases, health concerns may become central in patients' lives, overtaking their identity and straining their interpersonal relationships, as well as their relationship with their likely multiple medical providers. The symptoms may range from pain to fatigue to normal body perceptions, but the individual's suffering is genuine.

In contrast to patients with somatic symptom disorder, individuals with illness anxiety disorder are less concerned about somatic symptoms in and of themselves, but they may be convinced that they have acquired a serious and undiagnosed medical illness. In illness anxiety disorder, somatic symptoms typically either are not present or are mild in intensity. Thorough evaluations do little to quell the individual's concern, and the patient may, for example, continue to interpret a tension headache as evidence of a brain tumor or transient tinnitus as a clear sign of an impending stroke. These patients may engage in excessive and maladaptive behaviors such as repeatedly checking their body for signs of illness, extensively researching their suspected disease, seeking constant reassurance from others, and avoiding situations that they fear might jeopardize their health. If a diagnosable medical condition is in fact present, the patient's anxiety is often significantly out of proportion to the severity of the condition. Attempts by medical providers to provide reassurance or palliate symptoms do little to alleviate the patient's concerns and may even heighten them.

A patient with conversion disorder (functional neurological symptom disorder) may present to the emergency department with one or more symptoms of altered motor function (e.g., left-sided weakness) or sensory function (e.g., blindness). To support a diagnosis of conversion disorder, clinical findings must provide evidence of incompatibility between the symptom and established neurological or medical conditions (e.g., Hoover's sign, tunnel vision). The onset of symptoms in conversion disorder may be associated with acute stress or trauma, although this is not always the case. Conversion disorder is thought to be relatively common; however, the precise prevalence is unknown because symptoms are often transient.

A diagnosis of somatic symptom disorder, illness anxiety disorder, or conversion disorder does not preclude an individual from also having a separate medical (or psychiatric) condition, so the first step in evaluation, as with panic attack, is to rule out serious medical threats. This rule-out may include a focused physical examination while avoiding more invasive laboratory or diagnostic procedures, although clinical judgment should always dictate the extent of the workup.

The role of the emergency physician in managing somatic symptom and related disorders is to first assure the patient that there is no life-threatening pathology at play while also validating the patient's experience and maintaining a balanced emotional response (i.e., not blaming the patient for his or her somatic experience). Because patients who fall under this diagnostic category are likely to have been told by previous providers that their symptoms are imaginary, they are prone to feeling dismissed. The emergency room physician should emphasize that the patient's symptoms are real, that the condition is common and treatable, and that the brain has powerful influences over the body, especially during times of stress (Stephenson and Price 2006). This approach is sometimes termed the "good news" approach, which may improve a patient's willingness to engage in mental health evaluation and treatment (Thompson et al. 2013). Additionally, making the patient feel invalidated risks his or her abandonment of use of the emergency department, leaving the patient without a safety net should he or she experience a true medical emergency.

The most important therapeutic intervention the emergency physician can undertake is to arrange for outpatient follow-up with the patient's primary care provider. The primary care provider may then consider referral to a psychiatrist or to a subspecialty clinic that matches the patient's particular somatic complaints. In some tertiary centers, subspecialty clinics are developing integrated behavioral health programs for patients with functional bowel disorders, nonepileptic spells, and so forth. Somatic symptom and related disorders are best treated within one health care system so as to prevent unnecessary workup. Ideally, the patient will eventually be willing to follow up with a mental health professional, because individual and group psychotherapy has been shown to reduce these patients' health care costs by 50% (Sadock and Sadock 2003).

Other Anxiety Disorders and Related Conditions

Although panic and somatization have particular salience in the emergency department context, other types of anxiety-related conditions impact the likelihood and nature of patient presentations to the emergency room. All of the anxiety and anxiety-related disorders can contribute to heightened fear or worry in the face of physical symptoms and can increase the odds that a patient will appear for emergent care instead of pursuing help through less urgent avenues. Patients with obsessive-compulsive disorder may demonstrate a near-delusional level of concern about germs or infection. Patients with a blood-injection-injury phobia may faint when in the emergency department for another reason. Trauma is the triggering event for many psychiatric disorders, including PTSD, and trauma patients often first present for medical care in the emergency department. A full discussion of these conditions is beyond the scope of this chapter given that neither clinical experience nor research studies would support a particular approach for diagnostic or therapeutic interventions specific to an emergency department setting.

Key Clinical Points

- Anxiety is a common complaint in the emergency department, and anxiety disorders pose a significant burden to the medical system if they are not adequately recognized and treated.

- Panic attacks can be managed without medications, using cognitive and behavioral techniques.

- SSRIs provide relief from most anxiety disorders, although a slow titration to the target dose may be needed, given the propensity of SSRIs to cause anxiety-provoking physical symptoms during the medication-initiation phase.

- Somatic symptom and related disorders are characterized by pronounced somatic symptoms associated with significant distress and impairment that can prompt highly anxious patients to seek emergency care.

- The presence of severe anxiety does not reduce the likelihood of major medical problems requiring urgent attention and should not divert attention from necessary medical evaluation. High risk may remain even if life-threatening medical illness is ruled out, because anxiety may reflect an underlying psychiatric disturbance that carries a serious risk of self-harm or harm to others.

References

American Psychiatric Association: Diagnostic and Statistical Manual of Mental Disorders, 4th Edition, Text Revision. Washington, DC, American Psychiatric Association, 2000

American Psychiatric Association: Diagnostic and Statistical Manual of Mental Disorders, 5th Edition. Arlington, VA, American Psychiatric Association, 2013

Austin DW, Richards JC: The catastrophic misinterpretation model of panic disorder. Behav Res Ther 39(11):1277–1291, 2001 11686264

Barsky AJ, Orav EJ, Bates DW: Somatization increases medical utilization and costs independent of psychiatric and medical comorbidity. Arch Gen Psychiatry 62(8):903–910, 2005 16061768

Coley KC, Saul MI, Seybert AL: Economic burden of not recognizing panic disorder in the emergency department. J Emerg Med 36(1):3–7, 2009 17933481

Deacon B, Lickel J, Abramowitz JS: Medical utilization across the anxiety disorders. J Anxiety Disord 22(2):344–350, 2008 17420113

Fleet RP, Lavoie KL, Martel JP, et al: Two-year follow-up status of emergency department patients with chest pain: Was it panic disorder? CJEM 5(4):247–254, 2003 17472767

Huffman JC, Pollack MH: Predicting panic disorder among patients with chest pain: an analysis of the literature. Psychosomatics 44(3):222–236, 2003 12724504

Milner KK, Florence T, Glick RL: Mood and anxiety syndromes in emergency psychiatry. Psychiatr Clin North Am 22(4):755–777, 1999 10623969

Reiss S, Peterson RA, Gursky DM, et al: Anxiety sensitivity, anxiety frequency and the prediction of fearfulness. Behav Res Ther 24(1):1–8, 1986 3947307

Sadock BJ, Sadock VA: Synopsis of Psychiatry, 9th Edition. Philadelphia, PA, Lippincott Williams & Wilkins, 2003, pp 591–642

Schmidt NB, Zvolensky MJ, Maner JK: Anxiety sensitivity: prospective prediction of panic attacks and Axis I pathology. J Psychiatr Res 40(8):691–699, 2006 16956622

Stephenson DT, Price JR: Medically unexplained physical symptoms in emergency medicine. Emerg Med J 23(8):595–600, 2006 16858088

Thompson N, Connelly L, Peltzer J, et al: Psychogenic nonepileptic seizures: a pilot study of a brief educational intervention. Perspect Psychiatr Care 49(2):78–83, 2013 23557450

Wulsin L, Liu T, Storrow A, et al: A randomized, controlled trial of panic disorder treatment initiation in an emergency department chest pain center. Ann Emerg Med 39(2):139–143, 2002 11823767

Suggested Readings

Craske MG, Barlow DH: Master of Your Anxiety and Panic: Therapists Guide, 4th Edition. New York, Oxford University Press, 2006

Stein MB, Goin MK, Pollack MH, et al: Practice Guideline for the Treatment of Patients With Panic Disorder, 2nd Edition. January 2009. Available at: http://www.psychiatryonline.com. Accessed December 23, 2014.

Wells A: Cognitive Therapy of Anxiety Disorders. Chichester, UK, Wiley, 1997

7

The Agitated Patient

Gerald Scott Winder, M.D.
Rachel L. Glick, M.D.

Case Example

Mr. H is a 43-year-old single white man with a past psychiatric history of schizophrenia, cannabis use disorder, alcohol use disorder, and stimulant intoxication, as well as a past medical history significant for obesity, hyperlipidemia, hypertension, and prediabetes. He was brought to the emergency department by police after patrons in a local supermarket reported that he was exhibiting bizarre behavior on the premises. He quickly became belligerent and combative when approached by police and paramedics. He was seen in the emergency department under similar circumstances a year earlier and was admitted to inpatient psychiatry at an outside facility. No more recent documentation is available. Lab work is significant for positive urine toxicology for cannabis, a negative blood alcohol level, and a mild transaminitis. His current medications are unknown, and a previous note prominently states that he is generally noncompliant with psychiatric medications and that he does not follow up regularly with his primary care physician. The paramedics administered intravenous midazolam 2 mg en route to the hospital in response to Mr. H's persistent agitation while restrained on the gurney. His last set of vital signs is notable for a blood pressure of 182/98 mmHg and tachycardia into the 120s but is otherwise unremarkable. From the gurney, the patient continues to speak loudly to staff about his desire to leave. He mumbles under his breath even when not spoken to, and audible content of his speech includes ideas about "government nanotechnology." He is malodorous and disheveled, has poor dentition, and is wearing clothes inappropriate for the cold weather. (At the conclusion of this chapter, we present an approach to the assessment, diagnosis, and treatment of this patient.)

Agitation is a common symptom evaluated by emergency providers. Behavioral emergencies of various etiologies make up 6% of emergency department visits in the United States (Lukens et al. 2006). Agitation threatens the provider-patient relationship, a complete and accurate history, and patient and staff safety. The ability of emergency clinicians to intervene early and effectively is of immense importance.

A composite of fluctuating behaviors, agitation includes motor restlessness, stimulus sensitivity, irritability, and inappropriate verbal or motor activity (Lindenmayer 2000). It is classified into aggressive and nonaggressive forms of both physical and verbal phenomena (Cohen-Mansfield and Billig 1986). Its onset can lead to aggression and a behavioral emergency. Under certain conditions, agitation confers survival benefits (Buss and Shackelford 1997), but it becomes a clinical concern when it threatens the safety of the patient or staff, interferes with diagnosis and treatment, or leads to property damage. Personnel in the emergency setting are particularly vulnerable to injury from agitated patients (Gates et al. 2006).

Agitation arises from the complex interaction of biology and behavior. The neurophysiology is not well understood, in large part because of how poorly agitation lends itself to study (de Almeida et al. 2005). The existing literature indicates that aggressive behavior likely involves various genes, neurocircuitry, and neurotransmitters (de Almeida et al. 2005; Lindenmayer 2000). Compounding complexity, agitation also subsumes arrays of environmental factors and psychological constructs, which can lead to a varied presentation across patients. All of these factors combine to make agitation a challenging symptom to understand, diagnose, and treat.

A unique aspect of agitation is the strong emotion elicited from the treating clinician (Balducci 2013). Clinicians have differing levels of comfort with

Table 7–1.   Early signs of agitation

Speech	Loud speech volume
	Use of profanity
Interpersonal	Argumentativeness
	Uncooperativeness
	Excitability
	Expressed distrust of staff
	Threats (to self or others)
	Phobic reactions including poor eye contact
	Negativism
Psychomotor	Pacing
	Sleep disturbance
	Muscle tension
	Hyperkinetic movement (e.g., bouncing leg, changing positions)
	Tearing paper or clothing
	Wandering
	Repetitious mannerisms (e.g., asking questions, trying the doors)

Source.   Lindenmayer 2000; Richmond et al. 2012.

behavioral symptoms, and their comfort levels directly affect assessment and treatment. Clinical skill sets should include prevention strategies, a thoughtful diagnostic approach, and evidence-based treatment.

Prevention and Early Intervention

General Strategies

Personnel should be properly instructed in detection of agitation and early intervention techniques. Table 7–1 lists clinical signs that should alert staff to act. At the first sign of patient agitation, a staff member should connect empathically using open-ended questions to query for immediate needs and then follow up at appropriate intervals.

Agitated individuals display anxiety and inner turmoil in various ways, and proficient assessment using a reliable clinical scale (e.g., Behavioural Activity Rating Scale [Swift et al. 2002]) optimizes communication and documentation. Integrating courtesy, respect, and reliable detection strategies into the culture of an emergency department can decrease the incidence and severity of behavioral emergencies over time.

The Patient

Beginning with triage, the patient adjusts to new surroundings and processes. Emergency department staff can easily forget patients' nonmedical needs. Boredom, acclimation to the facility's temperature, and nutrition status are easily overlooked. Blankets, food, television, or reading materials increase comfort and convey attentiveness and concern. Introductions to staff members, an orientation to facility procedures, and a review of patient rights may ease tension arising from uncertainty and fear. In all interactions, staff should remain flexible, maintain a professional demeanor, and communicate with empathic dialogue.

As the clinical encounter progresses, several strategies reduce the likelihood of agitation. Clear instructions with careful attention to personal space are essential. The interview should take place in a quiet space, which is distinctly important for intoxicated patients. The room should allow maximal privacy and should be set up so both patient and provider have easy, unobstructed access to the room's exit. There should not be anything in the room that could be used as a weapon.

The provider should avoid prolonged eye contact with, touching of, or standing over the patient, to decrease perceived provocation. By positioning oneself at an angle alongside the patient (instead of standing directly in front of him or her), the provider shows alliance. Another staff member in the room can be a comfort to both patient and provider, while supporting the guideline of ready access to adequate trained staff at all times (four to six persons are recommended for a show of force). The provider's speech should be clear, gentle, and sincere. These measures may be insufficient, however, and the patient's behavior may remain a concern. There is always a low threshold to end the interview, involve security, and reconsider the course of the evaluation.

Family and Friends

Family and friends accompanying the patient can themselves escalate behaviorally given the time spent waiting. Emergencies rarely allow preparation for the hours spent in the hospital. Many individuals will neglect basic needs or arrive without supplies (food, cell phone, device for Internet connection, toiletries, medication) and will appreciate any accommodation. Providing interval updates to the family, while maintaining confidentiality, may alleviate their frustration stemming from the evaluation process.

Differential Diagnosis

Gathering Information

The cause of agitation will not often emerge from a single laboratory or radiographic finding. Instead, accurate assessment of the symptom and appropriate treatment depend primarily on how the provider accesses and assembles information. Collateral information is invaluable in formulating an accurate clinical assessment and plan. With severely affected patients, early pharmacological treatment may be needed to facilitate obtaining a history. Family members should be asked to provide details about the patient's recent behavior, any psychiatric and medical history, recent sleep patterns, and any known substance use. Emergency medical services and nursing home personnel are reliable sources in building a narrative and differential diagnosis.

The evaluating clinician needs to elicit and consider several aspects of the agitated patient's history. One important question is how the current constellation of symptoms compares with past behaviors. Abrupt differences may suggest an underlying medical cause. Regardless of setting, clinicians must always consider reversible causes underlying agitation. The onset of many psychiatric conditions usually occurs earlier in life, so new symptoms after age 45 should pique suspicion for a nonpsychiatric etiology. Medical causes of agitation are numerous and should be individually considered during acute evaluation. Table 7–2 lists several findings that if present at any point in the evaluation should prompt medical workup.

Medical Causes

There are several general categories of medical causes of agitation. Infectious processes, especially when present in the elderly, can disseminate as sepsis and/or directly involve the central nervous system (CNS), resulting in agitated delirium. These are accompanied by fluctuations in awareness, vital sign abnor-

Table 7–2.   When agitation requires a medical evaluation

General	Abnormal vital signs (pulse, blood pressure, body temperature)
	Difficulty rousing the patient (i.e., score of 1 on BARS) with poor attention
	Obvious bodily trauma and injury
	Slurred speech
	Suspicion of acute intoxication or toxin exposure
Cardiovascular	Chest pain
	Persistent tachycardia or palpitations
Metabolic	Unintentional weight loss
	Temperature intolerance
	High fever
Musculoskeletal	Extreme muscle stiffness or weakness
Neurological	Discordant pupil size
	Hemiparesis, hemiplegia
	Seizures
	Incoordination
	Severe headache
Psychiatric	New-onset psychosis
	Significant cognitive deficits (i.e., orientation, language, memory, executive function)
Respiratory	Difficulty breathing

Note.   BARS= Behavioural Activity Rating Scale (Swift et al. 2002).
Source.   Adapted from Nordstrom K, Zun LS, Wilson MP, et al.: "Medical Evaluation and Triage of the Agitated Patient: Consensus Statement of the American Association for Emergency Psychiatry Project BETA Medical Evaluation Workgroup." *Western Journal of Emergency Medicine* 13(1):3–10, 2012.

malities (e.g., hypotension, fever), and perceptual disturbances, including visual hallucinations. The co-occurrence of altered mental status, nuchal rigidity, and temperature change (hypothermia or fever greater than 38°C) are of immediate concern and may indicate a primary infection in the CNS. Agitated patients may exhibit seizures or focal neurological deficits when there is direct CNS involvement. For example, head trauma often presents with symptoms of amnesia, speech irregularities, discordant pupil size, headache, or decreased consciousness. If the patient has recently had a seizure, the postictal period is characterized by confusion and agitation. Primary degenerative neurological processes (i.e., neurocognitive disorders) often involve agitation as a primary symptom. Electrolyte disturbances (e.g., hyponatremia), abnormal glucose levels, hypoxia, hepatic encephalopathy, and thyroid axis irregularities may masquerade as behavioral symptoms. Each of these processes may alter the patient's sensorium and awareness sufficiently to cause agitation.

Medications

Routine doses of medications can account for agitation. Steroids for an inflammatory process (CNS or elsewhere) are associated with behavioral disturbances. Any use of anticholinergic agents, opioid painkillers, sedatives, psychiatric medications, or antiepileptics should be elicited in the history. Verification of drug adherence and serum drug levels are useful. Paradoxically, antipsychotic medications can worsen symptoms of agitation in some patients. Akathisia, an idiopathic inner sensation of restlessness, muscular discomfort, and the need to move, can be confused for persistent or worsening agitation. If not detected, a positive feedback loop of worsening symptoms and repeat antipsychotic dosing develops. Polypharmacy itself can lead to altered mental status, and medication interactions at the hepatic and renal levels should always be considered.

Substance Abuse

Agitated patients are frequently evaluated in the context of recreational drug use. Reliable history is often difficult to obtain from patients who have recently used substances. Attention to vital signs, physical presentation (sites of intravenous drug use, scars), treatment history, and belongings (for paraphernalia, odor) becomes important. The intoxication or withdrawal phase of multiple drugs can account for severe behavioral symptoms.

Psychostimulants (e.g., cocaine, amphetamine, synthetic cathinones), via their sympathomimetic effects on monoamine neurotransmitters, are well known for causing agitation. Hallucinogens, many with serotonergic action, may lead to aggression when patients misinterpret their surroundings, hallucinate, or harbor delusional beliefs. Phencyclidine (PCP), an N-methyl-D-aspartate receptor antagonist, is notorious for its association with violent behavior. When sedatives such as benzodiazepines or alcohol are involved, there should be a low threshold for medical stabilization because risks from an abrupt withdrawal include seizures and death. Altered mental status (disorientation, impaired memory), unstable vital signs, diaphoresis, neurological symptoms (tremor, seizures), and perceptual disturbances (hallucinations) are frequently observed in patients withdrawing from alcohol and benzodiazepines.

Psychiatric Illness

Many major psychiatric illnesses, including bipolar disorder (particularly the manic and mixed phases), major depressive disorder, and schizophrenia, are associated with acute agitation. Aggression is often related to disease course, nonadherence with prescribed treatment, or changes in a patient's personal life. Patients with personality disorders or developmental delays also experience agitation. Frequently, however, agitation and aggression exist independently of mental illness. (Chapter 3, "Violence Risk Assessment," provides helpful information.)

Evaluation and Workup

Transported Patients

Agitated patients often arrive via ambulance from residences, nursing homes, or other hospitals. To optimize care, paramedics and/or the facility of origin should provide descriptions of the patient's behavior along with other key history. This information is useful to ensure safety and a thorough evaluation in the event that an involuntary hold or hospitalization is indicated. Receiving clinicians should quickly ensure that they have a working understanding of the patient's medical and psychiatric history, current symptoms, and any treatments administered en route (including any medications administered or restraints applied), all of which are important for any quick treatment decisions that need to be made. If the patient arrives in restraints, prompt vital-sign assessment and laboratory assessment are essential (Chapter 11, "Seclusion and Restraint in Emergency Settings," includes additional relevant information).

Collaboration With General and Emergency Medicine

Care for the agitated patient frequently requires collaboration between medical and mental health professionals. The various factors contributing to or causing patient agitation span multiple disciplines and are approached differently across the divisions of medicine and psychiatry. These differences have monetary and clinical effects. For example, psychiatrists and emergency physicians may differ in the type and frequency of lab tests they order in cases of agitation. Whereas emergency department physicians may not consider urine toxicology to be immediately useful, psychiatrists may later use the results diagnostically (independent of its pertinence in the acute setting). In the emergency department, tests such as thyroid-stimulating hormone blood test or urinalysis may be done in anticipation of what an admitting psychiatric unit will want to see, not because the physician suspects abnormal results (Zun et al. 2004). Even if psychiatric admission requires *medical clearance*— a term with an unreliable and vague definition (Korn et al. 2000)—the process should avoid rote procedure and remain patient centered, utilizing a differential diagnosis. Detailed clinician-to-clinician handoffs optimize the patient's transition between caregivers of different disciplines.

Mental Status Examination

Physical examination of an agitated patient can be limited by the psychiatric symptoms, but mental status examination can begin in spite of them at the first moment of patient contact. Inviting a colleague into the room with an agitated patient can be a safety measure, an opportunity for collaboration, and a logistical strategy when multiple clinicians evaluate patients. Psychomotor activity is a key aspect of the patient's presentation to be examined early in the encounter. Questions or observations about any increased psychomotor activity may be an appropriate starting point for the patient interview (thus allowing the clinician to promptly discuss medications if needed). Information about cognitive function, including orientation, becomes directly and indirectly available as the interview progresses with questions about the history. Using a flexible approach to interview structure, the examiner can simultaneously allow the agitated patient to recount the events while gathering data about the patient's affect, insight, judgment, and executive functioning. Thought content, if not volunteered by the patient spontaneously, should be carefully examined for suicidal or homicidal ideation as part of fundamental risk assessment. Paranoia, hallucinations, and delusional systems are important to detect and understand early because they may impact how staff should interact with the patient. Combining multiple steps in this way ensures a timely, efficient interaction and can contribute to a reduction in the level of patient frustration that often accompanies a prolonged interview.

Intoxicated Patients

For patients intoxicated with alcohol, there is not a standard blood alcohol level below which a psychiatric interview can be conducted. The practice of routinely postponing examination of agitated and intoxicated patients until their blood alcohol level drops below a certain threshold is not literature based. Cognitive testing and the application of principles of capacity and informed consent to each case will ensure that the patient can meaningfully participate in the examination and that the results are reliable. Consent cannot be ethically obtained from a clinically intoxicated patient.

Physical Examination

Physical examination is essential regardless of the setting—medical or psychiatric. When performed, maneuvers used during the examination should answer clinical questions motivated by the history. It is important to include adequate examination of key organ systems—cardiovascular, respiratory, neurological, gastrointestinal, and skin—with additional evaluation depending on the history obtained. This is essential not only for the refining of the differential diagnosis but also for adequate documentation if the patient requires psychiatric admission.

Imaging and Laboratory Tests

If certain at-risk groups of agitated patients display abnormal vital signs or physical examination findings, the clinician's level of concern should rise accordingly. These groups include elderly patients, substance-abusing patients, individuals with no prior psychiatric history, and those of lower socioeconomic status (Lukens et al. 2006). The clinician may consider serum laboratory testing (urinalysis, toxicology, electrolytes, complete blood count, glucose, urea nitrogen, serum B_{12} levels), lumbar puncture, electrocardiogram, electroencephalogram, chest X ray, or computed tomography of the head, as appropriate.

The literature, however, is mixed on how this should be done if a patient in one of these groups requires further workup. Some authors argue for extensive testing, citing statistics that many patients have treatable medical reasons causing the agitation. Others caution against high costs and elevated rates of false positives. They assert that few lab findings are not predicted by the history and physical examination findings and believe that widespread labs and imaging are an expensive redundancy. The American College of Emergency Physicians recommends that the workup of behavioral symptoms, including laboratory assay and imaging, should be directed by history and physical examination and contends that routine lab testing is of low yield (Lukens et al. 2006).

Do No Harm

Treatment of behavioral emergencies is impacted simultaneously by what the clinician does and does *not* do. Whether the provider empirically treats or cautiously waits, the ethical principle of doing no harm is invoked. Both inaction and hasty intervention can adversely affect the outcome.

Current or historical agitation may make verbal de-escalation impossible and instead necessitate the use of medications. Forestalling medication may risk injury or property damage. Proper evaluation of the patient, including interview, laboratory testing, and physical examination, may not be feasible until medication has taken effect. However, routine and automatic medication use (especially involuntary, intramuscular injections) risks direct physiological and psychological side effects. Restraint and involuntary medication are frequently detrimental to the provider-patient alliance. Patients with a history of trauma are at particularly high risk of psychological side effects due to the arousal of past memories and behaviors.

Verbal De-Escalation

Although medications such as antipsychotics and benzodiazepines have traditionally been first-line treatments for agitation, recommendations now focus more on verbal de-escalation strategies with the goal of avoiding medication altogether. This approach improves the assessment and treatment of the agitated patient. There are several reasons why a noncoercive approach is in the interest of both providers and patients: 1) physical intervention may introduce or reinforce the idea that use of force solves problems, 2) restraining a patient increases the chances of a hospital admission and a prolonged length of stay, 3) the Joint Commission and the Centers for Medicaid and Medicare Services deem low rates of physical restraint to be a key indicator of quality care, and 4) the likelihood of staff and patient injury is reduced when physical management is avoided (Richmond et al. 2012).

The American Association for Emergency Psychiatry Project BETA (Best practices in Evaluation and Treatment of Agitation) De-Escalation Workgroup has put forth a practical, noncoercive, three-part overarching philosophy (Richmond et al. 2012) for patient de-escalation. It includes verbal engagement of the patient, establishment of a collaborative relationship with the team, and the actual verbal de-escalation out of the agitated state. Table 7–3 summarizes the group's domains of verbal de-escalation.

It is important that during the de-escalation process only one person at a time should verbally engage the patient. More than one communicator risks discontinuity, confusion, frustration, and potentially further escalation. Often, however, having several staff members present in a simultaneous display of concern for the patient in a show of force facilitates the de-escalation efforts of the leading clinician.

Medication Considerations

Inevitably, verbal de-escalation will be ineffective for a segment of agitated patients (e.g., patients who are too psychotic or cognitively impaired to be able to communicate effectively), and medications then become an important part of treatment. When medications are being considered, allergies should be reviewed in the chart and verified with the patient. With the first signs of agitation, offering the patient an oral formulation is ideal (oral agents should precede parenteral formulations). Simultaneously, the clinician should discuss why the recommendation is being made. Allowing the patient to participate in the selection of the drug maintains the clinical alliance and informed consent (Allen et al. 2005). Medications can be approached in an openended, nonthreatening way by asking about past medications that have helped.

Selecting the right agent with an appropriate onset of action and duration involves a series of psychiatric and medical considerations. This task under-

Table 7–3. American Association for Emergency Psychiatry Project BETA De-Escalation Workgroup's 10 Domains of De-Escalation

Respect personal space	Maintain two arms' lengths of distance (more if needed); heed and respond to any patient threats; be aware of patient vulnerabilities (past trauma, sexual abuse, homelessness) to avoid exacerbating symptoms
Do not be provocative	Use body language to convey empathy and safety; keep hands visible and unclenched; stand at an angle to avoid confrontation; maintain calm facial expression and demeanor; avoid challenging patient
Establish verbal contact	Have only one person interacting with patient at a time; introduce self; provide orientation for what to expect; ask how patient would like to be addressed and then use patient's preferred name
Be concise	Use short sentences and simple vocabulary; allow patient time to process and respond; repeat message until it is heard
Identify wants and feelings	Allow patient to share expectations and immediate needs; synthesize free information (trivial dialogue, body language, past encounters) to identify wants; frequently express desire to help
Listen closely to the patient	Use active listening (verbal acknowledgment, body language, conversation); use clarifying statements; assume that what patient says is true
Agree or agree to disagree	Agree with truths ("needlesticks are uncomfortable"), principles ("everyone wants to be respected"), and odds ("many people would also find that frustrating") while maintaining neutrality; be willing to agree to disagree
Set clear limits	Inform patient of acceptable behaviors; mention consequences as a matter of fact (not as a threat); acknowledge when patient causes fear and discomfort; limit violation results in reasonable consequence; use gentle confrontation
Offer choices and optimism	Offer things that can be perceived as kindness (blankets, magazines, phone, food); avoid deception; offer medications and allow patient to participate; do not rush to medicate but do not delay either; reaffirm belief that things will improve
Debrief patient and staff	Restore therapeutic alliance after involuntary action; explain why action was necessary; explore alternatives; teach proper expression of anger; touch base with family who may have witnessed the encounter; allow staff to express feelings and point out areas for improvement

Note. BETA= Best practices in Evaluation and Treatment of Agitation.

Source. Adapted from Richmond JS, Berlin JS, Fishkind AB, et al.: "Verbal De-Escalation of the Agitated Patient: Consensus Statement of the American Association for Emergency Psychiatry Project BETA De-Escalation Workgroup." *Western Journal of Emergency Medicine* 13(1):17–25, 2012.

scores the importance of gathering an accurate history and maintaining a wide differential diagnosis. The clinician should establish a provisional etiology for the agitation and target it with appropriate pharmacotherapy. Table 7–4 features several major classes of drugs that are used in treating agitation along with common agents that are used. For patients in whom medications may become a stable part of their ongoing treatment, establishing tolerability early is essential. Inducing severe side effects, such as a dystonic reaction with an antipsychotic, will decrease the likelihood of future treatment compliance from a pharmacotherapy perspective (if the patient fears taking medication again) and may damage the therapeutic relationship (Yildiz et al. 2003).

Approach to Involuntary Medication

If a patient is unable to participate in the selection and use of medication and the need for pharmacotherapy persists, then involuntary medication should be considered. Usage of involuntary medication does not preclude providing the patient with relevant information, however. Every effort should still be made to explain the rationale for proceeding in this way and to clearly describe how the treatment will be carried out. If the patient requires seclusion or restraint, medications should invariably accompany this intervention in an effort to facilitate rapid removal. It is important to note that medications should not be used as restraints themselves or to induce sleep. Oversedation increases the risk of falls, respiratory insufficiency, and aspiration, and thereby increases the burden on nursing due to the need for frequent monitoring and generally interferes with the clinical evaluation.

Substance Use Disorders

Agitation may originate from recreational drug use. The clinician should use the history (subjective and collateral), medical record (internal and external), and any available toxicology assay to discern which agents may be involved. Agitation resulting from the majority of recreational substances, especially stimulants, generally responds to benzodiazepines. When psychosis complicates the behavioral emergency, as frequently occurs in chronic amphetamine users, an antipsychotic is first-line treatment (it may be given along with a sedative as appropriate).

If the agitated patient is intoxicated with alcohol, minimal medication, if any, should be used due to the risk of respiratory depression with any increas-

Table 7–4. Useful medications in agitation

Drug class and name	Psychiatric FDA indications	Recommended acute dosing in adults	Metabolism/half-life	Notable adverse effects in acute setting	Formulation(s)	Absorption, T_{max}
Second-generation antipsychotics						
Risperidone[i]	Bipolar I disorder, schizophrenia	PO: initial dose of 1–2 mg; MAX: 4 mg/day	CYP2D6 3–20 hours (mean half-life of risperidone and active metabolites is 20 hours)	EPS, akathisia, NMS, cerebrovascular events in elderly patients, orthostatic hypotension	PO (tablet, disintegratin g tablet)	PO: 1 hour
Olanzapine[ii]	Bipolar I disorder (acute mixed or manic, maintenance, depression [with fluoxetine]), treatment-resistant depression, agitation (related to schizophrenia or bipolar I disorder)	PO: initial dose of 5–10 mg; MAX: 20 mg/day IM: 10 mg (5 mg or 7.5 mg when clinically warranted); MAX: 20 mg/day	CYP1A2, CYP2D6 (minor) 21–54 hours	Orthostatic hypotension, sedation, EPS, akathisia, constipation, dizziness, cerebrovascular events in elderly patients, NMS	PO (tablet, disintegratin g tablet), IM	PO: 6 hours IM: 15–45 min (peak concentration five times higher than PO)

Table 7–4.   Useful medications in agitation (continued)

Drug class and name	Psychiatric FDA indications	Recommended acute dosing in adults	Metabolism/ half-life	Notable adverse effects in acute setting	Formulation(s)	Absorption, T_{max}
Second-generation antipsychotics (continued)						
Ziprasidone[iii]	Bipolar I disorder (acute mixed or manic) monotherapy or adjunct, schizophrenia	PO: initial dose of 10–20 mg at 4-hour intervals; MAX: 80 mg/day IM: initial dose of 10–20 mg; can be given at 4-hour intervals; MAX: 40 mg/day	CYP3A4, CYP1A2 (minor) 7 hours	QT prolongation, EPS, akathisia, NMS, cerebrovascular events in elderly patients, sedation	PO, IM	PO: 6–8 hours (increased twofold in the presence of food) IM: 1 hour
Asenapine[iv]	Bipolar I disorder (acute mixed, manic) monotherapy or adjunct	SL: initial dose of 5 mg; MAX: 10 mg/day	UGT1A4, CYP1A2 24 hours	Somnolence, dizziness, EPS, akathisia, NMS	SL (avoid eating and drinking for 10 min after administration)	SL: 1 hour

Table 7–4. Useful medications in agitation *(continued)*

Drug class and name	Psychiatric FDA indications	Recommended acute dosing in adults	Metabolism,[f] half-life	Notable adverse effects in acute setting	Formulation(s)	Absorption, T_{max}
Second-generation antipsychotics (continued)						
Aripiprazole[v]	Psychomotor agitation (autism spectrum disorder, schizophrenia, bipolar disorder), schizophrenia, bipolar I disorder (adjunctive therapy, monotherapy of mixed or manic states), major depressive disorder (adjunctive therapy)	PO: initial dose of 10–15 mg once daily; MAX: 30 mg/day. IM: initial dose of 9.75 mg (dose range 5.25–15.00 mg); repeat dose can be given after 2 hours; MAX: 30 mg/day	CYP2D6, CYP3A4 75 hours	Somnolence, dizziness, akathisia, EPS, NMS	PO (tablet, disintegrating tablet, syrup), IM	PO: 3–5 hours IM: 1–3 hours
Benzodiazepines						
Lorazepam[vi]	Anxiety, insomnia	PO: initial dose of 1–2 mg; MAX: 8 mg/day. IM/IV: initial dose of 1–2 mg; MAX: 8 mg/day	UGT1A3, UGT2B15 12–14 hours	Excessive sedation, behavioral disinhibition, stupor, confusion, ataxia, anterograde amnesia, respiratory depression	PO, IM, IV	PO: 2 hours IM: 1.0–1.5 hours

Table 7–4.   Useful medications in agitation *(continued)*

Drug class and name	Psychiatric FDA indications	Recommended acute dosing in adults	Metabolism/ half-life	Notable adverse effects in acute setting	Formulation(s)	Absorption, T_{max}
Benzodiazepines *(continued)*						
Midazolam[vii]	Anxiety	IM: age<60: 0.07–0.08 mg/kg; MAX: 5 mg age≥60: 0.02–0.05 mg/kg (1 mg may suffice); MAX: 3.5 mg IV: age<60: start with 1 mg. MAX of 2.5 mg can be given over a period of at least 2 min. Wait additional 2 or more min to evaluate sedative effect. MAX: 5 mg age≥60: start with 1 mg. MAX of 1.5 mg can be given over a period of at least 2 min. Wait additional 2 or more min to evaluate sedative effect. MAX: 3.5 mg	CYP3A4; 1.8–6.4 hours	Excessive sedation, behavioral disinhibition, stupor, confusion, ataxia, anterograde amnesia, respiratory depression	IM, IV	IM: 30–60 min

Table 7–4. Useful medications in agitation *(continued)*

Drug class and name	Psychiatric FDA indications	Recommended acute dosing in adults	Metabolism/ half-life	Notable adverse effects in acute setting	Formulation(s)	Absorption, T_{max}
First-generation antipsychotics						
Haloperidol[viii]	Schizophrenia, Tourette's disorder	PO: initial dose of 2–5 mg, subsequent doses every 4–8 hours; MAX: 20 mg/day IM: initial dose of 5–10 mg; MAX: 20 mg/day	CYP3A4, CYP2D6 15–37 hours	QT prolongation (risk higher with IV administration), NMS, EPS, sedation, cerebrovascular events in elderly patients, orthostatic hypotension	PO, IM, IV (not recommended)	PO: 2–6 hours IM: 20 min
Chlorproma-zine[ix]	Bipolar mania, schizophrenia	PO: initial dose of 25–50 mg with 3–4 doses in 24 hours; MAX: 200 mg/day IM: initial dose of 25 mg IM; can give another 25–50 mg IM in 1 hour; MAX: 200 mg/day	CYP1A2, CYP3A4 6 hours	QT prolongation, orthostatic hypotension, anticholinergic effects	PO, IM, IV (not recommended)	PO: 2.8 hours IM: 2.8 hours

Table 7–4.   Useful medications in agitation (continued)

Drug class and name	Psychiatric FDA indications	Recommended acute dosing in adults	Metabolism/ half-life	Notable adverse effects in acute setting	Formulation(s)	Absorption, T_{max}
First-generation antipsychotics (continued)						
Fluphenazine[x]	Schizophrenia	PO: initial dose of 2–5 mg; MAX: 10 mg/day; IM: initial dose of 2–5 mg; MAX: 10 mg/day	CYP2C19, CYP2D6, CYP3A4; 33 hours	QT prolongation, NMS, EPS, sedation, cerebrovascular events in elderly patients, orthostatic hypotension	PO, IM	PO: 2.8 hours; IM: 1.5–2.0 hours

Note.   CYP = cytochrome P450; EPS = extrapyramidal symptoms; FDA = U.S. Food and Drug Administration; IM = intramuscular; IV = intravenous; MAX = maximum; NMS = neuroleptic malignant syndrome; PO = by mouth (oral); SL = sublingual; T_{max} = time to maximum absorption; UGT = uridine diphosphate glucuronosyltransferase.

Source.   Micromedex Healthcare Series. DRUGDEX System. Greenwood Village, CO: Truven Health Analytics, 2014. Available at: http://www.thomsonhc.com. Accessed March 27, 2014.

Drug information sources (accessed on May 21, 2014):
[i] Risperdal [package insert]. Titusville, NJ: Janssen. Revised April 2014. Available at: http://www.janssenpharmaceuticalsinc.com/assets/risperdal.pdf
[ii] Zyprexa [package insert]. Indianapolis, IN: Lilly, USA. Revised June 2013. Available at: http://pi.lilly.com/us/zyprexa-pi.pdf
[iii] Geodon [package insert]. New York, NY: Pfizer. Revised January 2014. Available at: http://labeling.pfizer.com/ShowLabeling.aspx?id=584
[iv] Saphris [package insert]. Whitehouse Station, NJ: Merck. Revised March 2013. Available at: http://www.merck.com/product/usa/pi_circulars/s/saphris/saphris_pi.pdf
[v] Aripiprazole. In: U.S. National Library of Medicine. Bethesda, MD: National Institutes of Health. Updated February 2011. Available at: http://dailymed.nlm.nih.gov/dailymed/lookup.cfm?setid=b624233-8846-4ea8-a2fa-a563e48fdc29#nlm34090-1
[vi] Lorazepam. In: U.S. National Library of Medicine. Bethesda, MD: National Institutes of Health. Updated October 2013. Available at: http://dailymed.nlm.nih.gov/dailymed/lookup.cfm?setid=ad2a0633-50fe-4180-b743-c1e49fc110c6#nlm34090-1
[vii] Midazolam. In: U.S. National Library of Medicine. Bethesda, MD: National Institutes of Health. Updated April 2010. Available at: http://dailymed.nlm.nih.gov/dailymed/lookup.cfm?setid=373fc1d0-9bd2-414b-8798-7bf04526a12e
[viii] Haloperidol. In: U.S. National Library of Medicine. Bethesda, MD: National Institutes of Health. Updated April 2009. Available at: http://dailymed.nlm.nih.gov/dailymed/archives/fdaDrugInfo.cfm?archiveid=14040
[ix] Chlorpromazine. In: U.S. National Library of Medicine. Bethesda, MD: National Institutes of Health. Updated May 2010. Available at: http://dailymed.nlm.nih.gov/dailymed/lookup.cfm?setid=33c01749-ef88-4e9c-8b45-0f026af1d5fd
[x] Fluphenazine. In: U.S. National Library of Medicine. Bethesda, MD: National Institutes of Health. Updated June 2011. Available at: http://dailymed.nlm.nih.gov/dailymed/lookup.cfm?setid=7b762f8b-86f7-46b0-8ace-83addaabe46b

ing sedative load. Antipsychotics are preferred in this instance, with haloperidol as a preferable choice, according to expert opinion (Wilson et al. 2012). Second-generation antipsychotic drugs can also be useful (Lukens et al. 2006).

When the patient is actively withdrawing from alcohol, as determined by laboratory and clinical examination, benzodiazepines are the treatment of choice to avoid life-threatening complications. Clonidine may be useful adjunctively due to its modulation of sympathetic activity in the CNS. In alcohol withdrawal, symptoms of autonomic instability (tachycardia, blood pressure fluctuations, fever), mental status changes (including seizures, hallucinations, disorientation), diaphoresis, and tremors always require immediate attention, and clinicians should consider consulting with medical colleagues.

Delirium

If a patient's agitation is thought to be secondary to delirium (not related to drugs and alcohol), the immediate priority lies in establishing a diagnosis and appropriate treatment. Proceeding with the physical and laboratory examination is prudent. If metabolic derangements (electrolytes, hypoxia, pH abnormalities, glucose irregularities) are discovered, their prompt correction may directly influence the patient's agitation symptoms. To manage problematic behaviors while the workup progresses, oral second-generation antipsychotics (olanzapine, risperidone) are first-line choices (Wilson et al. 2012). Medically ill patients may have higher rates of extrapyramidal symptoms, and avoiding first-generation antipsychotics (and parenteral administration) is advised but not always possible. Benzodiazepines are generally a poor choice for symptomatic treatment in this population because they can paradoxically worsen symptoms. Use of sedative-hypnotics for sleep is similarly ill advised.

Psychiatric Illness

In agitation arising from psychopathology, the clinician should focus on the patient's thought content. If psychosis is present, an oral second-generation antipsychotic (olanzapine, risperidone) as first-line treatment is optimal. Treatment should be directed at an underlying cause (Yildiz et al. 2003). First-generation agents (haloperidol) are appropriate second-line oral treatment. In the event that the initial dose of antipsychotic is ineffective, adding a benzodiazepine is more effective and generally recommended over additional doses of the same or a different antipsychotic (Yildiz et al. 2003).

If psychosis is absent, an oral benzodiazepine is first-line treatment. Use of an oral second-generation antipsychotic (olanzapine, risperidone) would be an appropriate next strategy if the benzodiazepine is ineffective. Whether or not psychosis is present in psychiatric patients, parenteral antipsychotic medication (olanzapine and ziprasidone are preferable to haloperidol) can be used if oral treatment is not feasible or indicated. With intravenous administration of highly specific dopaminergic agents (of which haloperidol is one), coadministration of an anticholinergic medication such as benztropine or diphenhydramine is useful prophylaxis for extrapyramidal symptoms and other neuromuscular side effects. If the cause for agitation is complex or unknown and the patient is not delirious, benzodiazepines are first-line agents; if psychotic symptoms are present, then second-generation antipsychotic medications would be recommended.

Conclusion to Case Example

In this section, we apply the principles discussed in this chapter to Mr. H from the case example at the beginning of the chapter. Mr. H's history suggests a primary thought disorder, and current mental status findings suggest psychotic ideation, including discrete paranoia. His verbalized threats raise concern for the possibility of his acting out were he not restrained. Substance use could be causal or contributory. Underlying cardiovascular, neurological, or infectious processes are considerations given his poor self-care, infrequent follow-up, and persistent hypertension after sedative administration.

It is prudent to transport Mr. H to a quiet room with restraints in place for the time being. Clear delineation of limits is essential for this patient, as well as a show of force and one clinician acting as leader. Standing at a distance, the clinician can provide an orientation to where the patient is, who the staff is, and what events will follow. Allowing the patient to decide how staff addresses him is ideal given that the clinician will want to refer to him frequently by name. Eye contact will be intermittent, body language open, and dialogue empathic. The patient is not wearing adequate clothing, and offering a blanket while asking about any other needs will ally the provider with the patient.

A rapidly dissolving oral medication will be important due to Mr. H's psychosis, probable nonadherence, and current state of agitation. An atypical antipsychotic would be the first choice due to presence of psychosis and the likelihood of drug continuity with his future regimen. If indicated, the decision about intramuscular medication would be made with available information about what prescriptions he is currently taking, whether he has any allergies, when his last dose was, and what has helped him in the past. Given the patient's nonadherence, there is value in selecting a medication with a variety of available formulations, allowing easy conversion from intramuscular to oral formulation. With the assistance of security staff, transitioning the patient to restraints in a hospital bed and medication administration should take place next. This would provide an opportunity for laboratory assessment, which should be considered given the fact that Mr. H may not provide reliable information about physical symptoms. Nursing will continue to monitor the patient's vital signs while he continues in restraints. Focused physical examination should be delayed but conducted when clinically appropriate. As the medication takes effect, every effort should be made to promptly remove restraints and then debrief the patient.

Key Clinical Points

- Agitation represents a challenging group of complex symptoms and behaviors that arise from numerous etiologies.

- Agitation frequently requires clinicians to make quick decisions (often with insufficient information) in diagnosis and treatment.

- Patient and staff safety are of utmost importance in every clinical encounter in which agitation occurs. In at-risk patients, a low threshold should be used to escalate the type, level, and strategy of care to prevent injury.

- Adequate clinician training accompanied by empathy and flexibility can reduce agitation in patients or prevent it entirely.

- Optimal assessment of agitation involves careful longitudinal assessment of the patient; collateral information from family, friends, and the medical record; physical, mental status, and laboratory examinations; and self-awareness on the part of the clinician.

- Each clinician should consider the possibility that a medical, reversible cause could be responsible for the agitation observed in the patient.

- Verbal de-escalation techniques are effective first-line interventions that can preclude or complement pharmacological treatment (which has been overprescribed historically).

- When medications are indicated, every effort should be made to use oral formulations before intramuscular injections. If a patient is placed in seclusion or restraints, appropriate medication should be given.

- Pharmacological treatment of agitation should take place only in the context of a working differential diagnosis. Awareness of the patient's particular set of symptoms (i.e., psychosis, delirium, substance use) helps in optimizing the clinician's medication selection.

References

Allen MH, Currier GW, Carpenter D, et al; Expert Consensus Panel for Behavioral Emergencies 2005: The expert consensus guideline series. Treatment of behavioral emergencies 2005. J Psychiatr Pract 11 (suppl 1):5–108, quiz 110–112, 2005 16319571

Balducci L: The "hateful" patient. Journal of Medicine and the Person 11(3):113–117, 2013

Buss DM, Shackelford TK: Human aggression in evolutionary psychological perspective. Clin Psychol Rev 17(6):605–619, 1997 9336687

Cohen-Mansfield J, Billig N: Agitated behaviors in the elderly, I: a conceptual review. J Am Geriatr Soc 34(10):711–721, 1986 3531296

de Almeida RM, Ferrari PF, Parmigiani S, et al: Escalated aggressive behavior: dopamine, serotonin and GABA. Eur J Pharmacol 526(1–3):51–64, 2005 16325649

Gates DM, Ross CS, McQueen L: Violence against emergency department workers. J Emerg Med 31(3):331–337, 2006 16982376

Korn CS, Currier GW, Henderson SO: "Medical clearance" of psychiatric patients without medical complaints in the emergency department. J Emerg Med 18(2):173–176, 2000 10699517

Lindenmayer JP: The pathophysiology of agitation. J Clin Psychiatry 61 (suppl 14):5–10, 2000 11154018

Lukens TW, Wolf SJ, Edlow JA, et al; American College of Emergency Physicians Clinical Policies Subcommittee (Writing Committee) on Critical Issues in the Diagnosis and Management of the Adult Psychiatric Patient in the Emergency Department: Clinical policy: critical issues in the diagnosis and management of the adult psychiatric patient in the emergency department. Ann Emerg Med 47(1):79–99, 2006 16387222

Richmond JS, Berlin JS, Fishkind AB, et al: Verbal de-escalation of the agitated patient: consensus statement of the American Association for Emergency Psychiatry Project BETA De-escalation Workgroup. West J Emerg Med 13(1):17–25, 2012 22461917

Swift RH, Harrigan EP, Cappelleri JC, et al: Validation of the Behavioural Activity Rating Scale (BARS): a novel measure of activity in agitated patients. J Psychiatr Res 36(2):87–95, 2002 11777497

Wilson MP, Pepper D, Currier GW, et al: The psychopharmacology of agitation: consensus statement of the American Association for Emergency Psychiatry Project BETA Psychopharmacology Workgroup. West J Emerg Med 13(1):26–34, 2012 22461918

Yildiz A, Sachs GS, Turgay A: Pharmacological management of agitation in emergency settings. Emerg Med J 20(4):339–346, 2003 12835344

Zun LS, Hernandez R, Thompson R, Downey L: Comparison of EPs' and psychiatrists' laboratory assessment of psychiatric patients. Am J Emerg Med 22(3):175–180, 2004 15138952

Suggested Readings

Richmond JS, Berlin JS, Fishkind AB, et al: Verbal de-escalation of the agitated patient: consensus statement of the American Association for Emergency Psychiatry Project BETA De-escalation Workgroup. West J Emerg Med 13(1):17–25, 2012

Wilson MP, Pepper D, Currier GW, et al: The psychopharmacology of agitation: consensus statement of the American Association for Emergency Psychiatry Project BETA Psychopharmacology Workgroup. West J Emerg Med 13(1):26–34, 2012

8

The Cognitively Impaired Patient

James A. Bourgeois, O.D., M.D., F.A.P.M.
Tracy McCarthy, M.D.

Case Example

Mr. C, a 75-year-old man with multiple vascular risk factors, presented to the emergency department a few days after having an outpatient cardiac catheterization that revealed severe coronary artery disease. The patient had no immediate complications following the procedure; however, shortly after his return home, he experienced motor agitation, confusion, and disorientation. He did not appear to have any new neurological deficits. When seen in consultation, he had a variable level of consciousness, was grossly confused and disoriented, and was seeing "animals." Collateral history from family members revealed a gradual onset of mild problems, including memory and word-finding difficulties, even prior to the catheterization. He also was "depressed" and had mild sleep, energy, and appetite disturbances.

Patients with cognitive impairment, such as Mr. C, present unique challenges in emergency psychiatry. Many discrete psychiatric illnesses are associated with cognitive impairment. Thus, the differential diagnosis of cognitive impairment is broad, covering many, often overlapping diagnostic categories

179

and forcing the physician to consider many possibilities. In addition, the "core deficit" of cognitive impairment may be less dramatic in its emergency presentation than the more "disruptive" clinical states (e.g., psychosis, mania, motor agitation, violence against self and/or others) that may be the initial focus of clinical attention. Therefore, the clinician encountering numerous disruptive clinical states in an emergency setting must keep in mind the possibility of an underlying cognitive disorder as explanatory for the bulk of the patient's clinical problems.

Prompt assessment requires an integrative approach, including analysis of the clinical history (from both the patient and collateral sources), clinical examination (including validated "bedside" formal cognitive testing), neuroimaging, clinical laboratory testing, physical examination, electrocardiogram, and, on occasion, electroencephalogram (EEG).

Clinical disposition of patients with cognitive impairment presenting for emergency care may be quite varied and sometimes challenging, and may include the emergent use of psychopharmacology, medical or surgical admission with psychiatric psychosomatic medicine consultation, medical-psychiatric unit admission, psychiatric unit admission, or placement in alternative models of supervised living. By necessity, the definitive psychiatric diagnosis and long-term management plan may not always be achievable in the emergency setting; initial assessment and intervention, however, remain crucial to the eventual definitive disposition of these cases.

As the population has aged, the prevalence of cognitive disorders has increased (Blennow et al. 2006). Simultaneously, increasing numbers of patients are not covered by appropriate health insurance, although this may be mitigated (in the United States) by the implementation of the Affordable Care Act in 2014. The convergence of these trends will inevitably lead to more patients with cognitive impairment being seen in emergency settings. Therefore, mastery of the emergency management of these patients is a clinical imperative.

Evaluation of the Patient

Safety and Restraint

Safety and restraint must be considered early in interactions with patients with cognitive impairment, often before a firm diagnosis is made. In addition to being a danger to themselves, patients who are agitated and cognitively im-

Table 8–1.   Components of the history in patients with cognitive impairment

History of present illness

Prior neuropsychiatric history

Prior non–central nervous system medical history

History of head trauma, seizures, stroke, other central nervous system events

Recent level of cognitive function

Substance abuse history

Highest level of educational and vocational attainment

Medications (prescription, over-the-counter, herbal supplements)

Family history of cognitive disorders and other psychiatric illness

paired are very disruptive to the operation of an emergency service (not to mention potentially dangerous to other patients). As a result, emergency departments must have well-developed as-needed procedures to provide sitters for, seclude, restrain, and medicate disruptive patients with cognitive impairments. Once safety is assured, clinical management may proceed.

Workup

The emergency workup of the patient with cognitive impairment is a graphic illustration of the integrative biopsychosocial approach. The triad of examination, laboratory, and neuroimaging should be kept in mind in these evaluations; EEG and lumbar puncture can be considered in certain situations.

Examination

As in other areas of clinical practice, examination begins with history taking. Because patients with cognitive impairments are invariably poor historians, collateral history from family, caregivers, other physicians, social service agencies, and others with an interest in the patient should be solicited (Robert et al. 2005), especially in an emergency setting. However, privacy regulations must be followed; the clinician must be circumspect about telling the collateral sources private information about the patient. Items to address in the history include but are not limited to those listed in Table 8–1.

The examination needs to include the physical and mental status items listed in Table 8–2. A number of brief cognitive screening tests are available to clinicians that can serve as useful tools in assessment and in following the course of cognitive disorders. The most popular instrument is the Mini-Mental State Examination (MMSE; Folstein et al. 1975). The MMSE is validated, has been translated into multiple languages, and is quick to administer. Disadvantages include the MMSE's limited ability to assess frontal lobe executive function and its inability to distinguish definitively between delirium and major or mild neurocognitive disorder (NCD). An instrument similar to the MMSE is the Montreal Cognitive Assessment (MoCA) (Nasreddine et al. 2005; www.mocatest.org). The MoCA is administered in a manner similar to the MMSE but has the additional value of testing visuospatial and executive functions. Clock drawing (Shulman 2000) is a useful screening test for cognitive impairment, particularly for patients with limited language capacity or other communication barriers. The Mini-Cog consists of the three-item recall from the MMSE and the clock draw (Borson et al. 2000). It can be a useful quick screening tool for major or mild NCD. Another commonly used tool is the Confusion Assessment Method (CAM; Inouye et al. 1990). Used in assessing delirium, the CAM can also be administered in very little time and is geared toward use by general medical clinicians for the evaluation of acute delirium. Based on DSM-III-R (American Psychiatric Association 1987), the CAM also is validated, with high sensitivity and specificity. Executive functioning can be evaluated with the Frontal Assessment Battery, which includes tests of motor sequencing, verbal fluency, response inhibition, and other functions (Dubois et al. 2000). Of note, these tests are often less useful in evaluating subcortical disorders. An oral version of the Trail Making Test—Part B, called the Mental Alternation Test, is more useful for patients with subcortical disorders and has been validated in major and mild NCD associated with HIV. This simple test requires the patient to alternate saying numbers and letters (1, A, 2, B, 3, C, etc.). The number of correct alternations in 30 seconds is the score, with a maximum score of 52 and a cutoff score of approximately 14 (Billick et al. 2001).

Laboratory Assessment

Laboratory assessment is crucial in the assessment of cognitive impairment. Because the acute presentation of cognitive impairment often represents overlapping syndromes of delirium and major or mild NCDs, a wide laboratory net needs to be cast for thoroughness. Table 8–3 lists laboratory tests com-

Table 8–2. Examination of patients with cognitive impairment

Physical examination

Vital signs

Pulse oximetry

Head, ears, eyes, nose, and throat (including thyroid)

Cardiovascular, pulmonary, and abdominal examination (including fecal occult blood)

Genitourinary and/or gynecological examination (as appropriate)

Neurological examination

Mental status examination

General appearance

Psychomotor activity

Speech

Mood and affect

Thought process and content

Psychotic symptoms, suicidality, and homicidality

Judgment and insight

Formal cognitive examination (e.g., MMSE, MoCA, clock drawing)

Frontal lobe testing

Note. MMSE = Mini-Mental State Examination (Folstein et al. 1975); MoCA = Montreal Cognitive Assessment (Nasreddine et al. 2005).

Table 8–3. Laboratory tests in cognitive impairment

Acetaminophen level	Creatine phosphokinase	Quantitative drug levels
Ammonia	Cultures	Rheumatological panel
Arterial blood gases	Heavy metal screen	Thyroid panel
Blood alcohol level	Hepatitis panel	Urinalysis
Chemistry panel	HIV	Urine drug screen
Chest X ray	12-Lead electrocardiogram	VDRL or RPR
Complete blood count	Liver enzymes	Vitamin B_{12}

Note. RPR = rapid plasma reagin; VDRL = Venereal Disease Research Laboratory.

monly used in patients with cognitive impairment; individual items on this list may be omitted if clinical suspicion is low.

Neuroimaging

Because the workup for altered mental status is in many cases the same as a workup for major or mild NCD, neuroimaging is increasingly commonly included. The debate of computed tomography (CT) versus magnetic resonance imaging is a useful one; however, for most emergency purposes, CT is easier to obtain, lower cost, easier for the patient to tolerate, and not subject to patient contraindications (e.g., claustrophobia, indwelling metallic devices). In addition, with CT there is usually no need for intravenous contrast dye to acutely evaluate cognitive disorders. Although the clinician needs to be mindful of repeated radiation exposure and thus not obtain CT scans excessively, the threshold for CT scanning in the emergency setting needs to be appropriately low so as not to miss reversible causes of cognitive impairment.

EEG and Lumbar Puncture

The EEG may be helpful in differentiating between delirium and NCDs, because it reliably reveals diffuse slowing in delirium cases and has a characteristic pattern in Creutzfeldt-Jakob disease (Engel and Romano 2004). However, because the EEG is not as useful in subtyping of delirium, it is not routinely obtained in typical delirium cases. Similarly, lumbar puncture is considered if there is high clinical suspicion of central nervous system (CNS) infection, but the yield is not adequately high for the procedure to be recommended routinely in all cases of altered mental status.

Case Example (continued)

Mr. C had admission scores of 12 on the MMSE and 14 on the MoCA, with clear impairments in attention span, orientation, and memory. His clock drawing revealed poor numeral and hand placement. He was diagnosed with delirium and was admitted to the medical service for further evaluation. On physical examination at admission, his catheter wound site was found to be surrounded by an erythematous ring and was warm and tender to touch. There was no pus from the wound. Complete blood count revealed a leukocytosis. Head CT did not demonstrate evidence of a recent infarct but did show some diffuse cortical atrophy and small vessel white matter disease.

Although Mr. C was initially diagnosed with delirium, the reports of gradual prehospitalization decline in cognitive functioning were concerning for a comorbid diagnosis of major depression or of major or mild NCD. Given the imaging findings, a diagnosis of major or mild vascular NCD was considered, but definitive diagnosis was deferred until Mr. C's delirium had a chance to clear.

Psychiatric Disorders Characterized by Cognitive Impairment

The issue of psychiatric diagnosis of cognitive impairments warrants a general discussion of semantics and classification. The formal diagnosis of cognitive disorder may not be adequately inclusive of all of the psychiatric disorders characterized by cognitive impairment seen in the emergency setting. The majority of patients who present with cognitive impairment in the emergency setting will have an illness classified in DSM-5 (American Psychiatric Association 2013) among the NCDs. This new classification system eliminates the previous diagnoses of amnestic disorders and introduces the various major and mild NCDs. Subclassification is according to specific neuropathological cause (e.g., major or mild NCD due to Alzheimer's disease, major or mild vascular NCD). The main distinction between major and mild disorders pertains to the greater cognitive decline and functional impairment in the major conditions. This classification can be applied elastically to conditions such as postconcussive syndrome and the psychiatric sequelae of traumatic brain injury (TBI), which may be subsyndromal for more impairing disorders or may present in a mixed picture that bridges the constructs of major or mild NCDs and delirium (Mooney and Speed 2001). A smaller percentage of patients with cognitive impairment, including adults, will have illnesses classified in DSM-5 among the neurodevelopmental disorders. Even these two broad categories, however, will not capture all cognitive impairments seen in an emergency setting, because some patients with psychotic disorders, dissociative disorders, and substance use disorders may also present with cognitive impairment.

Delirium

According to DSM-5, delirium is a subacute- to acute-onset condition characterized by disturbance in attention and awareness, circadian disturbances, cognitive impairment (e.g., memory deficit, disorientation, language disturbance, visuospatial impairment, perceptual disturbance), and a variable course. It is the psychiatric consequence of systemic disturbance(s) and may follow a myriad of systemic

Table 8–4. Common causes of delirium

Brain tumor	Infection
Cardiopulmonary disease	Kidney disease
Electrolyte or fluid imbalance	Liver disease
Head trauma	Seizures
Hypercarbia	Substance intoxication
Hypoalbuminemia	Substance withdrawal
Hypoglycemia	Thiamine deficiency
Hypoxia	Other systemic illness

disorders (see Table 8–4). The keys to a diagnosis of delirium are the acute or sub-acute onset and the fluctuating course. Although delirium is invariably the consequence of one or more systemic disturbances, the most important "static" risk factor for the development of delirium is the presence of a preexisting major or mild NCD, a concept that can be understood as the "vulnerable brain" or "decreased cognitive reserve" (Engel and Romano 2004). Even though delirium presents with an acute or subacute onset, it can become chronic if the underlying systemic cause is not reversed. Examples of conditions associated with chronic delirium include disseminated cancer and end-stage liver disease.

Although the patient with major or mild NCD is highly vulnerable to the development of delirium, delirium also occurs in patients without preexisting NCDs. Because delirium is the psychiatric manifestation of systemic illness and has myriad causes, emergency presentation of delirium mandates an efficient but thorough clinical search for the implicated systemic disturbance(s), covering many possible organ systems. The workup is ideally initiated in the emergency department. Although the underlying cause may not be evident initially, delirium should be managed actively and syndromally while the search for systemic precipitants proceeds apace. This holds true for both agitated and nonagitated delirious patients.

Prompt treatment of delirium is important for minimizing suffering and maximizing safety. Patients frequently remember the aspects of the delirium episode, and delirium is often quite frightening to family members as well.

Delirium Superimposed on Major or Mild NCD

A common presentation to the emergency room is the patient with premorbid major or mild NCD who subsequently develops acute delirium (Fick et al. 2002). Often, the premorbid major or mild NCD has not been clinically appreciated and treated. The delirium episodes may be recurrent, which may point to major or mild NCD as a risk factor.

Neuroleptic Malignant Syndrome

A particularly dangerous form of delirium is the iatrogenic syndrome of neuroleptic malignant syndrome (NMS). This constellation of delirium, rigidity, and increased creatine phosphokinase (CPK) should be suspected in any patient who presents with altered mental status and has had access to antipsychotic agents. In recent years, NMS has been increasingly commonly reported with the use of atypical antipsychotics. Prior episodes of validated NMS are an important part of the patient's history. Management requires an appropriately high index of suspicion, a prompt determination of CPK level, supportive care, and withholding of antipsychotics until the CPK has renormalized for at least 2 weeks, at which point antipsychotic therapy may be cautiously restarted with CPK monitoring. In some cases, dantrolene, bromocriptine, and electroconvulsive therapy may be considered.

Major or Mild NCD

Major or mild NCD is a syndrome of cognitive impairment that, according to DSM-5, includes decline from a previous level of performance in one or more cognitive domains ("mild/modest" decline in mild NCD; "significant/substantial" decline in major NCD) that is not solely due to delirium or another psychiatric illness. Patients with mild NCD maintain independent function, while patients with major NCD (formerly referred to as *dementia*) have interference with independent function. Major or mild NCD presents with full alertness, which is crucial in distinguishing major or mild NCD from delirium, with which it is frequently comorbid. Most major or mild NCD syndromes have insidious onset and a course characterized by slow progression, but the physician must bear in mind that this course, although prototypical for major or mild NCD and common in the majority of cases, is not uniform (Engel and Romano 2004). Acute presentation of a large decrement in cognitive function may result from a critically located CNS lesion (e.g., a dominant-hemisphere middle cerebral artery cerebrovascular accident [CVA] in a case of poststroke major or mild vascular NCD) (Román 2002). Major or mild NCD syndromes may be quite rapidly progressive (e.g., Creutzfeldt-Jakob disease) or may be somewhat reversible with clinical intervention (e.g., hypothyroidism, vitamin B$_{12}$ deficiency) (Boeve 2006; Engel and Romano 2004).

The distinction between major or mild NCD and delirium, although a crucial clinical concept, is in some ways a false dichotomy in clinical practice, because patients with previously undiagnosed major or mild NCD will often present with delirium simultaneously. Major or mild NCD is the most tangible and important risk factor for the later development of delirium. Many patients will experience several episodes of delirium during the tragic course of a degenerative major or mild NCD.

In addition, major or mild NCDs are associated with a range of other psychiatric comorbid conditions that episodically may dominate (and in a sense even define) the clinical picture. Mood disorders, most commonly depressive states, are very common in patients with major or mild NCD (Lyketsos et al. 2002; Robert et al. 2005). A patient who is acutely significantly depressed and has chronic mild dementia may well present to the emergency room with depressed mood, neurovegetative signs, and even suicidal crisis, even though the underlying psychiatric illness is major or mild NCD. Many patients with comorbid major or mild NCD and depression will experience an episode of depression more in the cognitive realm (e.g., decreased memory or concentration) than in the emotional realm, and may interpret their clinical situation as one of increasing cognitive impairment, likely triggering even more seriously depressed mood, and thereby setting up a vicious cycle.

Even more disruptive, and leading to many emergency presentations of patients with major or mild NCD, is the pernicious relationship between major or mild NCD and psychosis. Common comorbid psychotic symptoms in major or mild NCD include delusions, particularly paranoid delusions, and hallucinations (Leverenz and McKeith 2002). The delusions in major or mild NCD may be a defensive attempt to "cover up" cognitive impairment. For example, the patient who has lost a valued object because of cognitive impairment may instead believe that a family member has stolen the object. Indeed, the onset of psychotic symptoms in a patient with major or mild NCD is both disruptive and dangerous to the patient and the family, and is a common context of emergency presentation (Robert et al. 2005). Therefore, the differential diagnosis of acute psychosis must necessarily include a rule-out of major or mild NCDs. Less frequently, a patient with major or mild NCD may present to the emergency room with an episode of comorbid acute hypomania or mania (Román 2002).

Patients with major or mild NCD may present with the phenomenon of sundowning, wherein the patient develops increased confusion and motor agitation in the evening and at night. These patients may or may not meet criteria for an episode of comorbid delirium for these episodes; nonetheless, these patients can become very dangerous and unsafe to manage at home or in noncontrolled living situations.

Finally, the emergency presentation of patients with major or mild NCD may be due to social factors rather than clinical ones. Patients with mild to moderate impairment can usually live in the community, if they have adequate supervision and the provision of basic needs by helpful others. When a support person is ill or dies, however, the now-unsupervised patient with major or mild NCD may be brought to the emergency department solely because of the inability to care for himself or herself. The clinician should routinely inquire into the stability of the social system, especially the loss of primary support figures, in the timing of emergency presentation of a patient with major or mild NCD.

Major or Mild NCD Due to Alzheimer's Disease

Major or mild NCD due to Alzheimer's disease (referred to hereafter as NCD due to Alzheimer's disease) is the most common major or mild NCD subtype in Western societies. It represents the majority of dementing illness in the United States (Blennow et al. 2006). Onset of NCD due to Alzheimer's disease is generally after age 65, and the population incidence increases with age. NCD due to Alzheimer's disease is characterized by insidious onset and slow but steady loss of multiple domains of cognitive function. Clinically, patients may present with amnesia and various other cognitive deficits, including disorientation, aphasia, anomia, apraxia, disturbed executive functioning, and loss of capacity for activities of daily living. Presentation to the emergency room is rarely for loss of cognitive function per se, but more commonly for the onset of decreased self-care behavior or for psychiatric comorbidity (e.g., depression, psychosis, agitation, violence).

Major or Mild Vascular NCD

Major or mild vascular NCD results from CNS infarction(s) encountered in patients with multiple vascular risk factors, usually a combination of hyperlipidemia, hypertension, smoking, and/or diabetes mellitus. The pattern of cognitive deficits may resemble those in NCD due to Alzheimer's disease, although the course of illness tends to vary. Patients with major or mild vascular NCD may have relative stability of deficits over time, with occasional abrupt losses in cognitive function; this stepwise progression differs from the continuous progression in NCD due to Alzheimer's disease (Román 2002). Less frequently (e.g., following a dominant-hemisphere CVA), a patient with major or mild vascular NCD may present who has not had prior cognitive impairment but who is suddenly experiencing an acute loss of a substantial number of cortical functions. Although following large CVAs patients may present with delirium acutely, once the delirium has cleared these patients are best understood as having major or mild vascular NCD.

Major or Mild NCD With Lewy Bodies

Major or mild NCD with Lewy bodies (NCD with Lewy bodies) and the Lewy body variant of NCD due to Alzheimer's disease, although somewhat distinct conditions neuropathologically, are overlapping clinically. Neuropathologically, both NCD with Lewy bodies and the Lewy body variant of NCD due to Alzheimer's disease feature distinctive Lewy bodies; however, the Lewy body variant of NCD due to Alzheimer's disease has characteristic neuropathology of Alzheimer's disease as well. Both are clinically distinct from (and understood as being more severe than) NCD due to Alzheimer's disease. Compared with NCD due to Alzheimer's disease, NCD with Lewy bodies and the Lewy body variant of NCD due to Alzheimer's disease are characterized by a younger age at onset, a more rapidly progressive course, fluctuations in mental status, and early-onset and clinically prominent hallucinations, typically visual hallucinations (Boeve 2006; Leverenz and McKeith 2002). The emergency presentation of these patients is often driven by the disruption caused by the dramatic onset of the visual hallucinations, which is often a defining clinical feature.

Major or Mild Frontotemporal NCD

Major or mild frontotemporal NCD (frontotemporal NCD) is a major or mild NCD that, relative to NCD due to Alzheimer's disease, is characterized by more prominent frontal lobe deficit–related decrements in appropriate social behavior with relatively preserved memory function. These patients present early in their illness with disruptive social behavior, such as sexual inappropriateness, aggression, impulsivity, and emotional dysregulation (Boeve 2006;

Kertesz and Munoz 2002). All of these behaviors tend to be quite disruptive to the caregivers; indeed, a caregiver's distress is often much greater than that of the patient. When evaluated clinically, these patients have the above-noted frontal lobe deficit states but otherwise have a remarkably preserved cognitive examination, often including MMSE scores in the nonimpaired range.

Major or Mild NCD Due to HIV Infection

Major or mild NCD due to HIV infection (NCD due to HIV infection) may result from direct effects of the HIV virus on CNS tissue and does not necessarily require clinical evidence of immunosuppression in general, although HIV patients with systemic immunocompromise will be at risk of other opportunistic CNS infections (e.g., toxoplasmosis) and CNS lymphoma, which further complicate the clinical picture. Because patients with HIV may occasionally present a somewhat ambiguous picture, with concurrent signs of delirium and major or mild NCD, NCD due to HIV infection needs to be on the differential diagnosis of any new patient presenting with neurocognitive impairment (and HIV testing should thus be strongly considered for new major or mild NCD cases). New-onset cognitive impairment in a known HIV patient should primarily be considered to be NCD due to HIV infection until other causes can be definitively established. NCD due to HIV infection is important to identify early, because aggressive treatment with highly active antiretroviral therapy agents can result in some reversibility of neurocognitive symptoms. In addition, persistence of cognitive impairment can be a significant problem in established HIV patients, whose ability to self-manage their medications may be significantly affected.

Major or Mild NCD Due to Traumatic Brain Injury

TBI is a common injury in the emergency setting. Critical variables to address are the period of unconsciousness, degree of posttraumatic amnesia, and cognitive status at the time of evaluation. Acutely, TBI patients may present with a picture more consistent with delirium, whereas over time, some may maintain a clinical appearance of major or mild NCD. The major or mild NCD due to TBI may take extended periods of time to improve (even months to years), and precise estimation of prognosis is difficult. Many TBI cases have elements of both delirium and major or mild NCD that can be understood as existing on the boundary of major or mild NCD and delirium. Still other TBI cases are clinically milder and subsyndromal for other cognitive disorders; these are sometimes called postconcussion syndrome.

Major or Mild NCD Due to Other Neurodegenerative Illness

Neurodegenerative illness due to several causes is characterized by cognitive impairment. Graphically illustrating the whole-brain concept that "neurological" and "psychiatric" illnesses commonly co-occur in patients with CNS degenerative disease, familiar neurological illnesses with a progressive course (e.g., Parkinson's disease, Huntington's disease, multiple sclerosis) are associated with a significant risk of major or mild NCD (on the order of 50% or more at some time during the course of illness; Boeve 2006). Subsequently, these patients are prone to delirium as well. The presentation of cognitive impairment in a patient with known neurological illness should lead the clinician to make these connections; indeed, in cases of multiple sclerosis, in particular, acute mental status changes may reflect a "flare" of the background neurological illness.

Other Clinical Syndromes of Cognitive Impairment

Transient Global Amnesia

Transient global amnesia is an acute-onset global amnesia that is reversible. It usually occurs in middle-aged patients with no prior psychiatric history. Other aspects of cognitive function are unimpaired. The cause is unclear but may be a temporary disturbance in temporal lobe function. Because of its precipitously acute onset and the preservation of other cognitive function, transient global amnesia is very disturbing to the patient and often leads to an emergency presentation. Full workup, including neuroimaging and assessment for vascular disease, is needed. Whether these patients have increased risk of cognitive impairment in the future is unclear.

Korsakoff Syndrome

Korsakoff syndrome is a usually acute-onset amnestic disorder in the context of alcohol dependence. It is attributed to thiamine deficiency. It may occur in isolation or as part of a larger picture of alcohol-induced major or mild NCD. It is treated with intravenously administered thiamine and subsequent nutritional supplementation.

Carbon Monoxide Poisoning

Carbon monoxide poisoning may result in focal hippocampal injury and thus amnesia in the absence of more global cognitive impairment. It may be seen in patients who attempted suicide by rerouting of vehicular exhaust or in fire victims. If emergently available, hyperbaric oxygen treatment may be considered.

Dissociative Amnesia

In dissociative amnesia, one of the dissociative disorders listed in DSM-5, the clinical emergency manifestations are cognitive. A patient with this disorder will be an acutely amnestic patient who has experienced a psychologically troubling or even traumatic event and defends against this reality with a dissociative defense, resulting in amnesia for the painful aspects of the experience. This history, however, may not be in the patient's awareness, so a collateral source is needed to establish the temporal connection.

Subdural Hematoma or Subarachnoid Hemorrhage

Subdural hematoma (often following head trauma) and subarachnoid hemorrhage (often associated with untreated hypertension) are vascular lesions that may lead to changes in mental status, resulting in an emergency presentation. These lesions may present in an emergency picture consistent with acute delirium, progressive major or mild NCD, or a combination of both.

Alcohol and/or Drug Disorders

Various substance-related conditions may present with cognitive impairment. Alcohol or drug intoxication may result in temporary cognitive impairment. Alcohol "blackouts" (brief periods of amnesia associated with alcohol dependence) may lead to emergency evaluation. Withdrawal from alcohol, sedatives, or hypnotics may present with frank delirium and autonomic instability (Engel and Romano 2004).

Depressive Pseudodementia

The overlap of mood and cognitive function is dramatically illustrated by the condition of depressive pseudodementia. In this condition, which is usually seen in older patients, the manifestation of depression is primarily cognitive, not emotional. Patients are often quite distressed by the insidious onset of cognitive impairment and are concerned that they are developing major or mild NCD. Formal cognitive examination usually reveals mild deficits in orientation, recall, and concentration. In addition, other symptoms of depression may be elicited. Treatment with an antidepressant and reassessment of cognitive function and mood symptoms after the patient is at a therapeutic level for an adequately long clinical trial of antidepressant (which may take as long as 2 months) will often be associated with improved cognitive performance.

Childhood-Onset Syndromes Characterized by Cognitive Impairment

Although often relatively neglected in the adult psychosomatic medicine literature, several childhood-onset illnesses are discussed in this chapter because they are characterized by cognitive impairment. When patients with these illnesses are seen in the emergency room, their cognitive impairment will likely be an important clinical aspect of the case. In addition, because intellectual disability is a risk factor for the later development of major or mild NCD, all of the considerations of major or mild NCD may also apply to these patients.

Intellectual Disability

Although classified in DSM-5 as a neurodevelopmental disorder, intellectual disability (called *mental retardation* in earlier DSM editions) is by definition a disorder of cognitive impairment. In addition to having impairments due to the baseline cognitive deficits, patients with intellectual disability have increased risk of major or mild NCD (even from their impaired baseline) as they age. In addition, they may have other psychiatric comorbidity, such as autism spectrum disorder, which may cloud the clinical emergency presentation.

Down Syndrome

Down syndrome is due to trisomy 21. The majority of patients with Down syndrome will have mild intellectual disability. However, as they age, there is a high likelihood of major or mild NCD superimposed on their intellectual disability.

Fragile X Disorders

Fragile X syndrome is the most common cause of intellectual disability due to a single genetic defect. In addition to having cognitive impairment, patients with fragile X syndrome often have autism spectrum disorder with associated impaired social function.

Fetal Alcohol Syndrome

Fetal alcohol syndrome is an intellectual disability syndrome due to in utero exposure to alcohol in the children of alcohol-dependent women. These children may have the characteristic facial features of fetal alcohol syndrome and various degrees of intellectual disability.

Clinical Management

Treatment

The first step in treatment of cognitive impairment is the management of systemic factors, as guided by the results of physical examination, laboratory, and imaging results. To treat behavioral symptoms, a range of psychotropic medications are now in common use. Antipsychotics, both typical and atypical, are now standard in emergency care (Carson et al. 2006; Kile et al. 2005; Lacasse et al. 2006; Meagher 2001; Tune 2001; Weber et al. 2004). Most commonly used in emergency settings are the typical antipsychotic haloperidol (most other typical antipsychotics are rarely used in the emergency setting) and several atypical antipsychotics.

Due to their sedative-hypnotic properties, benzodiazepines alone should be used for delirium due to alcohol withdrawal or delirium due to sedative-hypnotic withdrawal, either of which is often associated with signs of autonomic hyperarousal. Benzodiazepines are often combined with typical or atypical antipsychotics for the management of delirium due to other causes (Meagher 2001). They should be used with caution, however, because they may exacerbate many cases of delirium and may increase cognitive impairment in patients with major or mild NCD. The most important difference among benzodiazepines is in their pharmacokinetic properties—short-half-life agents will work more quickly but require more frequent dosing than long-half-life agents.

Although less frequently used in the emergency setting to treat patients with cognitive impairment, other agents are sometimes useful. Anticonvulsants may be used in a supplemental fashion to control agitation. One useful agent is Depacon, an intravenous form of valproate, which can be loaded at 15–20 mg/kg/day with monitoring of liver function, platelets, serum ammonia, and valproate serum levels (Kile et al. 2005). If anticholinergic toxicity is confirmed and/or if a history of premorbid major or mild NCD can be established, early use of cholinesterase inhibitors (donepezil, rivastigmine, or galantamine) may be initiated (Coulson et al. 2002). Finally, in cases of cognitive impairment with dangerous agitation, anesthetic agents such as propofol can be used emergently for a brief period, but the patient receiving this agent must be in an intensive care unit and receiving close clinical observation and airway management.

An important consideration is that medications used to control agitation in a patient with cognitive impairment also risk contributing to delirium, thereby worsening the patient's cognitive functioning. Therefore, medications should be used cautiously, and the minimum effective dose should be used, especially in elderly patients.

Case Example *(continued)*

Mr. C was treated with a low-dose antipsychotic for agitation in his delirium. He received intravenous antibiotics for the wound infection. Opioids were minimized, and anticholinergic medications and benzodiazepines were held. Over the next several days, his delirium improved. His score was 22 when the MMSE was readministered, and family members assured the treatment team that he was at his recent cognitive baseline. He was discharged to the community for further outpatient workup for major or mild NCD and major depression.

Disposition

Disposition of patients with cognitive impairment, once they are stabilized, from an emergency setting can be accomplished to a number of receiving institutions. These disposition decisions are often complicated, and no one type of institution will optimally manage the needs of all of these patients (Meagher 2001). Table 8–5 summarizes some possible disposition options, with associated advantages and disadvantages.

Legal Issues in Cognitive Impairment

Although not always a critical concern while patients are in the emergency setting, many legal issues may arise in the management of patients with cognitive impairment (see Table 8–6). The clinician needs a useful methodology to address these issues in the acute presentation of cognitive impairment.

Table 8–5.   Considerations in disposition of patients with cognitive impairment

Disposition	Advantages	Disadvantages
Medical admission	Full medical workup Access to consultants	Limited psychiatric care
Psychiatric admission	Full psychiatric care 24-hour supervision	Limited medical care May refuse cognitive disorder patients
Medical-psychiatric admission	Comprehensive care 24-hour supervision	Rarely available May refuse cognitive disorder patients
Rehabilitation admission	Familiar with cognitive impairment	Limited medical care May not have comprehensive psychiatric care
Structured placement (skilled nursing facility)	Safe for impaired patients 24-hour supervision	Minimal medical care Minimal psychiatric care

Table 8–6.   Legal considerations in the management of patients with cognitive impairment

Decisional capacity for medical/surgical procedures, do-not-resuscitate orders, estate management, social placement, other decisions

Assignment of surrogate decision maker

Informed consent for off-label medications

Interface with social service agencies (e.g., adult protective services)

Participation in clinical trials

Confidentiality

Insurance issues

Financial issues

Key Clinical Points

- Cognitive disorders are among the most common categories of psychiatric illness in the emergency department setting.

- Patients with cognitive impairment may present with various behavioral symptoms (e.g., psychosis, agitation, violence) in the emergency department.

- Cognitive disorders are an important part of the differential diagnosis of the presentation of agitated states.

- The "smoke" of delirium often leads to the discovery of the "fire" of major or mild neurocognitive disorder.

- Thorough mental status examination and quantitative cognitive assessment are required for initial workup and serial assessments.

- Workup of the agitated patient with cognitive impairment requires neuroimaging, clinical laboratory, and physical assessment.

- Emergency department presentation of cognitive impairment is more often due to psychosis, agitation, and disruption in the care model than to progression of cognitive impairment per se.

- Acute management of the patient with cognitive impairment may require typical antipsychotics, atypical antipsychotics, benzodiazepines, and other sedatives; chronic management requires the use of many classes of psychopharmacology.

References

American Psychiatric Association: Diagnostic and Statistical Manual of Mental Disorders, 3rd Edition, Revised. Washington, DC, American Psychiatric Association, 1987

American Psychiatric Association: Diagnostic and Statistical Manual of Mental Disorders, Fifth Edition. Arlington, VA, American Psychiatric Association, 2013

Billick SB, Siedenburg E, Burgert W 3rd, et al: Validation of the Mental Alternation Test with the Mini-Mental State Examination in geriatric psychiatric inpatients and normal controls. Compr Psychiatry 42(3):202–205, 2001 11349238

Blennow K, de Leon MJ, Zetterberg H: Alzheimer's disease. Lancet 368(9533):387–403, 2006 16876668

Boeve BF: A review of the non-Alzheimer dementias. J Clin Psychiatry 67(12):1985–2001, discussion 1983–1984, 2006 17194279

Borson S, Scanlan J, Brush M, et al: The Mini-Cog: a cognitive "vital signs" measure for dementia screening in multi-lingual elderly. Int J Geriatr Psychiatry 15(11):1021–1027, 2000 11113982

Carson S, McDonagh MS, Peterson K: A systematic review of the efficacy and safety of atypical antipsychotics in patients with psychological and behavioral symptoms of dementia. J Am Geriatr Soc 54(2):354–361, 2006 16460391

Coulson BS, Fenner SG, Almeida OP: Successful treatment of behavioural problems in dementia using a cholinesterase inhibitor: the ethical questions. Aust N Z J Psychiatry 36(2):259–262, 2002 11982550

Dubois B, Slachevsky A, Litvan I, et al: The FAB: a frontal assessment battery at bedside. Neurology 55(11):1621–1626, 2000 11113214

Engel GL, Romano J: Delirium, a syndrome of cerebral insufficiency. 1959. J Neuropsychiatry Clin Neurosci 16(4):526–538, 2004 15616182

Fick DM, Agostini JV, Inouye SK: Delirium superimposed on dementia: a systematic review. J Am Geriatr Soc 50(10):1723–1732, 2002 12366629

Folstein MF, Folstein SE, McHugh PR: "Mini-mental state": a practical method for grading the cognitive state of patients for the clinician. J Psychiatr Res 12(3):189–198, 1975 1202204

Inouye SK, van Dyck CH, Alessi CA, et al: Clarifying confusion: the confusion assessment method. A new method for detection of delirium. Ann Intern Med 113(12):941–948, 1990 2240918

Kertesz A, Munoz DG: Frontotemporal dementia. Med Clin North Am 86(3):501–518, vi, 2002 12168557

Kile SJ, Bourgeois JA, Sugden S, et al: Neurobehavioral sequelae of traumatic brain injury. Applied Neurology 1:29–32, 2005

Lacasse H, Perreault MM, Williamson DR: Systematic review of antipsychotics for the treatment of hospital-associated delirium in medically or surgically ill patients. Ann Pharmacother 40(11):1966–1973, 2006 17047137

Leverenz JB, McKeith IG: Dementia with Lewy bodies. Med Clin North Am 86(3):519–535, 2002 12171059

Lyketsos CG, Lopez O, Jones B, et al: Prevalence of neuropsychiatric symptoms in dementia and mild cognitive impairment: results from the Cardiovascular Health Study. JAMA 288(12):1475–1483, 2002 12243634

Meagher DJ: Delirium: optimising management. BMJ 322(7279):144–149, 2001 11159573

Mooney G, Speed J: The association between mild traumatic brain injury and psychiatric conditions. Brain Inj 15(10):865–877, 2001 11595083

Nasreddine ZS, Phillips NA, Bédirian V, et al: The Montreal Cognitive Assessment, MoCA: a brief screening tool for mild cognitive impairment. J Am Geriatr Soc 53(4):695–699, 2005 15817019

Robert PH, Verhey FR, Byrne EJ, et al: Grouping for behavioral and psychological symptoms in dementia: clinical and biological aspects. Consensus paper of the European Alzheimer Disease Consortium. Eur Psychiatry 20(7):490–496, 2005 16310680

Román GC: Vascular dementia revisited: diagnosis, pathogenesis, treatment, and prevention. Med Clin North Am 86(3):477–499, 2002 12168556

Shulman KI: Clock-drawing: is it the ideal cognitive screening test? Int J Geriatr Psychiatry 15(6):548–561, 2000 10861923

Tune LE: Anticholinergic effects of medication in elderly patients. J Clin Psychiatry 62 (suppl 21):11–14, 2001 11584981

Weber JB, Coverdale JH, Kunik ME: Delirium: current trends in prevention and treatment. Intern Med J 34(3):115–121, 2004 15030459

Suggested Readings

Blennow K, de Leon MJ, Zetterberg H: Alzheimer's disease. Lancet 368:387–403, 2006

Kile SJ, Bourgeois JA, Sugden S, et al: Neurobehavioral sequelae of traumatic brain injury. Applied Neurology 1:29–32, 2005

Lacasse H, Perreault MM, Williamson DR: Systematic review of antipsychotics for the treatment of hospital-associated delirium in medically or surgically ill patients. Ann Pharmacother 40:1966–1973, 2006

9

Substance-Related Psychiatric Emergencies

Adam D. Miller, M.D.

Gerald Scott Winder, M.D.

Kirk J. Brower, M.D.

Case Example 1

Mrs. N is a 68-year-old previously healthy woman who was brought to the emergency department by her son over concern about flulike symptoms over the past 2 days. Symptoms included runny nose, nausea, sweating, and generalized body aches. It was noted during the interview that Mrs. N's husband of 40 years passed away 1 month earlier. Drug screen results were positive for opioids. When informed of the result, Mrs. N reluctantly divulged that she had been taking her husband's oxycodone for the past 10 years until running out 3 days ago.

Case Example 2

Mr. K, a 44-year-old man with a history of chronic depression, was sent to the emergency department by his primary care physician after the patient presented for his yearly physical exhibiting impaired orientation. Upon arrival the patient was disoriented and hallucinating. He was also noted to have elevated blood pressure with tachycardia and tremulousness. Through collateral sources it was discovered that Mr. K had been consuming six to eight alcoholic drinks daily for the past 10 years but had stopped drinking 3 days prior to his appointment in an effort to "get healthy."

In this chapter, we provide a review of substances of abuse commonly encountered in the emergency context to help the busy clinician work through a differential diagnosis of common syndromes. For a more in-depth review of mechanistic issues and pharmacology and specific up-to-date treatment algorithms, the reader is referred to textbooks of emergency medicine, psychiatry, toxicology, and addictions (e.g., Glick et al. 2008).

Epidemiology, Prevalence, and Impact of Substance-Related Emergencies

Emergency departments (EDs) throughout the United States manage over 129 million visits annually (Centers for Disease Control and Prevention 2010). Of these, 2.5 million are estimated to be related to drug abuse or misuse. Over 87,000 Americans lose their lives annually because of alcohol (Centers for Disease Control and Prevention 2013), and 38,000 die because of illicit drugs (Centers for Disease Control and Prevention 2012). A 2011 review of information obtained from EDs nationwide found that for visits related to substance use, 10% were for suicide-related reasons and 10% for substance dependence (Substance Abuse and Mental Health Services Administration 2013).

Assessment in emergency psychiatry, therefore, must encompass a systematic review of substances, including potential toxicities and withdrawal syndromes. Knowledge about substance-related psychiatric symptoms with their added risk of suicide is also essential. For many patients with substance use disorders, the ED visit may be the first and/or only chance to initiate a path to substance use treatment (Rockett et al. 2006).

Initial Evaluation of Patients

A high proportion of presentations in the psychiatric ED are due either entirely or in part to substance use. Therefore, consistent and structured substance use screening for all patients presenting to the psychiatric ED is highly recommended and potentially effective (Academic ED SBIRT Research Collaborative 2010; Madras et al. 2009). Screening for high-risk drinking includes this single item recommended by the National Institute on Alcohol Abuse and Alcoholism (Academic ED SBIRT Research Collaborative 2010): "How many times in the past year have you had…5 or more drinks in a day?" (for men) or "4 or more drinks in a day?" (for women). One or more times is a positive screen. The Alcohol Use Disorders Identification Test Alcohol Consumption Questions (AUDIT-C) is a self-administered three-item tool that screens for both high-risk drinking and alcohol use disorders in psychiatric and emergency populations (Dawson et al 2005; Sanjuan et al 2014). The 10-item Drug Abuse Screening Test (DAST-10) (Macias Konstantopoulos et al. 2014) screens for substances other than alcohol. Diagnosis requires a thorough history using available sources and performance of a physical and psychiatric examination of the patient. If screening is inconclusive but substances are still suspected, then a urine drug screen should be obtained. The clinician should inquire about the use and abuse of prescribed and over-the-counter drugs, as well as botanicals, dietary supplements, and substances obtained over the Internet. Physical examination may reveal signs of drug use, such as track marks over veins. The physical examination should be followed by the appropriate laboratory and imaging studies to rule out commonly encountered medical complications, such as subdural hematomas in alcohol intoxication.

The clinician should be aware of some variables that can predict a difficult course. In general, withdrawal and intoxication syndromes are more complex in medically compromised patients. Management is particularly problematic with specific substance–medical condition combinations, such as cocaine abuse with heart disease, alcohol dependence with seizure disorder, and opioid or sedative-hypnotic dependence with chronic obstructive pulmonary disease or sleep apnea.

Whenever possible, clinicians should approach patients about drug screening in a matter-of-fact manner and in the spirit of helping. Some ED clinicians do not order a screen because the results may not be back in time to change the disposition. Nevertheless, consideration should be given for testing even if results are not expected until after discharge. With a patient who is a repeat user of the ED or treated elsewhere in the ED's health care system, results can be invaluable for the next clinician who sees the patient. If a urine sample can be obtained with the patient's cooperation, then blood testing can be avoided. In a true medical emergency situation, it is not necessary to obtain the patient's consent for a drug screen.

Urine drug testing begins with an immunoassay screen that is more sensitive than specific. Practical constraints include a limited number of substances tested on most panels, false positives due to cross-reactivity, and false negatives due to noninclusion on the panel (e.g., buprenorphine, methadone, or fentanyl on most opioid screens) or substance concentration below the detection threshold. Clinicians should be familiar with which drugs are on the routine panel and their laboratory cutoff values. If a substance not on the panel is suspected, then it should be specifically ordered. Confirmation testing of positive screens involves gas or liquid chromatography–mass spectrometry.

Serum toxicology, often using gas chromatography–mass spectrometry, can be helpful in multidrug overdose and for some psychotropic medications (tricyclic antidepressants, lithium) but may require hours to days for the result, depending on the drugs tested and laboratory availability. This test should be reserved for situations in which certain results are essential, in which a positive finding is contested, or with a forensic interest. Drug screening results should be interpreted within the context of the overall presentation. Positive tests only signify recent use and are not diagnostic by themselves. Manipulation of samples by patients is possible, if infrequent, and steps should be taken to prevent this, such as not allowing personal items to be carried into the bathroom where the sample is collected.

The Suicidal Patient and Substance Use Disorders

One of the greatest challenges faced by emergency psychiatrists is the disposition of the patient who voices suicidal ideation while intoxicated (Rothschild 1997). The comments in this section are especially pertinent for patients with substance use disorders; for a more comprehensive risk assessment, the reader is referred to Chapter 2, "Suicide Risk Assessment and Management." Once sober, initially intoxicated patients often deny any thoughts of self-harm, yet the fact that they abuse substances adds to the risk that they will indeed take their own life. Patients with a substance use disorder are at 6.2 times greater risk of attempted suicide (Molnar et al. 2001). Moreover, their risk of an attempt increases with postdischarge substance use, which is highly likely if not addressed in the ED. Therefore, a patient's assurances while he or she is sober should not simply be taken at face value. The clinician should ask whether the patient has attempted suicide before. If the answer is yes, additional questions should be asked: Was the patient intoxicated at that time? Does the patient have a safety plan that includes staying sober? Is this plan realistic? Who can support the patient with this plan? A recent loss of social support (e.g., divorce or breakup, loss of job or housing) is a particularly pertinent risk factor for patients with substance use disorders. Regarding co-occurring psychiatric disorders, the clinician should keep in mind that substance-related mood changes as well as independent mood disorders separately increase the risk of a suicide attempt, so the former should not be discounted when assessing for safety.

Syndromes in Substance-Related Emergencies

Substance-related emergency presentations can be grouped in several ways. In this section, we discuss patients who are neurophysiologically depressed; who are agitated, aggressive, or psychotic; and who are seeking drugs. The key for the emergency clinician is maintaining a high level of suspicion and recognizing the patient's behavior as a syndrome of intoxication or withdrawal.

The Neurophysiologically Depressed Patient

Neurophysiologically depressed patients are those whose mental status and physiological states are mostly manifested by slowness or depression in the broad sense. This category refers not only to patients who are acutely sedated, lethargic, or even comatose, but also to those whose history suggests a recent downward trend in mental status. The common substance-related manifestations of depressed function are intoxication with central nervous system (CNS) depressants or withdrawal of CNS stimulants.

The most commonly abused CNS depressants are alcohol, barbiturates, benzodiazepines, other sedative-hypnotics, and opioids. Over-the-counter medications such as antihistamines, decongestants, dextromethorphan, and inhalants are frequently abused by adolescents.

Alcohol Intoxication

Primary alcohol intoxication accounts for more than 600,000 presentations to emergency departments in the United States per year (Pletcher et al. 2004). The onset of intoxication may be experienced as disinhibition, which can result in agitation, combativeness, and in rare cases psychosis. Intoxication results in an overall depression of CNS function, with a dose-dependent decrease in motor control, diminished coordination, slurred speech, ataxia, and finally respiratory depression and coma. Very high blood alcohol levels (BALs) can cause a lethal respiratory arrest (e.g., BAL>400 mg/dL in nontolerant individuals). Alcohol will usually cause vascular dilation, hypothermia, and lowered blood pressure with reflexive tachycardia. Although alcohol intoxication is easy to diagnose, some coma presentations (e.g., hyperglycemic coma with ketosis) can mimic it.

Treatment of alcohol intoxication is supportive (Reoux and Miller 2000). Gastric lavage is not useful because alcohol is rapidly absorbed from the gastrointestinal tract. Toxic levels should be monitored serially for an expected gradual drop. Chronic alcoholic patients may metabolize ethanol at a rate of 15–20 mg/dL/hour, which gradually results in decreasing signs of intoxication over a few hours. If this does not occur, the clinician should consider other explanations for alteration in consciousness, including other toxins, metabolic dysfunction, or subdural hematoma, which can present without any external evidence of trauma.

Alcohol is frequently consumed in overdoses with other substances. For example, tricyclic antidepressants not only enhance the CNS depression of alcohol but also delay its metabolism (Kerr et al. 2001). Concomitant use of cocaine can result in a metabolite (cocaethylene) that has three to five times the half-life of cocaine, increasing the risk of sudden death up to 20 times compared with when cocaine is used alone (Farré et al. 1997).

When alcohol is consumed in the presence of disulfiram, the history is obvious unless the patient was unaware that what had been consumed contained alcohol (Fuller et al. 1986). For example, so-called nonalcoholic beers still contain sufficient alcohol to precipitate a disulfiram reaction. Symptoms are attributable to an accumulation of acetaldehyde, a vasodilator, which can cause dangerous hypotension, tachycardia, intense flushing, chest pain and pressure, nausea and vomiting, and weakness. The combination can be life threatening in patients with serious underlying cardiac disease.

Benzodiazepine and Other Sedative-Hypnotic Toxicity

Benzodiazepine and other sedative-hypnotic toxicity develops not only in acute overdose but also in less obvious circumstances, such as when patients exceed their scheduled doses or when other CNS depressants (alcohol, opioids, or over-the-counter drugs) are used concomitantly. Accumulation can also result when long-acting benzodiazepines are injected intramuscularly or when metabolism of mainly oxidized benzodiazepines is affected by liver compromise, advanced age, or drug interactions, resulting in accumulation of active metabolites (D'Onofrio et al. 1999). Temazepam, oxazepam, triazolam, alprazolam, and lorazepam are metabolized primarily by conjugation (glucuronidation), making them less likely to accumulate in patients with liver impairment.

Benzodiazepines exhibit dose-dependent effects on coordination, memory, and cognitive functioning. They affect level of consciousness, leading to somnolence and, in the extreme case or in combination with other toxins, to coma. In some instances, paradoxical agitation and excitement can occur, but this is a manifestation of drug-induced disinhibition plus external "stimulating" factors. Gastrointestinal symptoms, such vomiting, diarrhea, and urinary incontinence, can occur and tend to differentiate benzodiazepine toxicity from opioid toxicity, which is associated with urinary retention and not with diarrhea.

Flumazenil, given intravenously in doses not to exceed 1 mg, acts quickly to reverse the effects of benzodiazepines. However, it should be administered with great caution to patients known to be physiologically dependent on benzodiazepines because of the likelihood of precipitating seizures.

Benzodiazepines are rarely lethal by themselves but can be lethal due to synergism with other respiratory depressants, especially alcohol, barbiturates, or opioids. Benzodiazepines can also worsen ventilation in patients who have preexisting serious underlying cardiorespiratory problems such as sleep apnea, chronic obstructive pulmonary disease, or congestive heart failure.

The clinician should maintain a high index of suspicion for concomitant benzodiazepine use in patients whose drinking exceeds moderate levels or who have a history of an alcohol use disorder, because these patients are highly susceptible to cross-dependence and the combination may result in an overdose. Patients dependent on opioids also misuse benzodiazepines, as do cocaine users to relieve cocaine-induced anxiety.

When an individual (especially female) takes ill during or after attending a party or a club gathering, the clinician should consider possible unknowing exposure to γ-hydroxybutyrate or flunitrazepam, so-called date rape drugs. These drugs can be lethal, particularly in combination with alcohol. Toxicity with these agents can be differentiated from other depressant toxicity by sudden awakening, myoclonus, hypothermia, fecal and urinary incontinence, and bradycardia. The coma induced by these substances is attended by episodic agitation upon stimulation. The main interventions are vigorous supportive care and monitoring for bradycardia, which is generally responsive to intravenously administered atropine (Robert et al. 2001).

Presentations to the ED related to barbiturates doubled from 2009 to 2011 (Substance Abuse and Mental Health Services Administration 2013). Barbiturate toxicity is more likely than benzodiazepine toxicity to cause coma and cardiac effects. Barbiturates are more lethal than benzodiazepines when taken as single agents due to respiratory depression, particularly if the dose is more than 10 times the hypnotic dose. Pupil size, blood pressure, nystagmus, and reflexes are variable, but with serious poisoning, most patients develop hypothermia, apnea, and shock. A distinctive feature is the relative preservation of protective reflexes, such as sneezing and coughing, despite obvious respiratory depression. Treatment is supportive, including warming for hypothermia, volume expansion for cardiovascular shock, and mechanical ventilation for apnea. Removal of drug can be hastened with alkalization of the urine and diuresis. CNS stimulants, flumazenil, and naloxone are not effective (Wilensky et al. 1982).

Opioid Toxicity

Opioid toxicity is readily recognizable by the feature of miosis in the presence of CNS and respiratory depression. This feature is persistent unless overdose results in significant hypoxia, in which case pupil dilation is possible. However, not all opioids cause significant miosis, and normal to even enlarged pupils have been reported with use of propoxyphene, meperidine, morphine, and pentazocine, in part due to the anticholinergic properties of some of these agents (Estfan et al. 2005). In intoxication, patients are minimally responsive or nonresponsive to physical stimulation and have slow, shallow respiration. Gastrointestinal sounds are absent, and urinary retention is common. Opioids can be especially dangerous in combination with other medications, such as monoamine oxidase inhibitors. Also, prescription opioid formulations are frequently combined with acetaminophen or nonsteroidal antiinflammatory drugs (NSAIDs). Therefore, toxicity in intoxication or overdose may come from these agents as well.

Naloxone is a specific antidote for opioid toxicity. It should be used with caution in patients known to be opioid dependent because it can precipitate acute withdrawal, resulting in agitation, confusion, or combativeness. Relatively high doses might be needed to treat long-acting oxycodone toxicity (Schneir et al. 2002), and repeated doses may be necessary due to naloxone's short half-life. In 2014, the U.S. Food and Drug Administration approved injectable (subcutaneous or intramuscular) naloxone to be dispensed directly to patients. Each injection contains 0.4 mg of naloxone hydrochloride (0.4 mL) to be given by anyone who discovers the patient in an emergent overdose situation. Consideration should be given to prescribing it in the ED as a take-home medication for patients at high risk of overdosing on opioids.

Over-the-Counter Cough and Cold Medications

Over-the-counter cough and cold medicines are frequently abused by adolescents and may contain mixtures of various antihistamines, sympathomimetics with or without dextromethorphan, and acetaminophen. They are used alone or in combination specifically to produce a mood change (a high) and to self-manage detoxification. They are difficult to detect in urine, but the presence of amphetamine analogs such as pseudoephedrine may screen positive for amphetamines.

Designer Drugs

Designer drugs are a diverse group of substances that are similar to widely used drugs of abuse and that are, through modern technology, widely manufactured and distributed. Users are able to experience the psychoactive properties of marijuana, for example, using a compound that may not have yet been scheduled by a government agency. Examples include synthetic cannabinoids ("K2," "spice") and synthetic cathinones ("bath salts") (Jerry et al.

2012). These drugs continue to evolve and remain widely available despite recent legislation by federal agencies (Nelson et al. 2014). Many are given attractive, flashy names ("Bliss," "Bombay Blue") or names of household products ("bath salts," "incense") and are marketed using deceptive phrases, such as "not for human consumption" and "legal highs."

Many designer drugs confer severe psychiatric symptoms (severe agitation, hallucinations, delusions, manic symptoms) and medical morbidity (delirium, electrolyte disturbances, serotonin syndrome). They are not detected on routine drug screens. Isolating them on toxicology assay is most often done through specialized labs. Results may not be available in the acute setting, but the results may ultimately be diagnostically useful to the admitting team and future providers.

The presence of a designer drug should be considered in a substance-using patient displaying significant psychiatric symptoms with an inconclusive medical workup accompanied by a negative toxicology screen. A thorough patient history with collateral information is especially important in this context. Treatment is largely supportive (intravenous fluids, vital signs, observation), with use of antipsychotics (for psychosis alone or with agitation) and benzodiazepines (for agitation without psychosis) as needed (Peglow et al. 2012; Winder et al. 2013).

Inhalant Intoxication

Inhalants include a wide variety of aliphatic, aromatic, and halogenated hydrocarbons. (Anesthetic gases [e.g., nitrous oxide] and short-acting vasodilators [e.g., amyl nitrite] are classified separately from inhalants in DSM-5 [American Psychiatric Association 2013].) Intoxication leads to disinhibition, excitement, or a sense of drunkenness. Mounting inhaled concentrations lead to restlessness, then decreased consciousness and ataxia, and then potentially coma, respiratory depression, and death. Acute hazards include myocardial sensitization to epinephrine, with risk of arrhythmias, possible hepatic injury, and longer-term effects on cognition and concentration.

CNS Stimulant Withdrawal

CNS depression that seems to have evolved subacutely can also be a manifestation of CNS stimulant withdrawal (e.g., the cocaine "crash"). The hallmark of withdrawal from CNS stimulants is severe depression that may be accompanied by suicidal ideation, dysphoria, and sleep disturbance, along with severe drug craving. Increased appetite may also be observed as a rebound effect to the appetite-suppressant effects of stimulants.

The Agitated, Aggressive, or Psychotic Patient

The range of agitated behavior in the ED is rather wide, spanning from belligerence to physical aggression, and at times complicated by full-blown psychosis. These problems can represent CNS stimulation or activation and can be caused by withdrawal from CNS depressants or intoxication with CNS stimulants. Paradoxical excitement can also be caused by intoxication with alcohol, cannabis, sedative-hypnotics, and inhalants.

Alcohol Withdrawal

Alcohol withdrawal is the most common cause of presentation in the ED of agitated, aggressive, or psychotic patients. Alcohol withdrawal may be complicated both by the possibility of high BALs and by concomitant stimulant use or simultaneous withdrawal from another substance. Combativeness and aggression can be seen in both alcohol intoxication and withdrawal, yet the typical return of stability as the BAL normalizes in a severely intoxicated alcohol-dependent patient is a familiar picture to those working in the ED.

The BAL at which withdrawal appears varies from patient to patient, and withdrawal can begin in as little as 6 hours from the last drink in chronic alcoholics. The withdrawal syndrome is characterized by autonomic instability, with elevated blood pressure, tachycardia, and profuse sweating; gastrointestinal symptoms, with nausea, vomiting, and diarrhea; and CNS activation, with anxiety and tremor. Hallucinations and seizures, typically single grand mal events, can herald more serious withdrawal complications. After 48–72 hours, about 5% of patients in alcohol withdrawal will develop delirium tremens (DTs), which includes hallucinations (usually visual), delirium, and severe autonomic instability. Early treatment of emerging alcohol withdrawal can prevent progression to DTs, which can be lethal in 5%–10% of patients despite treatment and in 20%–35% without treatment. Consumption of large quantities of alcohol, concomitant medical illness, and a history of DTs increase the risk that a patient will enter into DTs during the course of withdrawal (Ferguson et al. 1996).

The optimal strategy for treating alcohol withdrawal is substituting a physiologically equivalent agent, such as benzodiazepine or phenobarbital, and then gradually tapering it off. This avoids an abrupt shift in equilibrium from the compensated intoxicated state to the uncompensated abstinent state. Shorter-acting benzodiazepines, such as lorazepam, can be titrated to produce a mild state of sedation. Longer-acting benzodiazepines, such as chlordiazepoxide, have the advantage of being self-tapering but may also accumulate in the presence of significant liver impairment (Greenblatt et al. 1978). Benzodiazepine accumulation may, in turn, lead to a delirium that can be indistinguishable from the original presentation. Gabapentin has also shown effectiveness as a treatment for mild to moderate alcohol withdrawal. Gabapentin provides an appealing alternative to sedatives such as benzodiazepines and barbiturates in that it has a lower abuse potential, renal excretion, limited side effects, and decreased risk of overdose alone or in combination with alcohol (Myrick et al. 2009).

The use of an antipsychotic medication, usually one with low or no anticholinergic activity (e.g., haloperidol), can be used for hallucinations not responding to benzodiazepines or for severe agitation. Central α_2-adrenergic agonists such as clonidine or a β-blocker such as metoprolol can be used for hypertension or tachycardia if autonomic symptoms are prominent. All of these medications are capable of causing toxicity (Battaglia et al. 1997). Given the potential lethality of alcohol withdrawal, caution should be exercised to avoid overmedication but not to the point of risking undertreatment.

The common practice of hydrating patients and providing them with thiamine and folic acid has helped to decrease long-term functional and neurological consequences of alcohol dependence, such as Wernicke's encephalopathy and Wernicke-Korsakoff syndrome. Hence, these practices continue to be essential in the treatment.

Sedative-Hypnotic Withdrawal

Sedative-hypnotic (e.g., benzodiazepine) withdrawal occurs within the first few hours to days after discontinuation of a GABAergic agent. Phenomenologically, this withdrawal is very similar to that produced by alcohol withdrawal except that it can be extended over days to weeks (instead of hours to days), depending on the sedative-hypnotic's half-life. Patients may initially identify themselves as experiencing a withdrawal reaction involving mostly subjective complaints. The syndrome may progress from this anxious prodrome to include tremor, tachycardia, hypertension, diaphoresis, gastrointestinal upset, mydriasis, sleep disturbance and nightmares, tinnitus, and increased sensitivity to sound, light, and sometimes tactile stimulation. Confusion or frank delirium can develop along with hyperthermia if the reaction is severe. CNS irritability may progress to generalized tonic-clonic seizures, which can appear up to 2 weeks following the last dose. With severe withdrawal, delirium and seizures tend to occur more frequently than with alcohol, and once the syndrome is actively evolving, it can be difficult to restore CNS equilibrium despite large doses of sedatives.

Significant anxiety, sleep disturbance, and mild to moderate autonomic symptoms can occur with abrupt discontinuation of long-term therapeutic doses. These symptoms may persist at some level for many months, and can be indistinguishable from disabling generalized anxiety or panic symptoms. Because of these features, it is rarely if ever a good strategy to abruptly stop these agents after a long period of use.

Optimal management includes transition to an agent with a long half-life for stabilization, followed by very gradual taper as tolerated. Carbamazepine also has evidence to support its use in attenuation of protracted benzodiazepine withdrawal symptoms (Schweizer et al. 1991). Oxcarbazepine is less supported by evidence but has the advantage of being relatively nontoxic. Adjunctive treatment of protracted withdrawal symptoms with β-blockers such as propranolol has also been modestly helpful in some patients (Onyett 1989).

Opioid Withdrawal

Opioid withdrawal is a distinctive entity that rarely causes change in mental status. Common symptoms include the presence of pupillary dilation, lacrimation, rhinorrhea, diaphoresis, piloerection, arthralgia and/or myalgias (hyperalgesia and aches), diarrhea, yawning, and serious drug craving/drug seeking. These symptoms are best measured using verified tools such as the Clinical Opiate Withdrawal Scale (Wesson and Ling 2003).

Withdrawal is heralded by anxiety, craving/preoccupation, and vague discomfort (hyperalgesia). With short-acting agents, such as heroin, symptoms begin within 6–18 hours after the last dose. The syndrome reaches a peak at 2–4 days. Symptoms are usually minimal to absent after 7–10 days. Significant withdrawal from long-acting agents, such as methadone or buprenorphine, may not emerge for 1–3 days and may be prolonged in some cases.

Although not life threatening in an otherwise healthy patient, opioid withdrawal can be lethal in the presence of significant medical complications, such as recent myocardial infarction. Symptomatic treatment of withdrawal is appropriate because it is inhumane to insist that a patient quit cold turkey. Effective symptom relief promotes an alliance, thus opening a window for engagement in treatment.

Buprenorphine, a partial agonist for μ-opioid receptors with high affinity, will effectively treat acute opioid withdrawal. It can also be continued as a maintenance drug. Because it acts as a partial agonist in comparison with other opioids, buprenorphine can precipitate acute withdrawal if given to an opioid user who is not already in withdrawal. Given sublingually, buprenorphine can generate rapid and dramatic relief. However, the Drug Addiction Treatment Act of 2000 (P.L. 106-310) requires that patients receiving this drug for opioid withdrawal or maintenance of sobriety receive the prescription from a provider with special training and a waiver from the Drug Enforcement Administration. Outpatient follow-up after initiation or taper of buprenorphine is essential, as relapse rates due to noncompliance or lack of access to the medication are significantly higher among individuals who fail to become engaged in comprehensive outpatient addiction treatment (Brigham et al. 2007).

Other medications are useful for symptomatic relief from opioid withdrawal to varying degrees, but none is as effective as an opioid. Clonidine, a central α_2-agonist, reduces sympathetic outflow and can attenuate some symptoms. NSAIDs can help with myalgias. Loperamide is useful for diarrhea. Sedating anticonvulsants (gabapentin) or neuroleptics such as quetiapine are sometimes used for anxiety and restlessness, and trazodone at bedtime can aid sleep. Benzodiazepines or other controlled sedative-hypnotics should be used with great caution because they are readily abused, cause cross-dependence, interact with opioids, and tend to be difficult to discontinue once started in patients going through opioid withdrawal.

CNS Stimulant Intoxication

CNS stimulants, such as amphetamines, cocaine, and stimulant-hallucinogens such as 3,4-methylenedioxymethamphetamine (MDMA, commonly known as Ecstasy), cause a variety of symptoms, mostly varying in magnitude and duration as a function of potency, dose, and the user's susceptibility to the drug's effect. Other symptoms of intoxication that are more specific to the particular agent may occur, such as mild hallucinatory effects with MDMA and formication with cocaine and methamphetamine intoxication.

Physical signs of intoxication include tachycardia, tachypnea, hypertension, mydriasis, myoclonus, hyperreflexia, tremor, movement disorders, nausea and vomiting, possible seizures, increased respiratory rate, and hyperthermia. The distinctive presence of these signs can help differentiate between drug-related toxicity and primary psychotic states.

When psychotic content occurs, it is frequently confined to paranoid delusions. Hallucinations, if present, are typically tactile (e.g., formication) or visual (e.g., simple geometric patterns or shapes). Evidence of a formal thought disorder or severe, bizarre delusions is rare. The history and time course of psychiatric symptomatology can be helpful in differentiating substance-induced from primary psychiatric presentations, because substance-induced symptoms can appear abruptly and resolve quickly (i.e., within days). Substance users may be less likely to have a family history of psychosis and frequently have no significant prodromal symptoms. The results of a drug screen can also influence the clinician's suspicion that a psychosis is a result of a substance.

Stimulant toxicity can result in death in severe cases, often due to cardiovascular or cerebrovascular causes. When a patient has a neurological deficit, rapid imaging to rule out possible intracranial lesion or bleeding is essential. When a patient has chest pain, myocardial infarction needs to be ruled out.

Sedation with a benzodiazepine is an appropriate initial intervention for CNS stimulant intoxication. Sedation with benzodiazepines can help with seizures and confers some protection against the toxic effects of cocaine. To provide sedation in paranoid states, benzodiazepines are preferable to neuroleptics, which are usually contraindicated due to the potential for lowering the seizure threshold, precipitating disturbances in cardiac rhythm, and increasing the risk of hyperthermia due to their anticholinergic effects. Adequate sedation is usually sufficient to have a "peaceful" course in the ED.

For stimulant-induced tachycardia and hypertension, β-blockers should never be used. They tend to produce unopposed α-adrenergic effects.

Hallucinogen Intoxication

Physical symptoms resulting from the use of hallucinogens may include changes in body temperature and seizures (which may be resistant to treatment unless hyperthermia is treated). Hallucinations may be associated with insight, such that patients know they are due to the drug; however, frank psychosis does occur. Anxiety symptoms may be prominent with "bad trips" and include panic and fear of losing one's mind. The management of these reactions is similar to that for stimulant-induced psychiatric states: minimization of stimulation and the presence of calm, reassuring personnel are helpful. Exploration of a previous similar experience with hallucinogens that resolved later can be helpful both to reassure the patient and promote reality testing.

Marijuana Intoxication

A common presentation in chronic high-dose marijuana users is the experience of hypervigilance and depersonalization/derealization. The presence of conjunctival injection, orthostatic hypotension, dry mouth, and increased heart rate can help differentiate marijuana-related presentations from other causes of psychiatric symptomatology. The frequent use of marijuana in a patient having known psychiatric illness can cause a dramatic exacerbation of symptoms and may be a factor in poor response to medication management.

The Drug-Seeking Patient

The types of substances that patients seek during ED visits range from benzodiazepines for "anxiety" and opioids for the treatment of pain (often out of proportion to objective findings) to medicines for which the patient says the prescription was "lost" (usually over a weekend or after pharmacy hours).

A clinician should suspect drug-seeking behavior when a patient is specific about what medication he or she needs, stating that the provider is not immediately available, or claims to be allergic to a list of alternate medications that might otherwise treat the symptoms. If available, a statewide audit register, such as the Michigan Automated Prescription System, can help identify a patient's prescription-filling habits by generating a record of all controlled substance prescriptions that have been filled under that patient's identification within a 12-month period.

Drug-seeking behavior may represent either 1) treatment seeking for a legitimate medical disorder or 2) drug seeking to maintain an addiction. Although addiction is also a legitimate medical disorder, it requires a very different approach to treatment. Discerning the difference between treatment seeking for a nonaddiction disorder and drug seeking to maintain an addiction is not always easy. Even patients with legitimate pain, for example, may sometimes use pain medicine for emotional reasons. It is not unusual for those patients to ask for higher doses in a demanding or hostile manner. A patient who is anxious and depressed might be so fearful of receiving a reduced pain medication dosage that he or she will never report a pain score lower than 5–6.

Guiding Patients With Substance Use Disorders to Make a Change

Motivational interviewing is more a manner of approaching the patient than a specific technique. The essential feature is that the patient's own perceptions are used as a platform on which to build a treatment approach. Behavioral and attitudinal change in this model is approached as a goal that has meaning for the patient (Smedslund et al. 2011).

The following are essential elements of motivational interviewing:

- Understanding the patient's views of his or her situation, especially through use of reflective listening statements
- Maintaining affirmation and acceptance of the patient as the overriding tone of the conversation
- Eliciting and selectively reinforcing the patient's own descriptive statements of problem recognition, concern, desire to change, benefit to self through change, and so on
- Having patience and allowing the patient to come to the awareness of a problem, rather than telling, diagnosing, or describing a problem to the patient, which is likely to elicit resistance
- Affirming the patient's freedom to choose not only the problem(s) identified and the associated consequence(s), but also the treatment (requiring reflection on the outcome)

An excellent review of these techniques is provided by Miller and Rollnick (2012).

Disposition Issues

A working knowledge of recovery resources available for patients with substance use disorders and their families is essential for the clinician to take advantage of the window for intervention that the emergency encounter can produce. These resources might include social service agencies, child or adult protective services, charities within the community, shelters, and institutionalized treatment programs providing various levels of care. Local directories of Alcoholics Anonymous, Narcotics Anonymous, and Al-Anon meetings are helpful. Larger Alcoholics Anonymous communities coordinate service groups that can arrange for members to visit with the alcohol-dependent individual to share the experience of recovery (a Twelfth-Step call) (D'Onofrio et al. 1998).

Key Clinical Points

- Familiarity with acute presentations related to substance use disorders is an essential component of training in emergency psychiatry. Such training should include the general management of acute changes in behaviors, along with medical knowledge of complications associated with the habitual or occasional use of substances of abuse.

- In the initial evaluation, acute life support needs should be ensured, and a working diagnosis of major intoxication or withdrawal states can be made. The clinician can then make a decision regarding the appropriateness of treatment in a general emergency department (where medical equipment and expertise are immediately available) or a psychiatric emergency department (where expertise can focus on behavioral management and use of psychotropic drugs and/or seclusion).

- Judicious use of antidotes or detoxification agents as indicated for intoxication and aspects of withdrawal should be followed by an assessment of the patient and a determination regarding further disposition.

- Psychiatric emergency personnel should be familiar with community resources for individuals with substance use disorders.

- Psychiatric emergency staff should help patients begin the path to recovery.

- Safety issues for patients, family, and staff are paramount throughout the course of diagnosis, evaluation, and management.

References

Academic ED SBIRT Research Collaborative: The impact of screening, brief intervention and referral for treatment in emergency department patients' alcohol use: a 3-, 6- and 12-month follow-up. Alcohol Alcohol 45(6):514–519, 2010 20876217

American Psychiatric Association: Diagnostic and Statistical Manual of Mental Disorders, 5th Edition. Arlington, VA, American Psychiatric Association, 2013

Battaglia J, Moss S, Rush J, et al: Haloperidol, lorazepam, or both for psychotic agitation? A multicenter, prospective, double-blind, emergency department study. Am J Emerg Med 15(4):335–340, 1997 9217519

Brigham GS, Amass L, Winhusen T, et al: Using buprenorphine short-term taper to facilitate early treatment engagement. J Subst Abuse Treat 32(4):349–356, 2007 17481458

Centers for Disease Control and Prevention: Division of Health Care Statistics: National Hospital Ambulatory Medical Care Survey. Emergency department summary tables. 2010. Available at: http://www.cdc.gov/nchs/data/ahcd/nhamcs_emergency/2010_ed_web_tables.pdf. Accessed December 28, 2014.

Centers for Disease Control and Prevention: Wide-ranging Online Data for Epidemiologic Research (WONDER). 2012. Available at: http://wonder.cdc.gov/mortsql.html. Accessed December 28, 2014.

Centers for Disease Control and Prevention: Alcohol Related Disease Impact (ARDI) application, 2013. Available at: http://apps.nccd.cdc.gov/DACH_ARDI/Default.aspx. Accessed December 28, 2014.

Dawson DA, Grant BF, Stinson FS: The AUDIT-C: screening for alcohol use disorders and risk drinking in the presence of other psychiatric disorders. Compr Psychiatry 46(6):405–416, 2005 16275207

D'Onofrio G, Bernstein E, Bernstein J, et al; Society for Academic Emergency Medicine: Patients with alcohol problems in the emergency department, part 2: intervention and referral. SAEM Substance Abuse Task Force. Acad Emerg Med 5(12):1210–1217, 1998 9864135

D'Onofrio G, Rathlev NK, Ulrich AS, et al: Lorazepam for the prevention of recurrent seizures related to alcohol. N Engl J Med 340(12):915–919, 1999 10094637

Drug Addiction Treatment Act of 2000, Pub. L. No. 106-310, sec. 3501, 21 USC 801

Estfan B, Yavuzsen T, Davis M: Development of opioid-induced delirium while on olanzapine: a two-case report. J Pain Symptom Manage 29(4):330–332, 2005 15857733

Farré M, de la Torre R, González ML, et al: Cocaine and alcohol interactions in humans: neuroendocrine effects and cocaethylene metabolism. J Pharmacol Exp Ther 283(1): 164–176, 1997 9336321

Ferguson JA, Suelzer CJ, Eckert GJ, et al: Risk factors for delirium tremens development. J Gen Intern Med 11(7):410–414, 1996 8842933

Fuller RK, Branchey L, Brightwell DR, et al: Disulfiram treatment of alcoholism. A Veterans Administration cooperative study. JAMA 256(11):1449–1455, 1986 3528541

Glick RL, Berlin JS, Fishkind AV, et al: Emergency Psychiatry: Principles and Practice. Philadelphia, PA, Lippincott Williams & Wilkins, 2008

Greenblatt DJ, Shader RI, MacLeod SM, et al: Clinical pharmacokinetics of chlordiazepoxide. Clin Pharmacokinet 3(5):381–394, 1978 359214

Jerry J, Collins G, Streem D: Synthetic legal intoxicating drugs: the emerging "incense" and "bath salt" phenomenon. Cleve Clin J Med 79(4):258–264, 2012 22473725

Kerr GW, McGuffie AC, Wilkie S: Tricyclic antidepressant overdose: a review. Emerg Med J 18(4):236–241, 2001 11435353

Macias Konstantopoulos WL, Dreifuss JA, McDermott KA, et al: Identifying patients with problematic drug use in the emergency department: results of a multisite study. Ann Emerg Med 64(5):516–525, 2014 24999283

Madras BK, Compton WM, Avula D, et al: Screening, brief interventions, referral to treatment (SBIRT) for illicit drug and alcohol use at multiple healthcare sites: comparison at intake and 6 months later. Drug Alcohol Depend 99(1–3):280–295, 2009 18929451

Miller WR, Rollnick S: Motivational Interviewing: Preparing People for Change. New York, Guilford, 2012

Molnar BE, Berkman LF, Buka SL: Psychopathology, childhood sexual abuse and other childhood adversities: relative links to subsequent suicidal behaviour in the US. Psychol Med 31(6):965–977, 2001 11513382

Myrick H, Malcolm R, Randall PK, et al: A double-blind trial of gabapentin versus lorazepam in the treatment of alcohol withdrawal. Alcohol Clin Exp Res 33(9):1582–1588, 2009 19485969

Nelson ME, Bryant SM, Aks SE: Emerging drugs of abuse. Emerg Med Clin North Am 32(1):1–28, 2014 24275167

Onyett SR: The benzodiazepine withdrawal syndrome and its management. J R Coll Gen Pract 39(321):160–163, 1989 2576073

Peglow S, Buchner J, Briscoe G: Synthetic cannabinoid induced psychosis in a previously nonpsychotic patient. Am J Addict 21(3):287–288, 2012 22494236

Pletcher MJ, Maselli J, Gonzales R: Uncomplicated alcohol intoxication in the emergency department: an analysis of the National Hospital Ambulatory Medical Care Survey. Am J Med 117(11):863–867, 2004 15589492

Reoux JP, Miller K: Routine hospital alcohol detoxification practice compared to symptom triggered management with an Objective Withdrawal Scale (CIWA-Ar). Am J Addict 9(2):135–144, 2000 10934575

Robert R, Eugène M, Frat JP, et al: Diagnosis of unsuspected gamma hydroxy-butyrate poisoning by proton NMR. J Toxicol Clin Toxicol 39(6):653–654, 2001 11762678

Rockett IRH, Putnam SL, Jia H, et al: Declared and undeclared substance use among emergency department patients: a population-based study. Addiction 101(5):706–712, 2006 16669904

Rothschild AJ: Suicide risk assessment, in Acute Care Psychiatry: Diagnosis and Treatment. Edited by Sederer LI, Rothschild AJ. Baltimore, MD, Williams & Wilkins, 1997, pp 15–28

Sanjuan PM, Rice SL, Witkiewitz K, et al: Alcohol, tobacco, and drug use among emergency department patients. Drug Alcohol Depend 138:32–38, 2014 24594289

Schneir AB, Vadeboncoeur TF, Offerman SR, et al: Massive OxyContin ingestion refractory to naloxone therapy. Ann Emerg Med 40(4):425–428, 2002 12239500

Schweizer E, Rickels K, Case WG, et al: Carbamazepine treatment in patients discontinuing long-term benzodiazepine therapy. Effects on withdrawal severity and outcome. Arch Gen Psychiatry 48(5):448–452, 1991 2021297

Smedslund G, Berg RC, Hammerstrøm KT, et al: Motivational interviewing for substance abuse. Cochrane Database Syst Rev (5):CD008063, 2011 21563163

Substance Abuse and Mental Health Services Administration: Drug Abuse Warning Network, 2011: National Estimates of Drug-Related Emergency Department Visits. (HHS Publ No SMA-13-4760, DAWN Series D-39). Rockville, MD, Substance Abuse and Mental Health Services Administration, 2013

Wesson DR, Ling W: The Clinical Opiate Withdrawal Scale (COWS). J Psychoactive Drugs 35(2):253–259, 2003 12924748

Wilensky AJ, Friel PN, Levy RH, et al: Kinetics of phenobarbital in normal subjects and epileptic patients. Eur J Clin Pharmacol 23(1):87–92, 1982 7128675

Winder GS, Stern N, Hosanagar A: Are "bath salts" the next generation of stimulant abuse? J Subst Abuse Treat 44(1):42–45, 2013 22445773

Suggested Readings

Hawkins SC, Smeeks F, Hamel J: Emergency management of chronic pain and drug-seeking behavior: an alternate perspective. J Emerg Med 34(2):125–129, 2008

Moeller KE, Lee KC, Kissack JC: Urine drug screening: a practical guide for clinicians. Mayo Clin Proc 83(1):66–76, 2008; erratum in Mayo Clin Proc 83(1):851, 2008

Schanzer BM, First MB, Dominguez B, et al: Diagnosing psychotic disorders in the emergency department in the context of substance use. Psychiatr Serv 57(10):1468–1473, 2006

10

Child and Adolescent Emergency Psychiatry

B. Harrison Levine, M.D., M.P.H.

Julia E. Najara, M.D.

In a summary of statistics for pediatric psychiatric visits to U.S. emergency departments (EDs) between 1993 and 1999, Sills and Bland (2002) reported that a relatively stable number of patients ages 18 years and younger were seen for psychotic symptoms and suicide attempts or self-injury, but that an increase occurred in the number of nonurgent complaints. These complaints included substance-related disorders, anxiety disorders, and attention-deficit and disruptive behavior disorders, using criteria from DSM-IV-TR (American Psychiatric Association 2000), which have been retained with very little change in DSM-5 (American Psychiatric Association 2013). No significant change has occurred in the delivery of mental health care in the outpatient setting to offset this long-term rising trend in overutilization of the ED for disruptive behavioral issues. Consequently, the ED clinician is likely to be asked to evaluate children and adolescents with seemingly less acute symptoms in addition to the steady number of patients with more severe psychiatric complaints, such as suicidal ideation. The World Health Organization estimates that by the year 2020, the most prevalent causes of morbidity, mortality, and disability for children will be neuropsychiatric disorders (Dolan et al. 2011).

Goldstein et al. (2005) noted that children and adolescents present with psychiatric emergencies according to the academic calendar, suggesting that school stressors may be significant sources of stress or may exacerbate underlying premorbid psychiatric conditions in the child or adolescent. Although fewer young children may present to a psychiatric emergency service during summer months, adolescents, by nature of their age and the natural development of more serious psychiatric disorders, will present year-round.

Children and adolescents who presented repeatedly to a psychiatric emergency service were found to have diagnoses that included adjustment, conduct, or oppositional disorders, and to be under the care of a child welfare agency. Additionally, these patients were more likely to be noncompliant with treatment and outpatient follow-up, to be admitted to the hospital more frequently, to demonstrate need for additional social services, and to be unmanageable in residential treatment facilities where, for a variety of reasons, they were unable to remain (Cole et al. 1991). The problem of reduced access to appropriate emergency services has been repeatedly documented, beginning in 1958 by Shortliffe et al., and continues to worsen as a public health issue, leading to the American Academy of Pediatrics (2004) policy statement about ED overcrowding. The Committee on Pediatric Emergency Medicine of the American Academy of Pediatrics reported that whereas ED visits increased by 32% from 1996 to 2006, the number of EDs decreased by 5% during this period (Dolan et al. 2011). The Centers for Disease Control and Prevention (2013) have described the most common emergency psychiatric presentations by children and adolescents

Basics

In approaching the patient, the clinician needs to keep in mind that a child or adolescent is by definition a minor and should not be unaccompanied, so there will necessarily be collateral informants from whom to obtain history. Often, especially during standard working hours, collateral information must also be obtained from agencies or institutions that are stakeholders in the welfare of the child, such as the child's school, teachers, treating clinicians, foster agencies, or child protective services.

The mental status categories remain fairly consistent across the age span, although child psychiatrists may use somewhat different labels and, particularly with young children, rely more on observation of the child's spontaneously emitted behavior in interactions with people (parents and/or examiner) and play materials, as well as with materials specifically designed to facilitate the assessment of developmental level, such as the ability to make a block tower or perform pencil-and-paper tasks. Ideally, any child age 12 years or younger should be seen by or referred to a child and adolescent psychiatrist who would be better prepared than an adult psychiatrist to address developmental issues.

Essential Principles

The following are important principles of emergency psychiatry involving a child or adolescent (Allen et al. 2005):

1. The psychiatrist acts as the patient's advocate.
2. The assessment of safety is the chief goal of emergency evaluation.
3. Any intervention considered should be one that is appropriate to establish and maintain the safety of the patient and of those in the immediate surroundings of the patient.
4. Assessment tests, procedures, and interventions should be efficient, practical, and useful in contributing to establishment of the etiology of the patient's presentation, and in helping to establish the primacy of medical versus psychiatric conditions.

Safety First

To achieve safety, the evaluator must obtain knowledge of the following:

1. The population to which this patient belongs
2. Specific risk factors associated with this population
3. The appropriate level of intervention required to maintain both temporary and long-term safety

4. Resources available to the specific population served
5. State, federal, and regulatory agency mandates
6. Standard level of care

General Evaluation Considerations

Specific to child and adolescent patients, the evaluator must assess and consider three spheres of functioning: home, school, and social. Relevant questions regarding these spheres are listed in Table 10–1.

Initial Assessment

Establish and Maintain Temporary Safety

The first priority in evaluating a child or adolescent in the psychiatric emergency service is to rule out any nonpsychiatric, general medical conditions that might be responsible for the patient's altered mental status or psychiatric symptoms. The patient should be triaged to the most appropriate setting, and if that means to a medical emergency room rather than the psychiatric emergency room, this quick evaluation is potentially lifesaving, especially with certain conditions such as nonobvious head trauma, hypoglycemia, or other potentially reversible causes of mental status changes. Regardless of the diagnosis, it is good practice to assume that the child and the child's parents or caretakers are frightened, worried, and/or confused.

Clear and tactful communication is essential. The clinician not only must appear to be empathetic and caring, but also must actively listen to the patient and whoever brought the patient to the emergency room. The clinician must be very clear about communicating the process of the psychiatric evaluation and potential interventions before, during, and after they occur. A patient who feels mistreated or unheard could rapidly escalate symptomatically, and parents or caretakers who feel they have been marginalized or left out of the process are more likely to become adversarial rather than allied with the clinician.

Psychiatric Evaluation

The clinician must ensure that the patient is not a danger to self or others and must provide a safe and nonthreatening environment to avoid escalation of

Table 10–1. Spheres of functioning for child and adolescent assessment

Sphere of functioning	Assessment considerations

Home	**Nature of the patient's relationship with family/caretakers**
	
	1. Parents
	   a. Are they married? Recently separated? In new relationships?
	   b. Do they have socioeconomic issues or stressors?
	   c. Do they have psychiatric issues? Drug or alcohol abuse/dependence?
	   d. Is there a history of domestic violence? Has the patient witnessed this?
	   e. Is the patient afraid something bad will happen to his or her parents?
	   f. What is the family's source of income?
	   g. What is the nature of the patient's relationship with parents?
	
	2. Siblings
	   a. Are the siblings biological? Half-siblings? Foster or adopted siblings?
	   b. What are the age differences?
	   c. Where does the patient fall in the sibling hierarchy?
	   d. What is the nature of the patient's relationship with siblings?
	
	3. Caretakers
	   a. If the parents are not the primary caretakers, who are?
	   b. Are the caretakers relatives? Foster family? Adoptive?
	   c. Is the child being cared for in an institutional setting? Residential home? Group home?
	
	Patient's enjoyment and place within the family
	
	1. Is there any aspect of the family system that antagonizes the patient?
	2. Is the family system supportive of the patient? How?
	3. Who are the parents/caregivers of this child? Are they married, separated, divorced, remarried?
	4. Where does the patient consider his or her home? Does the patient divide time between homes? Is there a parenting arrangement?

Table 10–1.   Spheres of functioning for child and adolescent assessment *(continued)*

Sphere of functioning	Assessment considerations
Home *(continued)*	**Patient's enjoyment and place within the family** *(continued)*

5. Is the patient happy at home? Scared to be home? Does the patient experience any emotional, physical, or sexual abuse? How does the family spend time together?

6. Is the patient allowed to have friends outside the family circle?

7. Has the family experienced any recent relocations?

8. Has the family experienced any recent losses?

Supervision

1. Is there adequate supervision of the minors, including the patient, in this home?

Social supports for the family

1. Is the family system strict? Unsupervised?

2. If there is more than one caretaker/parent, are the caretakers/parents in agreement about issues of child rearing?

Bedtime/curfew

1. When is bedtime/curfew for the patient? Is it enforced?

2. How often does the patient use the computer, especially the Internet? Tablets? Video games? Smart phones?

3. Does the patient stay up all night playing on the computer and then feel fatigued and nonproductive the following day at school?

4. What is the average time the patient spends online per day? What is he or she doing?

    a.   Online academic work

    b.   Gaming (please specify types, such as first-person shooter, war games, fantasy games, construction games, etc.)

    c.   Texting (please specify to whom)

5. Is the patient spending on average more or less time gaming versus being face to face with peers (beyond issues of curfew)?

Table 10–1. Spheres of functioning for child and adolescent assessment *(continued)*

Sphere of functioning	Assessment considerations
School	**Academic performance**

1. Has there been a decline in functioning?
2. Have the patient's grades deteriorated?
3. Has the patient had excessive school absences?
4. Have there been phone calls home from teachers?
5. Has there been a recent change of schools? Repeating of grades? School suspensions? Transfers?

Friends

1. Does the patient have friends at school?
2. Is he or she a bully or the victim of bullies?
3. Does the patient isolate himself or herself? Does the patient belong to a group? A gang?

Teachers

1. Was a psychoeducational evaluation performed on the child?
2. Does the child have any learning disabilities or speech-language difficulties?
3. Is the child in an appropriate classroom setting?
4. Does the child require more structure or supervision? Further testing?

Caretakers

1. Are caretakers supportive of the patient's academic work?
2. Do caretakers help the patient with assignments? With remembering to do homework?
3. Are the caretakers involved in the patient's school?
4. What method(s) do the caretakers use to help the patient perform to his or her academic level or behave appropriately in school? Do they use positive reinforcement? Negative reinforcement?

Table 10–1.   Spheres of functioning for child and adolescent assessment *(continued)*

Sphere of functioning	Assessment considerations
School *(continued)*	Enjoyment/sense of achievement
	1. Does the patient enjoy school?
	2. Does the patient feel adequately challenged?
	3. Is the patient struggling to keep up with schoolwork?
Social	Friends
	1. Does the patient have friends outside of school?
	2. Does the patient find it "hard" or "easy" to make friends? To keep friends?
	3. What is the longest time the patient has "kept" a friend?
	4. Are you aware of any bullying involving the patient, whether as perpetrator, participant, or victim?
	5. Does the patient limit himself or herself to "virtual" friends (i.e., friends made through the Internet on video games, chat rooms, etc.)?
	Hobbies
	1. Is the patient involved in after-school or extracurricular activities? Sports? Clubs?
	2. Does the patient have particular interests? Computer or video games? Playing a musical instrument? Singing? Dancing?
	Enjoyment/frequency
	1. Does the patient enjoy social interaction with peers?
	2. How often does the patient see friends? Engage in social activities?
	3. Does the patient have a sense of mastery?
	4. What is this patient's self-image?
	5. What is this patient's future outlook? What does patient want to be when he or she grows up?

potentially dangerous behaviors. Providing a quiet, softly lit room may suffice; however, some patients may need to be treated with medications or physically restrained to calm their anxiety, reduce their psychotic symptoms, or help them to regain control of their potentially dangerous behavior. The interaction between a patient and his or her caretakers must be quickly evaluated to determine if their physical proximity is likely to hinder, worsen, or improve the ability of the patient to remain safe.

When obtaining history in the course of examining an adult patient, a clinician makes many observations regarding mental status. Only later does the clinician supplement or augment by asking specific questions (e.g., about orientation, memory, psychotic symptoms). The most skilled psychiatric interviewers try to embed specific clarifying questions in the flow of conversation with the patient. Thus, in the assessment of adults, the patient is the primary source of information, both about his or her history, illness, symptoms, and so on, and about his or her mental status.

The evaluation of children differs from that of adults in that the history is frequently obtained from others and the mental status examination is based on observations of the child and his or her interactions with the evaluator and, especially when the child is young, with the parent. The evaluation is the summation of subjective and objective findings provided by the patient, the parents, and other caretakers in the patient's life.

1. Chief complaint and history of present illness: Elicit the specific reasons why the patient is in the emergency room. Obtain details about acute and chronic stressors and their temporal relationship to the onset of acute or chronic symptoms. Explore patient's strengths and weaknesses.
2. Psychiatric history
3. Family history
   a. Current stressors
   b. Intrafamilial stressors
   c. Familial coping abilities and strategies including religious and spiritual beliefs
4. Developmental history (as relevant)
5. Medical history (as relevant)
6. Social history (as relevant)
7. Mental status examination

Medical Evaluation and Examination

Any change in a patient's mental status should alert the clinician to the possibly reversible causes of psychiatric symptoms, including delirium, drug intoxication or overdose, physical illness, trauma, child abuse, or a primary neurological disorder. Accordingly, the physical evaluations listed in Table 10–2 should be conducted as clinically indicated.

Common Presentations

Although children and adolescents present to the ED for various reasons, some of the most common are suicidality; psychosis, agitation, or aggressiveness; child abuse; and eating disorders. We discuss these common psychiatric issues in this section.

Suicidality

Assessment

Once safety has been established, the patient should be evaluated for suicidal ideation. Compared with adults, adolescents more commonly experience suicidal ideation and attempt suicide; they also account for a higher proportion of all deaths by suicide. Furthermore, disruptive behavior disorders increase risk, and contagion effects are more powerful among adolescents than among adults (Ash 2008). According to epidemiological and clinical studies, risk factors for suicidality in children and adolescents are often comorbid with other psychiatric disorders, such as depressive, disruptive, anxiety, or substance-related disorders. Other risk factors include adverse family circumstances, such as the caretaker's low satisfaction with the family environment, low parental monitoring, and parental history of psychiatric disorder. Low familial understanding of and use of current technologies (especially social media) are thought to undermine self-esteem and hinder the development of supportive social affiliations, and indeed, these factors have been found to be associated with suicidal ideation or behavior in offspring (King et al. 2001). Evaluation of the child's home environment and the parents' or caretakers' capacity to support an at-risk child is important, especially as the evaluation moves toward a disposition.

The clinician should keep in mind the suicide rates among adolescents while evaluating risk. Although completed suicide is known to be a rare event

Table 10–2.   Key laboratory studies in medical evaluation

Basic labs

To help rule out *potentially reversible causes of delirium or mental status changes,* or for baseline assessment before the initiation of medications:

Complete blood count with differential

Blood glucose

General chemistry screen

Liver function tests

Thyroid function tests

Urinalysis

Urine toxicology screen

Alcohol level (if indicated)

Pregnancy screen (if applicable)

Electrocardiogram

New-onset psychosis labs

If at risk, or for *new-onset psychosis and atypical psychosis,* all of the above plus:

Infectious disease screens: Lyme titers (endemic areas), HIV, rapid plasma reagin (if at risk, such as runaways, delinquents, children of substance abusers)

Rheumatoid factor

Antinuclear antibodies

Erythrocyte sedimentation rate

Vitamin B_{12}/folate (if at risk, such as patients who have anorexia, are strict vegetarian, or are malnourished)

Computed tomography, magnetic resonance imaging (if evidence of neurological dysfunction or new-onset psychosis)

Electroencephalography (if history is suggestive of seizures or seizure-like events)

Lumbar puncture (if history is suggestive of central nervous system involvement)

Special labs

If patient is taking *valproic acid:*

Amylase

Lipase

Valproic acid—to rule out toxicity; to establish therapeutic levels, obtain trough level in the morning before A.M. dose of valproic acid

Table 10–2. Key laboratory studies in medical evaluation *(continued)*

Special labs *(continued)*

If patient is taking *lithium:*

Lithium—to rule out toxicity; to establish therapeutic levels, obtain trough level in the morning before A.M. dose of lithium

If patient is taking *antipsychotics:*

Hemoglobin A_{1c} (if weight has increased)

Fasting blood glucose (if weight has increased)

Lipid profile (if already taking or if starting antipsychotics)

Prolactin levels

among preteen children, the risk begins to increase at age 13 years, and by the end of adolescence the rates are similar to those of young adults. Girls make more frequent attempts than boys, but boys are more likely to die by suicide. Rates of completed suicide among U.S. adolescents (ages 15–19 years) have generally shown little change during the time that researchers have been monitoring this problem. Although a major increase was noted in the last decade of the 20th century, rates subsequently decreased and have remained fairly stable, at approximately 8.5 suicide deaths per 100,000 population (Centers for Disease Control and Prevention 2012).

Assessing the intention of a youth to commit suicide is important. The clinician should ask questions related to the components listed in Table 10–3.

Interventions

The clinician needs to spend time educating the family and patient about suicide, suicide prevention, and mental illness. It is important for the clinician to listen carefully, reflect back concerns, and be sure the patient and his or her parents or caretakers fully understand everything the clinician wishes to convey.

If the patient's suicidal gesture seemed to be a cry for help, he or she may not require further hospitalization but rather close follow-up with an outpatient clinician. Determination about setting should be based on the individual case, the resources available, the willingness of the family to engage in treatment, and other considerations. For a youngster who has made an apparent nonlethal suicide attempt or who has passive suicidal ideation, further exploration of the home environment is essential to determining where the patient

Table 10–3.   Elements of the suicide assessment

Suicide component considerations	Evaluation questions
Wish to die	What does the patient expect will happen if he or she dies?
	How lethal are the means by which the patient chose to end his or her life?
Preparations	Was the attempt planned beforehand or impulsive?
	Did the patient write a note or make attempts to say good-bye?
Concealment	Did the patient plan the attempt in a manner by which he or she would not be found? (Investigate the timing of the attempt or selection of the location in terms of discovery by others.)
Communication	Did the patient make attempts to tell others, either directly or indirectly?
Precipitants	What led to the event or the wish to die?
	What degree of stress or anxiety preceded the event?
	Was there any relief of symptoms after the event?
	Was any degree of reconciliation between the patient and significant others achieved by the event?
	In the context of similar stressors or exacerbation of stressors, does the patient now deny suicidality?

will be safest. Alternative placements may be necessary if the parents or caretakers are unable to adequately monitor the youngster, are known to be dangerous or to abuse alcohol or substances, do not fully comprehend the discharge instructions, or are considered by the youngster to be significant enough stressors that his or her safety at home cannot be guaranteed. If the patient's safety at home is in any way in doubt, the first option is to find other family members who may be willing and able to take the child temporarily. If this is not possible, the child should be admitted until appropriate placement can be arranged in a residential crisis center, with a foster care agency, or with a similar social service agency.

In the psychiatric emergency service, antidepressants are not typically started because the patient is unlikely to be seen again.

Medicolegal Concerns

The clinician needs to keep in mind various medicolegal concerns. Psychiatrists are mandated reporters for child abuse, which includes medical neglect.

If the patient's legal guardians refuse to cooperate and the child is in danger of harming self or others, the clinician may be required to report the case. If faced with such a dilemma, the clinician should consult a supervisor regarding the reporting of the case. Additionally, although children may be signed into a locked unit without the need for legal commitment, if the guardians are not cooperative and the clinician believes the child is at risk of or has suffered child abuse, the clinician needs to know whether his or her state law allows for detention of the patient by way of commitment. If the patient was injured "accidentally," for instance, by ingesting drugs or alcohol or by using a firearm, this may substantiate child abuse by neglect (Dubin and Weiss 1991). According to the most recently available statistics, approximately 4.5 million cases of child abuse and neglect were reported in 2008, compared with 3 million in the year 2000. In 2010, the percentage of reported child abuse cases involving neglect was 78.3% (Dolan et al. 2011). The most important consideration for the treating clinician is what are the most likely circumstances that may have led to a child's presentation in the ED: the perpetrators are typically known to the victims, and quite often drugs of abuse are involved, taken by the allegedly responsible adults and/or the patient. Each case must be examined afresh, without preconceived notions about the individual. Knowing the context helps guide questioning, not conclusions.

Disposition

From what is learned about the patient in the ED, the clinician determines the next level of care. Possibilities include inpatient hospitalization; hospital emergency room–based services (crisis intervention); step-down programs such as a day treatment program, home-based crisis intervention, or intensive case management intervention; standard outpatient care; or no follow-up at all. Another option is to contact child protective services or another social service agency.

Psychosis, Agitation, or Aggressiveness

Assessment

For the child or adolescent who presents with psychosis, agitation, or aggressiveness, the clinician needs to consider several questions.

1. Does the patient have accompanying symptoms suggestive of a psychiatric disorder or of a medical or neurological disorder? The clinician should attempt to rule out any possibly reversible cause of the mental status change (e.g., pain, infection, confused state from the infection, partial complex seizures, toxic states, medication intoxication/withdrawal syndromes).
2. Is the behavior volitional or done for secondary gain?
3. Is the behavior secondary to fear or anxiety, or is it in anticipation of hospitalization?
4. What is the patient's cognitive level? Some children with neurodevelopmental disorders appear to be agitated when in fact their behavior is a reflection of a soothing strategy or a slight exacerbation of baseline stereotypes.
5. Does the patient have hallucinations? It is vital to consider the difference between developmentally appropriate (primary) hallucinations and hallucinations in the presence of psychiatric disorders. Aug and Ables (1971) listed five factors that may predispose a child to experience so-called primary hallucinations in the absence of any diagnosable disease or disorder:

- Age and limited intelligence are important factors. For a child, wish-fulfilling fantasy is a common mode of thinking. However, a child of average intelligence at age 3 years can usually distinguish between fantasy and reality.
- Emotional deprivation can lead to increased fantasy thinking, and perhaps hallucinations, as a way of providing the gratifications that reality cannot provide.
- Emphasis on a particular mode of perception may be important. Life experience may make it difficult to distinguish between vivid auditory imagery and auditory hallucinations in a child who is hearing impaired, or between visual imagery and visual hallucinations in a child who is visually impaired.
- Family religious and/or cultural beliefs may predispose children to have deviant perceptual experiences.
- Strong emotional states at times of stress may lead to regression, hallucinations, and/or dissociative states.

Primary hallucinations include the following:

- Hypnagogic or hypnopompic hallucinations (transient, occurring between true sleep and waking)
- Eidetic imagery (child's ability to visualize or "auditorize" an object long after it has been seen or heard; an ability typically lost by the time of puberty in a child with no developmental delays or history of trauma)
- Imaginary playmate (typical for children ages 3–5 years, and the child is aware that this companion is fantasy or not real)
- Dreams, nightmares
- Isolated hallucinations (fleeting illusions based on misinterpretations of shadows, colors, and movements)
- Hallucinosis (a number of hallucinations extending over a period of time but not related to any known cause)

To determine whether the patient has a secondary hallucination suggestive of a psychiatric or medical etiology, the clinician should consider the full context of the patient's presentation (Weiner 1961). Primary mood or psychotic disorders should be considered if the patient also presents with severe mood symptoms, either depressed or manic; if the patient's affect is incongruent, flattened, blunted, or grandiose; or if the patient has impaired memory, agitation, restlessness, disturbed sleep-wake cycle, or disturbances of memory, attention, or concentration. If the patient's hallucinations are accompanied by perceptual distortions, automatic and repetitive movements, partial loss of consciousness, or periods of confusion, or if they are preceded by a visual aura, then a primary neurological condition such as epilepsy or migraines should be considered.

Intervention

Because safety is of primary importance, the clinician should first de-escalate the environment. If possible, familiar persons should remain nearby, and the patient should be provided with food, fluids, and diversionary activities such as toys, games, or drawing materials.

When working with a cognitively limited patient who is verbally and physically aggressive, the clinician should try to ignore the patient (e.g., by avoiding eye contact, verbal responses, and touching). If the patient approaches a staff member while engaging in aggressive or disruptive behaviors, the staff member should move away from the patient to limit interaction but maintain supervision. However, the staff member must take immediate action if the situation is potentially dangerous to the patient or anybody else.

If the patient remains agitated, the clinician should consider one of the medications listed in Table 10–4. The following considerations should be taken into account in choosing medications:

- Other psychoactive medications or substances that the patient currently is receiving or has ever received
- The possible effect of psychotropic medication on the patient's medical illness
- The patient's psychiatric diagnosis and comorbidity (e.g., autism spectrum disorder, intellectual disability)
- Potential cross-reaction with patient's medications
- Route of administration
- Potential side effects and the patient's risk factors
- Desired rapidity of effect
- Dosing

The following important guidelines should also be followed:

- Do *not* order "as needed" (prn) medications without physician reevaluation.
- Do *not* mix different types or classes of antipsychotic medications.
- Do *not* mix different types of benzodiazepines.

At times, restraints may be considered for patients who are psychotic, agitated, or aggressive. The use of restraints should be limited, however, to cases in which all interventions have failed and should be considered only temporary until an adequate level of behavioral control is gained by the patient.

Medicolegal Concerns

All interventions that require sedation or restraints should follow regulatory guidelines specific to the hospital and state. Additionally, parents must be included in all decisions.

Table 10–4.   Commonly used psychotropic medications for the
pediatric population

Name	Dose	Onset of action	Elimination half-life (hours)
Lorazepam	0.25–2 mg po or im q 6–8 hours prn (maximum 2–3 doses in 24 hours)	im: 20–30 minutes po: 30–60 minutes	Children: 11 Adults: 13
Haloperidol	0.25–5 mg po or im q 2–4 hours prn (maximum 2–3 doses in 24 hours)	im: 20–30 minutes po: 2–3 hours	18–40
Risperidone	0.125–2 mg po q 4–6 hours prn (maximum 2–3 doses in 24 hours)	po: 1–3 hours	20
Olanzapine	Zyprexa 1.25–5 mg po q 4–6 hours (maximum 20 mg in 24 hours); Zyprexa Zydis is quick-dissolving oral option	im: 15–45 minutes po: 6 hours	30
Benztropine	0.25–2 mg po or im	im: ≤15 minutes po: ≤1 hour	6–48
Diphenhydramine	12.5–50 mg po or im q 4–6 hours prn (maximum 2–3 doses in 24 hours)	im: <2 hours po: 2–4 hours	2–8

Haloperidol and lorazepam

For extreme agitation, to achieve a higher level of sedation

Haloperidol, lorazepam, and benztropine or diphenhydramine

For extreme agitation, to achieve a higher level of sedation, and to prevent extrapyramidal symptoms (EPS)

Table 10–4. Commonly used psychotropic medications for the pediatric population *(continued)*

Haloperidol and diphenhydramine

To achieve a higher level of sedation and to prevent EPS

To prevent EPS or if patient develops EPS, provide oral dosage of diphenhydramine q 6–8 hours to cover up to 48 hours postexposure to one single dose of haloperidol.

Haloperidol and benztropine

To prevent EPS

To prevent EPS or if patient develops EPS, provide oral dosage of benztropine q 8–12 hours to cover up to 48 hours postexposure to one single dose of haloperidol.

Lorazepam

Associated with respiratory depression; use carefully if pulmonary functions are compromised. Also, lorazepam is associated with paradoxical reactions (increased agitation) in small children and children with neurodevelopmental disorders.

Other anxiolytic or antipsychotic medications

If patient is already receiving them with good results, consider giving an extra dose.

Use of antipsychotics in the emergency room should be restricted to actively psychotic, manic, or aggressive patients. Use the minimal amount needed to manage the target symptoms, and maintain high vigilance for adverse events.

Young children, patients naïve to psychotropics, and patients with comorbid intellectual disability or autism spectrum disorder are known to have increased sensitivity to adverse events and may respond poorly to medications. Use medications carefully and only if all environmental and behavioral interventions have failed.

Olanzapine (Zyprexa Zydis)

Off-label use is common in many emergency rooms as an oral alternative to injectable medication. Tablets come in 5 mg and must be cut with scissors using gloves to avoid inadvertent melting and absorbing of the medication. Emergency psychiatric protocol includes first offering an oral medication prior to requiring an injectable if the oral is refused or the patient is unable to consume it. For the drug to work, the patient must swallow saliva. Olanzapine is not absorbed by buccal mucosa.

Note.   im=intramuscular; po=per oral; prn=as needed; q=every.

Source.   Findling 2008; Schatzberg and Nemeroff 2004.

Disposition

Any patient who presents with symptoms suggestive of a prodromal psychotic state, first-break psychosis, or exacerbation of psychotic symptoms that were previously well controlled should be hospitalized for safety, further evaluation, and management of symptoms. On occasion, some patients may present with mild psychotic symptoms that could be managed safely at home. If the family is able to provide appropriate supervision and outpatient follow-up, the home environment may be preferable. Patients with new presentations of mood, anxiety, or disruptive behavior disorders should be assessed for safety as previously described, and the most appropriate level of care should be determined for disposition. Patients with neurodevelopmental disorders, however, do not respond well to changes in their environment and/or caretakers. The presence of a familiar caretaker at the point of arrival at the ED very often de-escalates the patient's agitation by quickly reestablishing known routines. If the agitation is quickly controlled, the patient can be discharged home and hospitalization is avoided. The emergency services psychiatrist should be familiar with resources available for patients with neurodevelopmental disorders, and applications for external supports at school and home should be initiated at this point. Inpatient hospitalization should be used only as a last resort unless a unit with specialized interventions for children with neurodevelopmental disorders is available. Specific therapeutic interventions catering to this population are limited or lacking in regular psychiatric units, and these patients, due to their behavioral difficulties, are too often isolated and overmedicated in this setting.

Child Abuse

Any behavior by an adult that harms the physical or psychological well-being or the normal growth and development of a child is considered child abuse. From October 2005 to September 2006, approximately 905,000 U.S. children were victims of maltreatment that was substantiated by state and local child protective service agencies (Centers for Disease Control and Prevention 2008). There are no specific ethnic or socioeconomic groups in which child abuse is more prevalent. Because child abuse typically occurs in the context of a family crisis, the clinician should be suspicious of the nature of the child's emergency but work hard to establish rapport with both the child and the

Table 10–5. Risk factors for child abuse

Parent or caregiver factors	Personality characteristics/mental health
	History of abuse
	Substance abuse
	Child-rearing approaches
	Teen parents
Family factors	Family structure
	Domestic violence
	Stressful life events
Child factors	Birth to age 3 years
	Disabilities
	Low birth weight
Environmental factors	Poverty and unemployment
	Social isolation and social support
	Violence in communities

parents, without demonstrating outwardly any preconceived thoughts or attitudes. A strong alliance will help the child to reveal sensitive information. Additionally, maintaining a professional stance will help if the intervention requires removal of the child from the family to the protective environment of an inpatient unit or other social service until details are evaluated.

According to the Administration for Children and Families, a division of the U.S. Department of Health and Human Services, risk factors for child abuse fall into the categories listed in Table 10–5 (Child Welfare Information Gateway 2013). In addition to recognizing the risk factors for child abuse, the clinician needs to know the types of child abuse and be aware of child abuse law. The clinician should also be aware of available hospital and community resources that deal specifically with this issue.

Types of Child Abuse

Child neglect. Child neglect is generally characterized by omissions in care that result in significant harm or risk of significant harm. Typically, child neglect is divided into three types: physical, educational, and emotional neglect. Neglect is frequently defined in terms of a failure to provide for the child's basic needs, such as adequate food, clothing, shelter, supervision, or medical care.

Sexual abuse. Sexual abuse includes both touching offenses (fondling or sexual intercourse) and nontouching offenses (exposing a child to pornographic materials) and can involve varying degrees of violence and emotional trauma. The most commonly reported cases involve incest—that is, sexual abuse occurring among family members, including those in biological families, adoptive families, and stepfamilies. Incest most often occurs within a father-daughter relationship; however, mother-son, father-son, and sibling-sibling incest also occurs. Other relatives or caretakers also sometimes commit sexual abuse.

Physical abuse. Although an injury resulting from physical abuse is not accidental, the parent or caregiver may not have intended to hurt the child. The injury may have resulted from severe discipline, including injurious spanking, or physical punishment that is inappropriate to the child's age or condition. The injury may be the result of a single episode or repeated episodes and can range in severity from minor marks and bruising to death.

Psychological maltreatment. On the "Emotional Abuse" page at the Child Welfare Information Gateway (2013) Web site, psychological maltreatment, or emotional abuse, is defined as "a repeated pattern of caregiver behavior or extreme incident(s) that convey to children that they are worthless, flawed, unloved, unwanted, endangered, or only of value in meeting another's needs." That Web site lists six categories of psychological maltreatment:

- Spurning (e.g., belittling, hostile rejecting, ridiculing)
- Terrorizing (e.g., threatening violence against a child, placing a child in a recognizably dangerous situation)
- Isolating (e.g., confining the child, placing unreasonable limitations on the child's freedom of movement, restricting the child from social interactions)
- Exploiting or corrupting (e.g., modeling antisocial behavior such as criminal activities, encouraging prostitution, permitting substance abuse)
- Denying emotional responsiveness (e.g., ignoring the child's attempts to interact, failing to express affection)
- Mental health, medical, and educational neglect (e.g., refusing to allow or failing to provide treatment for serious mental health or medical problems, ignoring the need for services for serious educational needs)

Evaluation

The patient's mental status examination may reveal a frightened youngster who may have unrealistic expectations about reunions with an abusive family or family member, or who may describe magical thinking about undoing the abuse. The child or adolescent may present in a variety of ways, such as being overly responsible, being impulsive, displaying extreme mood swings, misunderstanding personal boundaries, or being shy or withdrawn. The younger patient may experience nightmares or night terrors, and may be extra clingy with one person but refuse to be near another. Older children, especially adolescents, may become more withdrawn, change their clothing style to one that is more sexually provocative, or make efforts to hide their sexual development and attractiveness. The older child may also develop promiscuous behaviors or deviant sexual behaviors, run away, develop alcohol or substance abuse problems, or attempt suicide.

A child who is a suspected victim of abuse should be examined carefully by a pediatrician in the medical ED for signs of abuse. Labs, cultures, swabs, and imaging studies may be warranted to substantiate clinical findings.

Intervention

As always, in working with potential abuse victims, the clinician should maintain a professional stance, which requires being sensitive, thoughtful, empathetic, objective, and goal and action oriented. Child abuse cases may bring up strong countertransferential feelings in the clinician, who may feel anger toward the alleged offender and sympathy for the victim; however, the clinician must refrain from being confrontational or accusatory, and must maintain a sense of calm and safety within the ED. The clinician should learn from both the patient and the patient's parents or caretakers the details of the alleged abuse and then consult with other members of the psychosocial team, members of the hospital child abuse assessment team, or supervisors to determine appropriate disposition.

Medicolegal Concerns

Whether there is suspected or confirmed child abuse, two reports must be filed: 1) a written legal form documenting the examination findings and 2) a telephone report to the child protective services agency to begin the disposition process and treatment plan for the child and family. The protective services agency will subsequently manage further disposition issues once the patient is discharged from the hospital. Usually, when the family of an at-risk child must be investigated by child protective services, a full evaluation is conducted within 24 hours. On occasion, the clinician may need to provide courtroom testimony, or hospital administrators may need to step in and use legal authorities to protect or hospitalize a child or to remove family members who are threatening and violent.

In any event, the family members must be informed of their rights and responsibilities, including the right to a full court hearing with legal representation and their continued duty to protect the child from further abuse (Ludwig 1983). In cases where suspected abuse is substantiated by physical findings (sexual or physical), the child may be admitted to the hospital and the appropriate investigative authorities may become immediately involved. If the state in which the abuse occurs has appropriate non-hospital-based outpatient facilities or specialty group homes, disposition to one of these facilities may be preferable. Investigative authorities may include a hospital-based child abuse assessment team, the local social services office, or, at the very least, law enforcement. If there are no physical findings and the abuse is alleged by the child, the aforementioned investigative authorities must be contacted and the allegations reported. Typically, these officials will direct the clinicians regarding how to proceed.

Disposition

If the child's safety is of primary concern, he or she should be hospitalized to control his or her environment, provide safety and consistency, and facilitate further evaluation of the child and the allegations. Once the diagnosis of abuse is made, the parents or caretakers should be informed immediately and the disposition plans described.

Eating Disorders

Some of the more common reasons for young patients with anorexia nervosa to present to the emergency room include recent dizziness, fainting spells, or seizures in school or at home; a parent's or caregiver's suspicion of an eating disorder after the patient is observed vomiting or heard complaining of a gastrointestinal illness; or a parent's or caregiver's observation that the patient is dangerously restricting intake. A 2008 study found that about 16.9% of patients with anorexia nervosa attempted suicide (Bulik et al. 2008).

For the emergency psychiatrist, the question of whether to admit a patient with an eating disorder to either a medical unit or a psychiatric unit will be based on the available resources in the clinician's hospital. Following completion of a full physical and psychiatric evaluation, including a necessary evaluation of the family, inpatient medical hospitalization may be warranted. Due to either the availability of or lack of resources for illnesses related to feeding and eating, each facility will likely have its own criteria for whether or not to hospitalize a patient with a suspected or known eating disorder. At Children's Hospital Colorado, the following criteria must be met for a patient with an eating disorder to be admitted to a medical unit:

- Patient's weight is less than or equal to 75% of ideal body weight (patient in gown after voiding)
- Heart rate is lower than 45 beats per minute (bpm), after patient has been lying down for at least 5 minutes
- Hypokalemia (on evaluation of plasma electrolytes)
- Hyponatremia (on evaluation of plasma electrolytes)

Given the significantly high suicide rate for patients with anorexia nervosa, some of their presentations will be similar to those of other psychiatric patients who require immediate hospitalization for stabilization and safety (American Psychiatric Association 2006):

- Severe suicidality with high lethality or intention (which under any circumstances warrants hospitalization).
- Worsening ability to control self-induced vomiting, increased binge eating, use of diuretics, and use of cathartics that may be considered life threatening.
- Weight changes related to altered or changed mental status due to worsening symptoms of mood disorder, suicidality, or psychotic decompensation.
- Preoccupation with weight and/or body image accompanied by food refusal, or obsessive thoughts about body image or weight that cause the patient to be uncooperative with treatment and require a highly structured setting for rehabilitation.

Other presentations may *not* warrant inpatient hospitalization, depending on the entire clinical picture and full psychiatric evaluation (American Psychiatric Association 2006):

- Recent precipitous or steady drop in weight and/or total body weight that is less than 85% of normal healthy body weight. Body mass index (BMI; calculated as [weight in kilograms/height in meters]^2) is less useful in assessing children than adults and should not be used to estimate, except at extremes, a patient's nutritional status. Age-adjusted BMIs are available (Centers for Disease Control and Prevention 2006). Children below the fifth percentile are considered underweight. However, other factors, such as abnormal muscularity, body frame status, constipation, and fluid loading, will influence these results and may be misleading. Additionally, specific individual BMIs may be better understood according to ethnic groups (Lear et al. 2003).
- Metabolic disturbances, including hypophosphatemia, hyponatremia, hypokalemia, or hypomagnesemia; elevated blood urea nitrogen in the context of normal renal function.
- Hemodynamic disturbances in children and adolescents: heart rate in the 40s; orthostatic changes (>20-bpm increase in heart rate or >10–20 mmHg drop); blood pressure below 80/50 mmHg.

A careful clinician will examine the patient's medication list very closely to make sure that the reason for the patient's presentation is not the direct result of medications prescribed for the patient. For example, a combination of drugs may cause unwanted and unknown side effects; the quantity of a medication may be excessive, leading to side effects; and the patient may not be able to tolerate a medication for allergic or other metabolic reasons. The clinician needs to have an understanding of all psychotropic or potentially psychotropic medications to better understand a patient in his or her full context. This investigation must also include over-the-counter medications and supplements that the patient may not even consider to be actual drugs but that could have very significant interactions with other over-the-counter or prescribed medications.

Key Clinical Points

- Temporary safety is the chief goal of emergency evaluation.

- Any intervention considered should be one that is appropriate to establish and maintain the safety of the patient.

- Assessment tests, procedures, and interventions should be efficient, practical, and useful for establishing the primacy of medical versus psychiatric conditions.

- In management of acute agitation, environmental de-escalation should be attempted first, before medications or physical restraints are used.

- In assessment of a patient for medication-caused or withdrawal conditions, it is necessary for the clinician to have a full understanding of all of the patient's current or recently ingested prescribed, over-the-counter, or otherwise procured medications.

- Acute crisis intervention requires the clinician to maintain a professional stance while demonstrating empathy, actively listening, and appropriately delivering education and instruction.

- Provisional psychopharmacological management should be attempted for patients with acute behavioral dyscontrol, agitation, aggressiveness, or psychosis.

- With children, especially those who are naïve to psychotropic medications, medications should be used only if necessary, starting with low doses.

- If a patient does not respond as expected after one or two doses, the clinician should discontinue the medication and review the case in detail.

- A provisional diagnosis should be established to guide treatment and preliminary disposition of the patient.

- The clinician should foster a sense of trust and alliance with the patient and his or her family. The clinician should avoid promising something he or she is unsure of or cannot deliver.

References

Allen MH, Currier GW, Carpenter D, et al; Expert Consensus Panel for Behavioral Emergencies 2005: The expert consensus guideline series. Treatment of behavioral emergencies 2005. J Psychiatr Pract 11 (suppl 1):5–108, quiz 110–112, 2005 16319571

American Academy of Pediatrics Committee on Pediatric Emergency Medicine: Overcrowding crisis in our nation's emergency departments: is our safety net unraveling? Pediatrics 114(3):878–888, 2004 15342870

American Psychiatric Association: Diagnostic and Statistical Manual of Mental Disorders, 4th Edition, Text Revision. Washington, DC, American Psychiatric Association, 2000

American Psychiatric Association: Practice guideline for the assessment and treatment of patients with eating disorders, third edition. 2006. Available at: http://psychiatryonline.org/pb/assets/raw/sitewide/practice_guidelines/guidelines/eatingdisorders.pdf. Accessed May 20, 2015.

American Psychiatric Association: Diagnostic and Statistical Manual of Mental Disorders, 5th Edition. Arlington, VA, American Psychiatric Association, 2013

Ash P: Suicidal behavior in children and adolescents. J Psychosoc Nurs Ment Health Serv 46(1):26–30, 2008 18251349

Aug RG, Ables BS: Hallucinations in nonpsychotic children. Child Psychiatry Hum Dev 1(3):152–167, 1971 5163289

Bulik CM, Thornton L, Pinheiro AP, et al: Suicide attempts in anorexia nervosa. Psychosom Med 70(3):378–383, 2008 18256339

Centers for Disease Control and Prevention: Tools for calculating body mass index (BMI). March 22, 2006. Available at: http://www.cdc.gov/nccdphp/dnpa/growthcharts/bmi_tools.htm. Accessed January 2, 2015.

Centers for Disease Control and Prevention: Nonfatal maltreatment of infants—United States, October 2005–September 2006. MMWR Morb Mortal Wkly Rep 57(13):336–339, 2008 18385640

Centers for Disease Control and Prevention: Injury Prevention and Control; Data and Statistics (Web-based Injury Statistics Query and Reporting System [WISQARS])—National Violent Death Reporting System: Violent Deaths 2003–2012. 2012. Available at: http://www.cdc.gov/injury/wisqars/nvdrs.html. Accessed June 18, 2015.

Centers for Disease Control and Prevention: Mental health surveillance among children—United States, 2005–2011. MMWR Surveill Summ 62 (suppl 2):1–35, 2013 23677130

Child Welfare Information Gateway: What is child abuse and neglect? Recognizing the signs and symptoms. Washington, DC, U.S. Department of Health and Human Services, Children's Bureau, 2013. Available at: https://www.childwelfare.gov/pubpdfs/whatiscan.pdf. Accessed May 20, 2015.

Cole W, Turgay A, Mouldey G: Repeated use of psychiatric emergency services by children. Can J Psychiatry 36(10):739–742, 1991 1790520

Dolan MA, Fein JA; Committee on Pediatric Emergency Medicine: Pediatric and adolescent mental health emergencies in the emergency medical services system. Pediatrics 127(5):1356–1366, 2011 21518712

Dubin WR, Weiss KJ: Handbook of Psychiatric Emergencies. Springhouse, PA, Springhouse, 1991

Findling RL: Clinical Manual of Child and Adolescent Psychopharmacology. Washington, DC, American Psychiatric Publishing, 2008

Goldstein AB, Silverman MA, Phillips S, et al: Mental health visits in a pediatric emergency department and their relationship to the school calendar. Pediatr Emerg Care 21(10):653–657, 2005 16215467

Human Rights Watch: U.S.: Number of Mentally Ill in Prisons Quadrupled: Prisons Ill Equipped to Cope. September 6, 2006. Available at: http://www.hrw.org/news/2006/09/05/us-number-mentally-ill-prisons-quadrupled. Accessed May 20, 2015.

King RA, Schwab-Stone M, Flisher AJ, et al: Psychosocial and risk behavior correlates of youth suicide attempts and suicidal ideation. J Am Acad Child Adolesc Psychiatry 40(7):837–846, 2001 11437023

Lear SA, Toma M, Birmingham CL, et al: Modification of the relationship between simple anthropometric indices and risk factors by ethnic background. Metabolism 52(10):1295–1301, 2003 14564681

Ludwig S: Child abuse, in Textbook of Pediatric Emergency Medicine. Edited by Fleisher GR, Ludwig S. Baltimore, MD, Williams & Wilkins, 1983

Schatzberg AF, Nemeroff CB: Textbook of Psychopharmacology, 3rd Edition. Washington, DC, American Psychiatric Publishing, 2004

Shortliffe EC, Hamilton TS, Noroian EH: The emergency room and the changing pattern of medical care. N Engl J Med 258(1):20–25, 1958 13493729

Sills MR, Bland SD: Summary statistics for pediatric psychiatric visits to U.S. emergency departments, 1993–1999. Pediatrics 110(4):e40, 2002 12359813

Weiner MF: [Hallucinations in children]. Arch Gen Psychiatry 5:544–553, 1961 14042371

Suggested Readings

Allen MH, Currier GW, Carpenter D, et al; Expert Consensus Panel for Behavioral Emergencies 2005: The expert consensus guideline series. Treatment of behavioral emergencies 2005. J Psychiatr Pract 11 (suppl 1):5–108, quiz 110–112, 2005

Findling RL: Clinical Manual of Child and Adolescent Psychopharmacology. Washington, DC, American Psychiatric Publishing, 2008

Tardiff K: Medical Management of the Violent Patient: Clinical Assessment and Therapy. New York, Marcel Dekker, 1999

11

Seclusion and Restraint in Emergency Settings

Heather E. Schultz, M.D.
Divy Ravindranath, M.D., M.S.

Case Example 1

Mr. E is a 33-year-old single, unemployed white man who was brought to the emergency department by police after being found walking in the middle of the street. His past medical history is significant for hepatitis C and bipolar disorder. A brief review of his medical records reveals three prior hospitalizations for cocaine intoxication and rhabdomyolysis. Police report that the patient has a history of violence. Per recent psychiatry records, he has a pattern of limited medication adherence.

This chapter was adapted from Mohr WK, Lucas G: "Seclusion and Restraint in Emergency Settings," in *Clinical Manual of Emergency Psychiatry.* Edited by Riba M, Ravindranath D. Washington, DC, American Psychiatric Publishing, 2010, pp. 233–259.

On arrival, he was combative, disoriented, and responding to visual hallucinations. Multiple intravenous (IV) puncture sites were noted. His urine drug screen was positive for cocaine. In the emergency department, the patient was calmed after being treated for acute agitation with haloperidol 5 mg and lorazepam 2 mg. He was admitted to the medical ward due to elevated creatine phosphokinase and creatinine.

On awakening, Mr. E pulled out his IV line and spat at and threatened to bite staff. His nurse paged the physician and then attempted to engage the patient with calming verbal de-escalation techniques. However, when the patient's physician arrived to the bedside, the patient continued to escalate and threw his urinal across the room. The nurse had alerted hospital security, who quickly arrived to the patient's room. The physician ordered four-point leather restraints, and the patient was taken down and restrained by a team of security guards. Mr. E's physician ordered intramuscular olanzapine, and the patient became calm over the course of the next hour. He was then able to receive IV fluids and supportive care. Mr. E was restarted on divalproex (Depakote) for bipolar disorder and met with a hospital social worker. After a 3-day admission and no further episodes of agitation or aggression, outpatient psychiatric follow-up was arranged, and Mr. E was discharged home with his brother, who agreed to stay with him temporarily.

As described in the clinical vignette, agitation requiring the use of restraints is encountered in both medical and psychiatric emergency departments. Emergency department patients may be intoxicated, delirious, manic, psychotic, cognitively impaired, and so on; to complicate matters, little may be known about their past medical history. For instance, the patient may have a history of responding to a particular medication in the past. All attempts should be made to calm the patient verbally and to offer medications voluntarily prior to physically restraining patients. However, in cases of continued agitation that puts the patient, staff, or other patients at risk, the use of restraints can be essential to maintain safety.

In the United States, two national organizations regulate and set standards for the uses of seclusion and restraint: the Centers for Medicare and Medicaid Services (CMS) and The Joint Commission (TJC; formerly the Joint Commission on Accreditation of Healthcare Organizations). Various definitions of the terms *seclusion* and *restraint* are used by different state and federal regulatory agencies and professional organizations. In short, *physical restraints* are procedures or devices that are employed to limit a person's mobility. These can range from the precautionary raising of a bed rail to prevent an incapacitated person from falling out of bed, to holding a person, to mechanical modalities of arm and leg cuffs (four-point restraints) and addition of a fifth point by tying a sheet across the person's midsection. Patients must always be physically restrained only in devices manufactured expressly for the purpose of restraining patients and approved by the U.S. Food and Drug Administration. A number of devices have been made from a variety of different materials, such as leather or polyurethane with buckles or Velcro closures.

Most commonly in psychiatric settings, a *restraint* consists of trained people taking patients to the floor and holding them until they are calm. In the case of children, restraint may include something euphemistically called a "therapeutic hold." This refers to a brief physical holding technique used to restrict a child's freedom of movement for reasons of safety (Berrios and Jacobowitz 1998).

Seclusion refers to the temporary, involuntary confinement of a patient in a room or area from which the person is physically prevented from leaving. Either locked or unlocked seclusion might be used. Seclusion does *not* refer to a time-out intervention that may be consistent with a patient's treatment plan; a time out should not exceed 1 hour.

Chemical restraint is an out-of-favor term that has historically referred to the administration of a medication that is used to control behavior or freedom of movement but that is not a part of a patient's daily medication regimen. Medications should not be used to restrain a patient, because oversedation is associated with increased risk of falls, respiratory insufficiency, and aspiration.

Indications

According to Centers for Medicare and Medicaid Services guidelines (Centers for Medicare and Medicaid Services, U.S. Department of Health and Human Services 2006), seclusion or restraint is to be used only in an emergency situation to ensure a patient's physical safety and after less restrictive interventions have been determined to be ineffective to protect the patient or others from harm. The guidelines of the Joint Commission on Accreditation of Healthcare Organizations (2000) are similar but include the phrase "where there is imminent danger." Both bodies prohibit seclusion or restraint used as a means of coercion, punishment, discipline, convenience, or retaliation by staff.

At this writing, the position statements of both the American Academy of Child and Adolescent Psychiatry (AACAP; Masters et al. 2002) and the American Psychiatric Association (1984) declare that the indications for the use of seclusion and restraint are for reasons of safety. Each organization also includes a statement indicating that restraint or seclusion may be used to prevent serious disruption of the treatment milieu or damage to property. The patient must present as a clear danger to self or others, and less intrusive measures to control such behavior must have failed. Therefore, medical providers facing an agitated patient who may harm self or others must quickly assess the imminent safety of both patient and provider(s).

Bioethicist George Annas (1999) opined that restraint use can only be justified in emergency situations to prevent patients from hurting selves or others, and then for the shortest time and with the least restriction possible.

The decision to place a patient in restraints should be made by a qualified staff member. TJC and CMS regulations regarding seclusion and restraint orders are summarized in Table 11–1.

Patient Assessment

A proper initial assessment of psychiatric patients should include identifying causes of violence (including a thorough differential diagnosis), history of violent behavior, early warning signs and triggers, relevant trauma history, and preexisting medical conditions that place individuals at risk of injury or death should safety measures such as seclusion, chemical restraint, and/or physical restraint be needed.

Choosing Seclusion or Physical Restraint

The treatment of acutely agitated individuals is a major issue in emergency psychiatry. The initial treatment of patients who are agitated or exhibit aggressive behavior should focus on calming them through a quiet and empathic approach, while remaining firm about issues regarding safety. Such patients may elicit fear in staff members, making treatment and communication difficult. However, empathy is the most useful tool in clinicians' armamentaria.

Published standard practices include limited information of an empirical nature to guide clinical decisions regarding seclusion and restraint; no overall

Table 11–1.   Regulations regarding seclusion and restraint orders

MD/LIP to order [CMS]

Qualified trained staff may initiate before order obtained [TJC]

MD/LIP to see patient
  Within 1 hour [CMS]
  Within 4 hours (or less for children) [TJC]

Re-evaluation and renewed order by primary treating MD/LIP [CMS and TJC]
  Every 4 hours for adults
  Every 2 hours for patients ages 9–17 years
  Every 1 hour for patients under age 9 years

MD/LIP in-person re-evaluation every 24 hours thereafter [CMS]

MD/LIP in-person re-evaluation thereafter [TJC]
  Every 8 hours for adults
  Every 4 hours for patients under age 18 years

No as-needed medications or standing orders [CMS and TJC]

Can "reuse" existing order if it has not expired [TJC]

Note.   CMS = Centers for Medicare and Medicaid Services (2006); MD/LIP = physician or licensed independent practitioner; TJC = The Joint Commission (Joint Commission on Accreditation of Healthcare Organizations 2000).

benchmarks for their use; and no data about the appropriate mix of seclusion, restraint, and medication for various kinds of patients. Controversy exists across different settings concerning the proper use of emergency measures with patients who pose a threat to themselves or others. In emergency departments, physicians most often use physical restraints or medications for agitation in the course of treating violent patients. In examining evidence for the treatment of patients in the emergency department, Zun (2005) concluded that some studies had examined the use of medications for agitation, but studies of the use of restraints/seclusion/medication—alone or in various combinations—were sorely lacking.

It is important to note that each state, although covered by federal law, has its own set of laws governing the rights of patients. Also, each hospital has its own "restraint policy," which should be reviewed by all physicians and staff, because it may be very specific about how to restrain patients and who needs to be informed that the patient has been restrained.

Figure 11–1 is an algorithm, based on review of various descriptive literatures in this area, that reflects clinical consensus of how decisions to restrain or seclude normally take place.

Contraindications to Seclusion and Restraint

Nonphysical safety measures are always preferable to seclusion and restraint. Above all, no form of restraint should be used in the absence of rigorous staff training in some formal type of crisis prevention or management program, as well as cardiopulmonary resuscitation. The presence of an automatic external defibrillator in psychiatric settings is advisable, and staff should know when and how to operate the device. According to the American Psychiatric Association (1984), the psychiatric use of seclusion and restraint is relatively contraindicated in patients with any unstable medical conditions, those with delirium or dementia, and those who are overtly suicidal. The AACAP parameters warn that the use of restraints in children who have been sexually abused should be avoided (Masters et al. 2002). Mohr et al. (2003) suggested that prone restraint in particular should be avoided in patients who have increased abdominal girth, a condition common in patients who have been treated with atypical antipsychotics. According to TJC (Joint Commission on Accreditation of Healthcare Organizations 2000), smokers are at higher risk of death when put in restraints; restraints should not be used with patients who have physical deformities that preclude the proper application of a restraint device; and prone restraints may predispose patients to asphyxia, and supine restraints may predispose them to aspiration.

Procedure

There are no overall professional standards that are empirically validated on how to deal with situations in which patients are violent. The psychiatric specialty organizations, nursing organizations, and emergency department physician organizations have issued consensus statements and parameters on the issue of seclusion and restraint; however, there are no guidelines as to how to handle such situations, and despite regulations, not all hospitals provide training in violence and aggression prediction (Peek-Asa et al. 2007). In general,

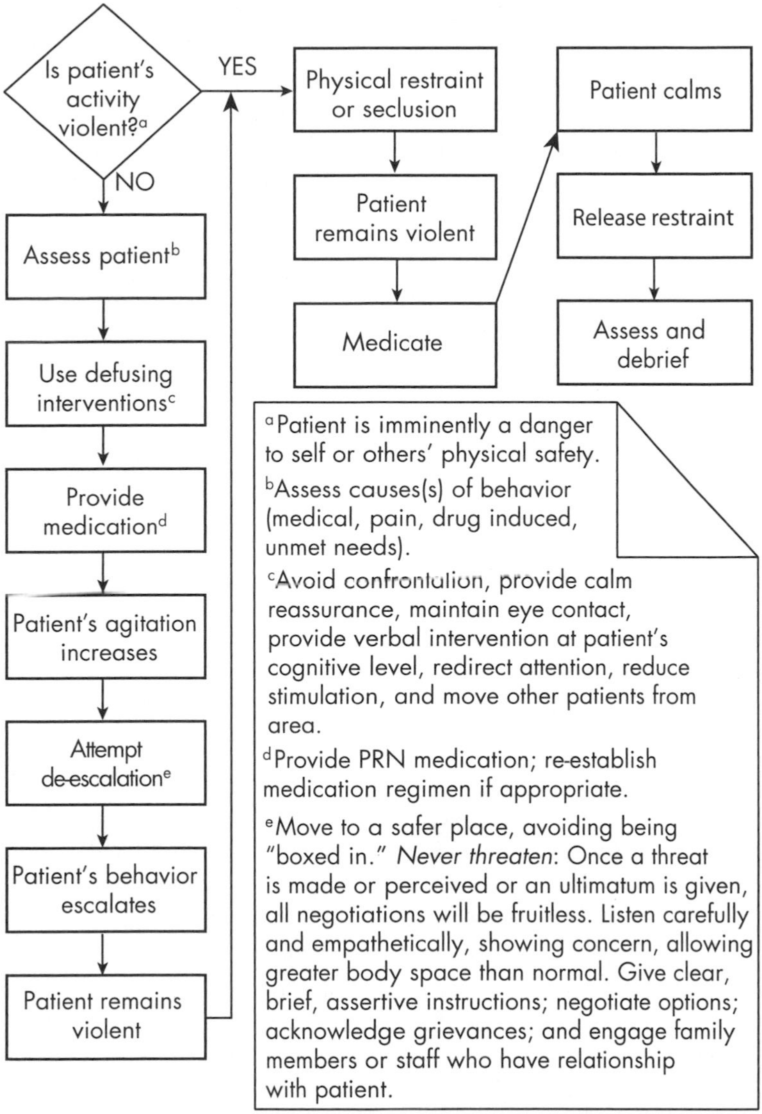
Is patient's activity violent?[a]
YES
NO
Physical restraint or seclusion
Patient remains violent
Medicate
Patient calms
Release restraint
Assess and debrief
Assess patient[b]
Use defusing interventions[c]
Provide medication[d]
Patient's agitation increases
Attempt de-escalation[e]
Patient's behavior escalates
Patient remains violent
[a]Patient is imminently a danger to self or others' physical safety.
[b]Assess causes(s) of behavior (medical, pain, drug induced, unmet needs).
[c]Avoid confrontation, provide calm reassurance, maintain eye contact, provide verbal intervention at patient's cognitive level, redirect attention, reduce stimulation, and move other patients from area.
[d]Provide PRN medication; re-establish medication regimen if appropriate.
[e]Move to a safer place, avoiding being "boxed in." *Never threaten*: Once a threat is made or perceived or an ultimatum is given, all negotiations will be fruitless. Listen carefully and empathetically, showing concern, allowing greater body space than normal. Give clear, brief, assertive instructions; negotiate options; acknowledge grievances; and engage family members or staff who have relationship with patient.

Figure 11–1. Algorithm for decision making regarding use of seclusion and restraint.

the following scenario occurs in clinical situations: When a patient's behavior begins to escalate such that he or she is in imminent danger—for example, if a patient becomes verbally threatening or moves to hurt himself or herself in any way—a staff member activates some sort of code established by the institution. Such codes are similar to those used for cardiac emergencies. This code triggers a response from trained designated staff, usually four or five people, who come to see if they can assist and de-escalate the patient. One person is designated as the leader of this team. If physical restraint is necessary, the leader directs the restraint and talks with the agitated person. Each staff member is assigned an extremity, and together they hold the person, carry the person to a seclusion room, or apply mechanical restraints.

Observation (Including the 1-Hour Rule)

Both TJC and CMS require that when patients are restrained by staff members using any technique, a staff member be designated to observe the patient continually for any signs of physical distress. Staff members must be directed never to disregard a patient's statement that he or she cannot breathe or to explain away such statements as manipulation. Too often, such pleas have been disregarded with tragic consequences (Nunno et al. 2006).

CMS requires that when a patient is in restraint or seclusion, the patient needs to be continually monitored face to face. TJC states that patients who are in seclusion should be continually monitored face to face, but that after the first hour in seclusion, patients may be monitored continually using video and audio equipment. TJC directs that a patient should be monitored every 15 minutes while in either restraint or seclusion for readiness to discontinue the procedure and to assure his or her comfort. Comfort refers to, among other things, vital signs, range of motion, proper body alignment, circulation, and need for toileting and/or hydration, as well as psychological comfort. Such monitoring should be conducted by a qualified staff member who is able to recognize when to contact a medically trained licensed independent practitioner or emergency medical service. Restraint use should also be documented. Clinicians are cautioned that it is imperative that patients be continually monitored and that the "15-minute checklist" should not be used as a pro forma exercise in paperwork.

The clinician, either a physician or other licensed independent practitioner, works with the staff and patient to identify ways to help the patient gain behavioral control. A new order is provided for seclusion and restraint if necessary. These orders must adhere to the regulations as explicated in Table 11–1.

Within 1 hour of the application of a restraint or a patient's placement in seclusion, a physician or a licensed independent professional must conduct a face-to-face evaluation of the patient. This "1-hour rule" was promulgated by CMS at the urging of professionals and advocates who were concerned about the misuse and overuse of seclusion and restraint, and about the number of deaths and injury that were accompanying them (see later section "Death and Other Adverse Effects").

Release from Restraint and Debriefing

When patients are calm and no longer pose a threat to themselves or others, they should be released from restraints. Early in the restraint process, patients should have been apprised of the rationale for the restraint and the criteria for release. This information should be clearly communicated to patients and should be reiterated when they are less agitated (usually after receiving medication for acute agitation). Before release, patients should be oriented to the environment and should have ceased verbally threatening the staff. Facilities may have specific behavioral criteria articulated in operational terms to provide guidance to staff; some facilities may also require that a patient contract verbally for safety. Most facility policy and procedure manuals and training programs have specific procedures for releasing patients from mechanical restraints.

CMS regulations require that a facility conduct an incident debriefing with staff and patient within 24 hours of the patient's release from restraint. The purpose of such a debriefing is to determine how to avoid a similar event in the future. Discussion should focus on the circumstances resulting in the seclusion and restraint (e.g., a precipitant), methods for more safely responding, helping staff to understand the precipitant, and developing alternative methods for helping patients and staff to cope and avoid future seclusion and restraint. The most important outcomes of such a debriefing should be a reexamination of the treatment plan, an assessment of whether the procedure was done safely and was consistent with training, and a determination of whether the procedure was necessary.

Death and Other Adverse Effects

The most commonly used physical restraint is holding of the patient by staff members until the patient becomes calm or transitions into more mechanical restraints. There is no preferred position in which to hold a person. All restraints have morbidity and mortality risks. Prone restraints seem to bear the greatest risk. TJC reviewed 20 cases of death in restraints; in 40% of the cases, the cause of death was asphyxia, most often resulting from factors such as placing excessive weight on the patient's back or obstructing the airway (Joint Commission on Accreditation of Healthcare Organizations 1998).

Mohr et al. (2003) identified asphyxiation as the most common reported cause of restraint-related death, but other causes included death by aspiration, blunt trauma to the chest (commotio cordis), malignant cardiac rhythm disturbances secondary to massive catecholamine rush, thrombosis, rhabdomyolysis, excited delirium with overwhelming metabolic acidosis, and pulmonary embolism. In a retrospective investigation of death certificates and records, Evans et al. (2003) identified a large number of restraint-related deaths, further underscoring that restraint is not a benign procedure.

In an executive summary by Equip for Equality (2011), 61 deaths were identified in connection to the use of restraints. These deaths occurred in small and large communities in both rural and urban settings. Whereas 26% of the deaths occurred in psychiatric settings, the rest occurred elsewhere, such as in medical units, emergency rooms, schools, nursing homes, and wilderness camps. Individuals who died ranged in age from 9 to 95 years, and 75% had a psychiatric diagnosis. Nearly half of those who died had limited or no communication capacity (due to medical circumstances that limited consciousness/awareness). Nearly all of the deceased had a preexisting medical condition such as cardiac or respiratory compromise or obesity. Two issues were of particularly high concern in this report: 1) the apparent connection between deaths and unsafe restraint methods and 2) the lack of evidence that the use of restraints met legal standards. Given these startling statistics, it was recommended that institutions establish policy and procedures to regulate dangerous restraint practices, that clinicians be trained to recognize contraindications that may increase the risk of death, and that staff be educated to identify signs of distress that must immediately be addressed. In addition, close supervision and clinical expertise during restraint and examination of incidents will also likely reduce future episodes of restraint.

Nunno et al. (2006) found 45 child and adolescent fatalities related to restraints in institutions between 1993 and 2003. In over half of the deaths, asphyxia was the cause. O'Halloran and Frank (2000) discussed 21 asphyxial deaths that occurred during prone restraints in health care facilities, detention centers, or jails; restrainers included police officers, security personnel, laypersons, custodial officers, and firefighters. One to seven persons were engaged in each restraint, and the time of restraint from initiation to death was estimated to be 2–12 minutes.

Case Example 2

F., 9-year-old girl weighing 56 pounds, fell asleep in her chair at a therapeutic school. She was awakened by staff and told to sit up and sit straight, without feet crossed. F. had been restrained for "oppositional behavior" twice that week for an hour each time; in her frustration, she kicked her foot, sending her shoe across the room. Staff members deemed her to be "out of control" and took her to the floor, restraining her in a prone position. A 250-pound staff member put the weight of his body over her torso. The child struggled against the restraint for 1 hour, during which time she cried that she could not breathe. She lost control of her bladder and bowels. When staff members regarded her to be quiescent, they turned her over. She was blue. Efforts at resuscitation were not successful. The cause of death was compressional asphyxia, and the manner of death was ruled homicide.

The negative psychological impact of restraint and seclusion has been well documented. Studies conducted of patients' subjective experiences of restraints found that the experiences were generally viewed as punitive and coercive, had a negative impact on the therapeutic alliance, and were counterproductive in that they promoted unwanted behaviors (Kahng et al. 2001; Magee and Ellis 2001; Zun 2005). When in seclusion, patients described feeling neglected, fearful, isolated, vulnerable, and punished (Martinez et al. 1999).

Staff members are also injured during restraint. In states and institutions that have reduced their restraint use, not only have staff injuries decreased, but the institutions have realized significant financial savings because each restraint episode represents a good deal of expense (LeBel et al. 2004).

Reporting Patient Death

On July 2, 1999, the Patients' Rights Interim Final Rule was published (Centers for Medicare and Medicaid Services, U.S. Department of Health and Human Services 1999), requiring that a hospital report to a CMS regional office any patient death that occurs while the patient is restrained or in seclusion for behavioral management. The CMS also stipulates that such reporting must include each death that occurs within 24 hours after a patient has been removed from seclusion and restraint and every death that occurs within 1 week of seclusion and restraint, if it is reasonable to assume that restraint use or placement in seclusion contributed directly or indirectly to a patient's death. The number of deaths reported from 1999 to 2002 was 75 (Centers for Medicare and Medicaid Services, U.S. Department of Health and Human Services 2002). This number undoubtedly does not reflect the complete picture, because only institutions receiving CMS funding are required to report these deaths.

Documentation

Documentation serves as an important source of information for other professionals. It is imperative that clinicians document as clearly and accurately as possible the rationale for restraint or seclusion and chronicle precisely what has transpired. The documentation should include the nature of the emergency or the reason that restraint was considered necessary, the measures enacted to de-escalate the patient to prevent the need for restraint, antecedents to the violent behavior if assessed by staff, the type of restraint employed, the staff members who were involved, the length of time of the restraint, and the patient's condition both during and after the restraint. Although some of this documentation may be delegated to staff members, physicians should keep in mind that many clinical staff, even those with college education, have little formal education in clinical psychiatry, and the only training they may have in restraint and seclusion is what they have been taught "on the job." Many staff members may not understand the proper way to document incidents appropriately in the medical record. Even with checklist documentation, which is becoming increasingly popular, they may not have a good understanding of the terms that are presented in the checklist. This can pose potential difficulties should legal problems arise (Mohr 2006).

Legal Considerations

Clinicians should be aware of legal considerations pertaining to restraint of psychiatric patients. Physicians are especially vulnerable from a legal standpoint because they have ultimate responsibility for patients' treatment, they must write the order for restraint or seclusion, and they must narrate the course of a patient's history and treatment, as well as the rationale for and outcomes of treatment (Northcutt and Shea 2006).

In the past, claims of constitutional violations were a common response to systemic overuse of seclusion and restraint. Constitutional claims include violations of the Fourteenth Amendment right to freedom from restraint and the Fourth Amendment right to freedom from unreasonable search and seizure. The use of restraints is supported by the Supreme Court decision in *Youngberg v. Romeo* (1982), which affirmed that a patient could be restrained to protect others or self. Challenges to this decision may re-emerge, because professional judgment in the field strongly supports significant reduction in the use of restraint.

In recent years, forensic pathologists have developed the following as a conventional standard: if an asphyxial death happens during a restraint episode, the manner of death is always listed as homicide, regardless of the intent of the procedure (National Association of Medical Examiners 2002). This has prompted criminal investigations that might not have happened in the past. Tort claims have also been more common. They can involve a number of different causes of action: excessive force, medical malpractice, failure to protect, assault and battery, and failure to maintain a safe environment. Attorneys are also examining the application of the Americans with Disabilities Act of 1990 to the use of seclusion and restraint under the *Olmstead v. L.C.* (1999) decision, in which the U.S. Supreme Court ruled that unjustified isolation of individuals with disabilities is regarded as discrimination based on disability.

Key Clinical Points

- Behavioral emergencies are dynamic, complex events requiring timely assessment and rapid intervention.

- Seclusion and physical restraints are tools in the arsenal for managing acute agitation when there is a high risk that a patient might harm self or others. However, these tools should be used only after attempts at verbal de-escalation have failed and after offering medication for agitation.

- Use of seclusion and physical restraints is regulated by the Centers for Medicare and Medicaid Services and The Joint Commission, and regulations vary from state to state.

- The use of physical restraints is fraught with risks for staff and patients, including death.

- High-quality empirical data on effective management of behavioral emergencies are lacking.

References

American Psychiatric Association: The American Psychiatric Association Task Force Report 22: The Psychiatric Uses of Seclusion and Restraint. Washington, DC, American Psychiatric Association, 1984

Americans with Disabilities Act of 1990, 42 U.S.C. § 12101 et seq.

Annas GJ: The last resort—the use of physical restraints in medical emergencies. N Engl J Med 341(18):1408–1412, 1999 10536135

Berrios CD, Jacobowitz WH: Therapeutic holding: outcomes of a pilot study. J Psychosoc Nurs Ment Health Serv 36(8):14–18, 1998 9726081

Centers for Medicare and Medicaid Services, U.S. Department of Health and Human Services: 42 CFR Part 482. Medicare and Medicaid programs; hospital conditions of participation: patients' rights; interim final rule. Fed Regist 64(127):36070–36089, July 2, 1999

Centers for Medicare and Medicaid Services, U.S. Department of Health and Human Services: 42 CFR Part 482. Medicare and Medicaid programs; hospital conditions of participation: clarification of the regulatory flexibility analysis for patients' rights. Fed Regist 67(191):61805–61808, October 2, 2002

Centers for Medicare and Medicaid Services, U.S. Department of Health and Human Services: Medicare and Medicaid programs; hospital conditions of participation: patients' rights. Final rule. Fed Regist 71(236):71378–71428, December 8, 2006 17171854

Equip for Equality: National Review of Restraint Related Deaths of Children and Adults With Disabilities: The Lethal Consequences of Restraint. Equip for Equality, 2011. Available at: http://www.equipforequality.org/wp-content/uploads/2014/04/National-Review-of-Restraint-Related-Deaths-of-Adults-and-Children-with-Disabilities-The-Lethal-Consequences-of-Restraint.pdf. Accessed January 3, 2015.

Evans D, Wood J, Lambert L: Patient injury and physical restraint devices: a systematic review. J Adv Nurs 41(3):274–282, 2003 12581115

Joint Commission on Accreditation of Healthcare Organizations: Preventing restraint deaths. Joint Commission Sentinel Event Alert. November 18, 1998. Available at: http://www.jointcommission.org/assets/1/18/SEA 8.pdf. Accessed January 3, 2015.

Joint Commission on Accreditation of Healthcare Organizations: Comprehensive Accreditation Manual for Hospitals: The Official Handbook. Oakbrook Terrace, IL, Joint Commission on Accreditation of Healthcare Organizations, 2000

Kahng S, Abt KA, Wilder DA: Treatment of collateral self-injury correlated with mechanical restraints. Behav Interv 16:105–110, 2001

LeBel J, Stromberg N, Duckworth K, et al: Child and adolescent inpatient restraint reduction: a state initiative to promote strength-based care. J Am Acad Child Adolesc Psychiatry 43(1):37–45, 2004 14691359

Magee SK, Ellis J: The detrimental effects of physical restraint as a consequence for inappropriate classroom behavior. J Appl Behav Anal 34(4):501–504, 2001 11800190

Martinez RJ, Grimm M, Adamson M: From the other side of the door: patient views of seclusion. J Psychosoc Nurs Ment Health Serv 37(3):13–22, 1999 10098107

Masters KJ, Bellonci C, Bernet W, et al; American Academy of Child and Adolescent Psychiatry: Practice parameter for the prevention and management of aggressive behavior in child and adolescent psychiatric institutions, with special reference to seclusion and restraint. J Am Acad Child Adolesc Psychiatry 41 (2 suppl):4S–25S, 2002 11833634

Mohr WK: Psychiatric records, in Medical Legal Aspects of Medical Records. Edited by Iyer P, Levin BJ, Shea MA. Tucson, AZ, Lawyers and Judges Publishing, 2006, pp 691–705

Mohr WK, Petti TA, Mohr BD: Adverse effects associated with physical restraint. Can J Psychiatry 48(5):330–337, 2003 12866339

National Association of Medical Examiners: A Guide for Manner of Death Clarification. Atlanta, GA, National Association of Medical Examiners, 2002

Northcutt CL, Shea MA: Generating and preserving the medical record, in Medical Legal Aspects of Medical Records. Edited by Iyer P, Levin BJ, Shea MA. Tucson, AZ, Lawyers and Judges Publishing, 2006, pp 3–10

Nunno MA, Holden MJ, Tollar A: Learning from tragedy: a survey of child and adolescent restraint fatalities. Child Abuse Negl 30(12):1333–1342, 2006 17109958

O'Halloran RL, Frank JG: Asphyxial death during prone restraint revisited: a report of 21 cases. Am J Forensic Med Pathol 21(1):39–52, 2000 10739225

Olmstead v L.C. 527 U.S. 581 (1999)

Peek-Asa C, Casteel C, Allareddy V, et al: Workplace violence prevention programs in hospital emergency departments. J Occup Environ Med 49(7):756–763, 2007 17622848

Youngberg v Romeo, 457 U.S. 307 (1982)

Zun LS: Evidence-based treatment of psychiatric patient. J Emerg Med 28(3):277–283, 2005 15769568

Suggested Web Sites

American Academy of Child and Adolescent Psychiatry (AACAP; http://www.aacap.org): Presents issue briefs on the use of seclusion and restraint with children and adolescents, and summaries of proposed legislation.

American Academy of Physician Assistants (AAPA; http://www.aapa.org: Includes position statement on reducing seclusion and restraint usage.

American Nurses Association (ANA; http://www.nursingworld.org): Contains position statement on reducing seclusion and restraint usage from the nursing perspective.

Judge David L. Bazelon Center for Mental Health Law (http://www.bazelon.org): Provides current information on legislation and court decisions affecting the use of seclusion and restraint in psychiatric facilities. Also contains information on the Americans with Disabilities Act and *Olmstead v. L.C.*

National Alliance on Mental Illness (NAMI; http://www.nami.org): Features position statement on seclusion and restraint and chart summarizing abuse of restraint usage across the country from October 1998 through March 2000.

National Association of Psychiatric Health Systems (NAPHS; http://www.naphs.org): Provides guidelines on the use of seclusion.

National Association of State Mental Health Program Directors (NASMHPD; http://www.nasmhpd.org/): Features a position statement, legislative updates, and free online publications.

National Disability Rights Network (NDRN; http://www.ndrn.org/index.php): Offers information on federally mandated protection and advocacy programs that protect the rights of persons with disabilities, including psychiatric disabilities. Also contains a special report on seclusion and restraint.

National Mental Health Consumers' Self-Help Clearinghouse (http://www.mhself-help.org): Includes information on restraint reduction and other issues from a consumer advocate perspective.

12

Legal and Ethical Issues in Emergency Psychiatry

Debra A. Pinals, M.D.

Nancy Byatt, D.O., M.B.A., F.A.P.M.

Emergency psychiatry departments can be exciting, fast-paced settings in which medical decisions are often made without the luxury of long periods of time for deliberation. From the moment a patient presents to a psychiatric emergency service (PES) setting, important issues surface that are critical for mental health staff to understand so that they operate within the constraints of law, ethics, and regulations. For example, a duty of care exists for patients who present themselves to the emergency room. Refusing care could incur allegations and liability related to patient abandonment. A patient who walks into a lobby but decides not to register may not fall under this duty of care. Once a patient is known to have presented, the mental health staff may have certain obligations related to treatment. From that point forward, legal, regulatory, and system issues related to confidentiality, informed consent, emer-

271

gency restraint, and utilization management are commonplace. Having an understanding of common legal and ethical underpinnings of emergency psychiatric practice is important in the PES setting. In this chapter, we review some of the common legal themes encountered in emergency psychiatry and provide information on their management.

Confidentiality

Case Example

While working as a mental health professional in the psychiatric emergency department, you answer an outside call. A woman on the line states, "I think my sister, Ms. P, is in the psychiatric emergency room. How is she doing?" How do you respond?

Trust is the foundation of a therapeutic relationship. A physician's maintenance of confidentiality assures patients that their autonomy is respected and valued. In adolescent populations, the lack of willingness to seek medical care and to disclose pertinent history has been linked directly to perception and fear of disclosure (Mermelstein and Wallack 2008) and may be linked to social anxiety as well (Colognori et al. 2012). Patients have also reported choosing to change or withhold pertinent clinical information due to fear of a breach in confidentiality (Mermelstein and Wallack 2008). It is incumbent on psychiatrists to respect patients' confidentiality by making every effort to ensure the highest degree of privacy possible.

One might argue that in no other field of medicine is the need for confidentiality as paramount as in psychiatry. Psychiatrists ask patients not only to reveal their innermost feelings but also to discuss problems that many people may find shameful or stigmatizing. Patients are placed in the precarious position of being vulnerable and dependent on psychiatrists to protect the information that needs to be shared so that treatment can take place.

The importance of confidentiality in psychiatric communication has been recognized in case law and codified in statute (Mermelstein and Wallack 2008). In the landmark case *Jaffe v. Redmond* (1996), the U.S. Supreme Court recognized the importance of a psychotherapist-patient privilege. Other legal actions regarding medical privacy have also been taken. For example, the

Health Insurance Portability and Accountability Act of 1996 (HIPAA; U.S. Department of Health and Human Services 1996) is a set of rules enacted by the federal government to systematically respond to threats to medical privacy. HIPAA mandates that patients authorize release of information and be informed as to how their medical information will be used.

Exceptions

Although important, the right to privacy is not absolute; exceptions arise that require confidentiality to be broken. Even though it may be clinically necessary and legally sound to break a patient's confidentiality in certain circumstances, one must carefully consider and document the necessity to do so for patient care, the effect of the communication, and the benefit-risk ratio of and alternatives to any such approach. A common example in the emergency department involves the need to contact family or other treatment providers to gather information about a patient who has presented. If a patient consents to such communication, the issue of breach of confidentiality is moot. However, emergency psychiatrists and clinicians often need to contact family members, friends, or other persons, without patient consent, to ascertain clinical background information that could ultimately help mitigate risk of harm to the patient or others. In an emergency, the PES clinician should proceed with obtaining the needed information and be sure to explain to the family member or other collateral contact the rationale for requesting the information without patient consent (Mermelstein and Wallack 2008).

A risk of harm to a third party raises another important potential exception to the obligation to maintain confidentiality of patient information (Herbert 2002). Most states have adopted legal rules, either through case law or legislation, that impose provisions stemming from California's Supreme Court decision in *Tarasoff v. Regents of the University of California* (1976; see case description in Chapter 3, "Violence Risk Assessment"). States vary in how they adopt legal rules regarding taking action to protect a potentially at-risk third party. Some states impose an actual and explicit duty to protect a potential third party who may be at risk of being harmed by a person under the care of a psychiatrist or other mental health clinician, whereas other states are more permissive and have less specific requirements, and these laws evolve over time. Taken separately, local laws may or may not impose a liability protection against claims of breach of confidentiality in such circumstances. At times, actions a clinician may ethically or legally take, depending on the clinical scenario and jurisdiction, include warning third parties of the potential for harm, but at other times, and important to the final California Supreme Court analysis of the original *Tarasoff* case (*Tarasoff v. Regents of the University of California* 1974), actions may need to extend beyond warning the potential victim toward taking actions to more specifically protect the potential victim. California, for example, recently adopted legislation that clarifies a duty to protect beyond the case law from the *Tarasoff* language; this legislation recognizes immunity from civil liability for issuing warnings, but also notes that warnings in and of themselves may raise other risks without as many benefits of protection of potentially at-risk individuals (Weinstock et al. 2014). For example, protection of a third party in a given circumstance may be better executed by taking other actions, such as hospitalizing the patient (Herbert 2002).

Sharing Information With Providers and Emergency Department Staff

PES staff often struggle to maintain confidentiality while obtaining information from or giving information to other providers and emergency department staff in the interest of patient care. Additional challenges result when certain components of the information in the mental health record are to be shared with other general health care providers, whose limitations related to confidentiality may not be held in the same regard. A bidirectional flow of necessary information between providers is essential because it allows PES staff to work in a patient's best interests and to maintain a collaborative relationship with other providers. Free sharing of information cannot, however, be done merely for staff convenience. An emergency exception to confidentiality allows for the communication to occur (Appelbaum and Gutheil 2007).

PES staff generally follow a crisis model that focuses on acute issues, such as safety and symptom relief, with the goal of transferring the patient to an inpatient hospital setting for stabilization or return to outpatient care. PES staff, therefore, should concentrate on obtaining and sharing information needed for acute patient care. In PES settings, where mental health clinicians work side by side with other clinicians, it is important to consider the physical setting and risk of incidental disclosure when discussing cases with referring clinicians (Mermelstein and Wallack 2008).

Asking for Releases, Time Permitting

HIPAA addresses authorization for release and permits disclosure of medical information in the interest of providing appropriate care for patients, unless requested otherwise. If time permits, PES staff ideally should educate the patient about the relevant issues and request consent before releasing information. In the case of Ms. P, one should obtain patient consent before acknowledging to others that the patient is in the emergency department. Given that this is often not feasible in the PES setting, staff should use discretion and limit what they discuss to what is necessary for acute patient care (Mermelstein and Wallack 2008). For example, although it may be important to share with certain family members that a patient is in the emergency room so staff can gather information from them, it may not be reasonable to share with them all patient information (e.g., the circumstances of a patient's recent breakup of a relationship).

Hospitalization

Case Example *(continued)*

Ms. P has been evaluated in the PES, and it is abundantly clear that she would benefit from a psychiatric hospitalization given the lack of outpatient psychiatric and psychosocial support available for her, as well as her severe depression, passive suicidal ideation, and psychotic symptoms that are significantly impacting her ability to function. You are, however, reassured because she is denying any intent or plan to act on her suicidal thoughts and states many reasons why she would not want to die. Also, although her family members are concerned about her functioning and prefer a psychiatric hospitalization, they feel that she would be safe if discharged home. Based on your assessment, you feel that a psychiatric hospitalization is indicated but do not feel that Ms. P meets criteria for involuntary commitment because she does not appear to be at imminent risk of harm to self or others. How do you proceed?

Psychiatric hospitalization is generally intended to stabilize and provide a therapeutic environment for patients, yet it can be perceived as a violation of one's civil liberty when done involuntarily. Psychiatry is distinct from other specialties in that it routinely uses involuntary civil commitment as a means to provide intensive, hospital-level care in certain circumstances when persons are in need of such intervention but are refusing voluntary hospitalization. PES staff must ensure that proper restrictions on hospitalization are used to preclude the abuse of power related to civil commitment (Lidz et al. 1989; Pinals and Mossman 2012).

Voluntary Admissions

Voluntary admission is preferred over involuntary because it can foster the development of a therapeutic alliance and recognizes an individual's autonomy. Regarding voluntary psychiatric admissions, some states have as part of statutory language the requirement that the facility is capable of providing care and that the patient is in need of psychiatric care. As in the case of Ms. P, PES clinicians must assess whether a voluntary admission is clinically indicated or whether a less restrictive alternative for psychiatric treatment (e.g., a crisis stabilization placement) would be appropriate and more therapeutic (Simon and Goetz 1999).

There are different types of voluntary status: pure voluntary status, conditional voluntary status, and emergency holds/detention. The procedure for discharge varies with each type (Appelbaum and Gutheil 2007).

Pure Voluntary Status

Under a pure voluntary status, the patient is free to leave the hospital at any time, much as in medical settings. Many states limit pure voluntary status in psychiatric settings, given the higher likelihood that patients who exercise their right to leave might raise enough clinical concern to warrant petitioning for their civil commitment (Appelbaum and Gutheil 2007).

Conditional Voluntary Status

The conditional voluntary status allows the admitting facility to detain patients in the hospital for a period of time, often up to several days, after the patient has announced his or her desire to leave. This period of detainment may be used to allow the patient to change his or her mind, for evaluation of the patient and a determination about whether it is clinically indicated to initiate proceedings for involuntary commitment, or for discharge planning. If the facility decides to seek commitment, the patient can be held in the hospital until the hearing takes place. If a patient decides to leave and criteria for involuntary commitment are not met, then the patient is free to go, even if further inpatient treatment is clinically indicated (Appelbaum and Gutheil 2007). The discharge in such a case is often granted against medical advice and documented as such, after a discussion with the patient that involves an attempt to address the patient's reasons for leaving and reviews risks for leaving versus benefits of further hospitalization. Regardless of whether the patient leaves against medical advice, follow-up treatment and referrals should be provided (Brook et al. 2006).

Although patient advocates have articulated concern that vulnerable persons with mental illness may be coerced into a conditional voluntary admission, research indicates that the legal status on admission is not a reliable indicator of whether patients experience coercion during the hospital admission process (MacArthur Research Network on Mental Health and the Law 2001; Pinals and Mossman 2012). PES clinicians, however, should be cautious not to coerce patients into agreeing to a voluntary hospitalization when there is no intention or rationale that would justify hospitalizing the patient involuntarily. In *Zinermon v. Burch* (1979), a person was committed to a state hospital voluntarily although he lacked the capacity to give informed consent to the hospitalization. The U.S. Supreme Court held that the failure to identify patients who lack the capacity to give informed consent is a violation of patients' rights. What this means in clinical practice is complex, because capacity to consent to inpatient psychiatric hospitalization may require a low threshold (Hoge 1994). In assessing a patient's competence to consent to psychiatric hospitalization, PES clinicians balance on the one hand the desire to make voluntary hospitalization and its benefits widely available (even to those who may have limited capacity for making a choice toward voluntary hospitalization) and on the other hand the need to ensure that patients without decisional capacity are not hospitalized involuntarily without appropriate legal grounds to do so (Lidz et al. 1989; Simon and Goetz 1999).

Emergency Holds/Detention

Psychiatric patients presenting to the emergency department are often escorted against their will by police officers. In many states, police officers have the power to transport patients involuntarily based on information obtained from a treating professional or family member that indicates that the patient is at imminent risk of harming self or others. Jurisdictions often have statutes allowing police officers to "emergency petition" patients to be transported to the nearest emergency department for further evaluation. Some emergency holds can last hours, some longer. While evaluating patients, PES clinicians need to consider how the petition was obtained and the circumstances that led to the petition. The PES evaluation is often the first step toward treatment or discharge after the initial holding mechanism was activated, and these initial legal holds, depending on clinical factors and whether they meet legal criteria, could result in downstream involuntary civil commitment (Pinals and Mossman 2012).

Persons who have ingested substances may present to the emergency department in an apparent state of acute psychiatric decompensation. Individuals who are intoxicated or abusing substances, for example, are often brought to the emergency department secondary to dangerousness to self or others. Patients with alcohol dependence and a high tolerance for alcohol may not present with slurred speech or ataxia and may disclose suicidal intent while appearing sober. A toxicology screen and cognitive screening examination should be completed to ensure that such a patient, and patients who have less tolerance, are not evaluated for involuntary psychiatric hospitalization while still intoxicated. Once sober, these patients may not fit the criteria for an involuntary psychiatric hospital admission (Pinals and Mossman 2012; Simon and Goetz 1999). Mental health statutes vary with regard to how substance use is factored into commitment criteria (Christopher et al., in press; Williams et al. 2014).

Involuntary Hospitalization

The power to commit a patient to the hospital involuntarily represents a significant limitation on the individual's liberty and should only be used with extreme care (Byatt et al. 2006; Pinals and Mossman 2012). Involuntary hospitalization should be sought only when less restrictive means are not available (Pinals and Mossman 2012).

The standards that the patient, as a result of having a mental illness, must meet to be committable generally include some combination of several of the following criteria: 1) danger to others, 2) danger to self, 3) inability to care for self, 4) danger to property, 5) need of psychiatric treatment, and 6) risk of deterioration. The emphasis on the dangerousness criteria—the first three criteria listed here—since the mid-1970s has created a tension related to trying to hospitalize patients who are in need of treatment but who are not putting themselves or others at risk. Some states have expanded commitment parameters, therefore, to allow especially the latter two possible criteria, although this is less common.

A state's general power to use civil commitment for psychiatric hospitalization is described as primarily limited to individuals who have at least a mental disorder, often itself defined by state regulations, statutes, or case law. The debate about the scope of civil commitment is at times posed as a problem of defining the kind of mental disorder that is required to justify commitment (Byatt et al. 2006; Pinals and Mossman 2012; Williams et al. 2014). Patients who are determined to be potentially violent toward others but who do not have mental illnesses do not generally meet criteria for involuntary commitment to a psychiatric hospital (Pinals and Mossman 2012; Simon and Goetz 1999).

Although engaging patients in voluntary care should always be an important goal in treatment, the ability to institute involuntary short-term psychiatric hospitalization for patients with mental illness who are declining care and who present with risks that cannot otherwise be mitigated in emergency situations is an important intervention to be used until a court hearing can be held. The period that a person can be held involuntarily varies across jurisdictions. The criteria that must be met to continue to hold a psychiatric patient are often those required for court-ordered commitment. At the end of the emergency commitment period, facilities must decide whether to discharge the patient or to petition for court-ordered hospitalization. The strict time limits on emergency commitment are sometimes subverted secondary to delays in scheduling hearings at the court level. As a result, patients may be involuntarily held for psychiatric reasons for weeks or longer before a hearing (Byatt et al. 2006).

Capacity to Make Medical Decisions

Case Example *(continued)*

A brief mental status examination completed on Ms. P reveals attention and memory deficits consistent with delirium. Discharge home no longer seems a possibility given her delirium and the fact that her mental status appears significantly different from her baseline. Ms. P is now demanding to leave. How do you proceed?

Assessment

Determining whether patients have the capacity to make medical decisions involves respecting the autonomy of patients who are capable of making decisions and protecting those who are not (Appelbaum 2007). Competence is usually presumed, and patients are afforded autonomy in their decisions to accept or reject recommended medical treatment unless their competence is questioned. The terms *capacity* and *competency* are often interchanged; however, capacity is based on a clinical judgment, whereas competence is a legal determination made by a judge (Appelbaum 2007; Byatt et al. 2006).

Capacity Versus Commitment

Frequently, patients who are hospitalized involuntarily in the emergency department or medical inpatient unit have acute medical problems and desire to leave or attempt to leave but lack the capacity to decide to leave against medical advice. To have decision-making capacity related to medical decisions, one must be able to appreciate the reasonably foreseeable consequences of a decision or lack of decision. Capacity is specific to particular decisions and can change over time. Patients who lack the capacity to make medical decisions may reject recommended treatment. In such cases, clinicians need to determine the appropriate course of action. Approaches to assessment and treatment planning should take into consideration what is the expectation of recovery and whether some type of advance directive for health care decisions may come into play (Byatt et al. 2006). It is important to consider that a patient who lacks capacity to make medical decisions is not necessarily committable to a psychiatric inpatient setting. Similarly, patients who appear to meet criteria for civil commitment due to risk of harm to themselves or others may not lack the capacity to make medical decisions.

Patients must be allowed to leave against medical advice if they have decisional capacity and choose to forgo recommended treatment. A patient who has such decisional capacity cannot be forced to accept unwanted treatment even if the treatment being refused could save the patient's life. The medical team, however, must take the necessary steps to keep a patient in the emergency department if the patient lacks decisional capacity and wants to leave against medical advice. At times, the steps needed to ensure that such patients stay in the hospital are not clear. Documents to initiate psychiatric civil commitment may not be appropriate for retaining in the emergency department those patients who do not fit criteria for commitment to a psychiatric facility (Byatt et al. 2006).

As with Ms. P, when a patient requests to leave the emergency department against medical advice, the emergency department team should contact appropriate consultants as needed to help ascertain a patient's decision-making capacity and appropriateness for civil commitment. Documentation should ideally include a general psychiatric evaluation and a capacity evaluation, indicating whether the patient has a primary psychiatric issue or a psychiatric issue secondary to a general medical condition. The involvement of next of kin is helpful to obtain guidance in making medical decisions. Unless a health care proxy or equivalent type of authorization is in place, next of kin cannot legally override a patient's refusal to stay in the hospital but can provide guidance with treatment decisions. Where there is no legal authority for family to make decisions for the patient, it is important to balance confidentiality and attempts at obtaining guidance in the particular emergency by providing family with only the information needed to manage the medical situation (Byatt et al. 2006).

The medical team may need to hold patients who lack decisional capacity involuntarily in an emergency department or on a medical floor but may not be able to treat patients against their will except in acute emergency situations where lack of treatment may result in a hastening of death or result in serious deterioration of health.

The medical or psychiatric team should try to use the least restrictive methods to keep the patient in the emergency department (Knox and Holloman 2012). Approaches to treatment should be trauma informed, because of the high prevalence of trauma histories among psychiatric patients (Alvarez et al. 2011). General restraint practices can represent failures in utilizing more effective, less restrictive alternatives to behavioral challenges. The medical or psychiatric team should only call the police or security to restrain the patient so as to mitigate safety risks after attempts to manage the patient without physical or mechanical restraints fail. Initiation of legal or administrative review can help attend to the legal rights of patients when the need for mechanical restraints arise and can also serve to address ethical concerns related to possible inappropriate coercive treatment of patients. Input from hospital legal, administrative, or ethics personnel can be critical when sorting through issues related to coercion in treatment. The medical treatment team may consider pursuit of guardianship if lack of capacity is suspected to persist; while guardianship is pending, the medical or emergency team may engage in emergency-based treatment (Byatt et al. 2006).

Informed Consent

Case Example *(continued)*

Ms. P's delirium cleared after a brief admission. She has returned to the emergency department a week later. She continues to be depressed and is reporting auditory hallucinations and delusions that parts of her body are rotting. The physicians indicate that she is in need of antipsychotic medications. How do you proceed?

Elements of informed consent include disclosure, competence, and voluntariness (Appelbaum and Gutheil 2007; Pinals 2009). The doctrine of informed consent requires that a physician disclose certain information to a patient so that the patient can make a decision about his or her own care. Determining how much information to disclose can be complicated; in general, topics should include information related to risks and benefits of the recommended treatment and alternatives to that recommended treatment, as well as risks of no treatment (Murray 2012). In addition, for a valid informed consent process to unfold between a doctor and a patient, the patient must be in a situation in which he or she is making a voluntary choice among alternatives and in which coerced treatment, except under certain legally and ethically permissible circumstances, would not be reasonable.

The doctrine of informed consent also is premised on the idea that a valid informed consent requires the patient to be competent to make treatment decisions. Persons are presumed to be competent to make decisions about their medical and psychiatric care unless certain circumstances exist whereby they are thought to lack capacity to make these decisions for themselves (see above for specific situations relevant to the emergency department). Laws related to health care proxies, for example, generally allow a previously designated health care proxy or person with durable power of attorney to make medical decisions for a patient who is assenting to treatment once a physician determines that the patient no longer has the capacity to make decisions for himself or herself. Guardianship may be sought for patients who lack capacity to make treatment decisions; in this case, the court makes a formal adjudication around the patient's capacity and approves a formal surrogate decision maker to make medical decisions on behalf of the patient whether or not the patient is assenting to the proposed treatment. Guardianship determinations often take time to obtain, but they can also be obtained in emergency medical situations. In an emergency room setting, it is important to identify whether a patient has a previously designated health care proxy or guardian who is legally authorized to make medical decisions on behalf of the patient. The involvement of family, if available, can also be helpful in the informed consent process, especially when the emergency department patient lacks the capacity to make decisions autonomously. As noted above (see "Capacity to Make Medical Decisions"), there may be ethical and legal limitations to the role of family that require balancing.

An exception to the requirements of informed consent is the emergency exception. A physician is permitted to medicate a patient involuntarily and without engaging in a full informed consent dialogue in a situation that involves a psychiatric emergency in which 1) risk of harm to self or others could not be averted in the absence of this intervention and 2) less restrictive alternatives to emergency medication would not be sufficient (Appelbaum and Gutheil 2007; Pinals 2009).

Another exception to the requirement for an informed consent dialogue with the patient is after a guardian has been appointed for the patient. However, even in situations where a patient is under guardianship, a discussion about treatment recommendations with an incompetent patient can still be an important component of psychiatric care in the emergency department setting. Such a discussion can also alleviate a patient's concerns and work toward building a foundation of a therapeutic alliance for a patient who may need long-term treatment and may return to the emergency room for treatment in the future. To the extent that such dialogue may need to be carried out in terms understandable to the incompetent patient, the information provided may be offered in a more limited manner to the ward, although full disclosure to the guardian would be part of the informed consent process (Pinals 2009).

A complicated exception to providing informed consent involves a therapeutic waiver whereby a competent patient states that he or she is agreeing to treatment but does not wish to hear the information about the treatment that the physician would be providing. Such an exception to informed consent would generally require documentation that the patient waived the informed consent process and was capable of doing so.

Another complicated exception is that of therapeutic privilege, which is when a physician elects not to provide a full informed consent disclosure because the physician believes that the information would be harmful in and of itself or create a situation for the patient wherein the opportunity for rational dialogue would be foreclosed if a disclosure related to the medical condition and recommended treatment is given in full. This exception is considered to be very narrow and should not be exercised simply because one believes that a patient would refuse a particular treatment if he or she heard about all the risks involved (e.g., see Murray 2012). In fact, the belief that psychiatric patients will refuse treatment if its risks are disclosed can be a problematic assumption. One study, for example, showed that information related to tardive dyskinesia did not specifically harm patients or even lead to refusal of treatment (Munetz and Roth 1985). Although this exception is not commonly used, if the therapeutic privilege exception is being considered, the rationale for not providing informed consent for the particular patient situation should be contemporaneously documented.

In the case of Ms. P, the clinician should recommend the needed medication, using language that the patient will understand about the condition that is being treated. The emergency department physician should also review with the patient the recommended treatment's risks and benefits, the risk of no treatment, and any alternative treatments available. If Ms. P is unable to engage in the discussion, the clinician should consider and document if any of the above exceptions to informed consent apply, prior to administering the recommended medication.

Transfer of Care

Case Example *(continued)*

A few hours later, the emergency department physician states that Ms. P has been medically cleared for transfer to a nearby freestanding psychiatric hospital. Ms. P has not had labs drawn and now appears confused. Is it appropriate to transfer Ms. P at this time?

In the past decade, much attention has been paid to creating legislation and policies to protect patients and health care providers from the financial, institutional, and political pressures that may interfere with the ability to evaluate and treat patients in a PES setting (Quinn et al. 2002; Saks 2004).

Abandonment

In the 1980s, reports emerged of inappropriate transfers of medically unstable patients, with a resultant increase in morbidity and mortality. Such inappropriate transfers were believed to occur in response to increasing financial pressures, motivating private hospitals to discharge patients to the streets or to public hospitals before adequate evaluation or stabilization. In response, Congress initiated the Emergency Medical Treatment and Active Labor Act of 1986 (EMTALA; for overview, see www.cms.hhs.gov/EMTALA) as part of the Consolidated Omnibus Budget Reconciliation Act of 1985 (COBRA). EMTALA mandated that all hospitals receiving Medicare funds must adequately screen, examine, stabilize, and transfer patients, regardless of the patients' ability to pay. Prior to transfer, patients must be evaluated and stabilized, and the receiving hospital must agree to the transfer and have the facilities to provide needed treatment. According to EMTALA, it would not be appropriate to transfer Ms. P given that she has not been adequately evaluated and she is not stable for transfer. EMTALA applies to both medical and psychiatric conditions; therefore, PES staff would benefit from education to ensure that legal and ethical standards of care are upheld (Quinn et al. 2002; Saks 2004). One preliminary review of cases noted that lawsuits claiming EMTALA violations in the care of patients in the psychiatric emergency department are uncommon and rarely successful (Lindor et al. 2014). However, standardized screening examinations demonstrating that there was no emergency condition that needed stabilization were helpful in defending psychiatric liability actions based on EMTALA (Lindor et al. 2014).

Communication

Appropriate transfer of patients requires proper documentation of medical and/or psychiatric evaluation and communication with the receiving facility.

The transferring facility must ensure that the receiving facility has the appropriate space and personnel, that it is agreeing to accept the patient, and that all relevant records are sent. In addition, a transfer certificate clearly documenting the risks and benefits considered in the transfer decision must accompany the patient and must be signed by the physician authorizing the transfer (Quinn et al. 2002; Saks 2004).

Transfer Problems

EMTALA requires hospitals with specialized capabilities, such as acute psychiatric units, to accept patients regardless of the patients' ability to pay, if the receiving facility has the capacity (Quinn et al. 2002; Saks 2004). Heslop et al. (2000) noted that psychiatric staff and patients are often frustrated with unacceptable standards of care due to the difficulties and delays encountered in securing access to suitable care.

Care may be hampered by stigmatization of certain psychiatric populations, such as those with personality disorders, agitated psychosis, or substance abuse, as well as by financial and practical problems, including lack of insurance and comorbid medical issues (Bazemore et al. 2005). It is being increasingly recognized that hospital ownership and market factors may impact transfer of psychiatric patients to certain settings (Shen et al. 2008). Heslop et al. (2000) commented on the lack of communication and coordination of care between emergency services and psychiatric inpatient units. Further exacerbating the problem, delays in transfer often result in longer waits for other waiting patients (Heslop et al. 2000). If an identified hospital refuses to accept a patient when it has the capability and capacity, then EMTALA has been violated. If the statute is violated by physicians or an institution, civil liability can be imposed, possibly resulting in termination of the institution's Medicare provider agreement. This is noteworthy given the negative impact that refusal of transfer has on standard of care in PES settings (Quinn et al. 2002; Saks 2004).

Liability Management

Case Example *(continued)*

Ms. P's medical workup is complete, and she appears medically stable for a psychiatric admission. She acknowledges suicidal ideation, obsessive thoughts about death, and feeling hopeless, helpless, and overwhelmed. Ms. P's family requests urgent psychiatric treatment, yet they do not feel that she is at acute risk of harm to self. Ms. P is requesting to leave the PES, denies any intent or plan for self-harm, and reports that she can maintain her safety outside the department. Although Ms. P is requesting discharge and denying any intent or plan for self-harm, you remain concerned about her welfare and feel strongly that an inpatient admission is indicated. How do you approach the patient and document your decision making?

Uncertainty is inherent in the practice of psychiatry, particularly in PES settings, and psychiatrists are understandably concerned about facing malpractice lawsuits. Although negative outcomes often result in tragic suffering and harm, such outcomes are not synonymous with malpractice. Malpractice is a negligent civil (noncriminal) wrong committed by a physician that leads to damage. Even when outstanding care is provided, malpractice lawsuits remain a risk, and it behooves the PES clinician to anticipate and prepare for such lawsuits by practicing professionally, seeking consultation in difficult cases, documenting clearly, using adequate risk assessment, and arranging clear follow-up (Appelbaum and Gutheil 2007).

Documentation

Almost as important as the dictum to "do no harm" is the requirement to "write it down," because countless acts of litigation provide evidence that documentation is the primary determinant of legal outcome. Writing more does not necessarily decrease liability. Efficient documentation that entails risk-benefit analysis, reasoning for clinical decisions, and assessment of the patient's capacity to participate in treatment planning is most effective (Gutheil 1980). When a thoughtful risk-benefit analysis is documented, a claim of negligence is more likely to be refuted even if a negative outcome proves that the decision was wrong. PES clinicians should attempt to succinctly summarize their decision-making process, and not merely the final decision, in the medical record. At times, PES clinicians may feel they are expected to read minds or predict future events in order to reduce harm. Documentation of the risks and benefits of the decision at hand and the patient's capacity to participate in treatment is critical. Brief quotes from the patient regarding his or her views of the treatment decisions may be helpful in demonstrating that an informed consent discussion took place (Appelbaum and Gutheil 2007).

Trend Toward Standard Risk Assessment Tools

A trend is growing toward a multidimensional approach to suicide and violence risk assessments commonly conducted in PES settings. The traditional approach has involved a clinical interview and clinical judgment, without as much attention to a standardized mechanism to consider risk factors that are shown to be statistically associated with increased suicide and violence risk. This approach has limitations given the complexity of risk assessment and the individual nature of each patient. Although the field is still evolving, some evidence suggests that formal risk assessment tools may reduce suicide risk by providing an assessment template that can assist with the vital aspects of the assessment (Cutcliffe and Barker 2004). Similar tools have also been developed for violence risk assessment (Lamberg 2007). Before using such instruments, however, the clinician needs to know whether they are appropriate for the emergency department context.

Planning for Aftercare

Adequate arrangement and documentation of follow-up are powerful as a liability and risk prevention tool. Follow-up recommendations should include, where appropriate, measures to mitigate ongoing risks that did not rise to the level of warranting voluntary or involuntary hospitalization. Options for various level of care (e.g., respite beds, crisis stabilization beds, partial or day treatment options) should also be explored. If such options are considered, the rationale for choosing or not choosing such options should be documented. Documentation of therapeutic approaches, interventions, and arrangement for follow-up after discharge can demonstrate the ongoing quality of patient care. PES clinicians should be careful to identify appropriate aftercare when this is thought to be indicated after a careful evaluation, and to carefully document the rationale if no aftercare is recommended (Appelbaum and Gutheil 2007).

Managed Care

Case Example *(continued)*

After you meet with Ms. P and her family, Ms. P agrees to a voluntary psychiatric admission. The PES clinician obtaining insurance approval informs you that Ms. P's insurance company will not approve an inpatient psychiatry admission without a doctor-to-doctor discussion. What will you tell the reviewer so that Ms. P gets the treatment you feel is warranted?

Financial Considerations

Managed care has had a dramatic impact on psychiatry and has led to unique ethical problems. A large proportion of insurance companies have mental health benefits managed under carve-out behavioral health care companies that contract to provide all mental health services and often substance abuse services. Many behavioral health care companies also provide services based on risk or capitations. In the risk model, payment or authorization of clinical services is approved only if there is evidence of enough acuity and risk to necessitate such treatment. Capitated services predetermine the hospital or clinical provider regardless of clinical situation, further exacerbating the issue (Lazarus and Sharfstein 2002).

Ethical and Legal Considerations

The financial arrangements associated with managed care prospective utilization review create unparalleled ethical dilemmas for health professionals. Clinicians often find themselves struggling with conflict of interest posed by utilization review, payers' focus on cost containment, and the demands of external regulatory bodies. Psychiatrists may encounter challenges when providing patient care because of the recent emphasis on patient autonomy and informed consent as opposed to the previous more authoritarian physician role (Lazarus and Sharfstein 2002). Legal liability toward clinicians working within the constraints of managed care is important to understand, especially in the face of limited liability for managed care organizations (Appelbaum 1993).

Utilization Review

Utilization review creates many ethical dilemmas that raise issues related to confidentiality, conflict of interest, and informed consent. The process itself can also interfere with the doctor-patient relationship. Third-party reviewers ask psychiatrists to reveal patient information that can compromise confidentiality. It may be unclear whether the information requested is overly inclusive or unnecessary given that cost containment is the primary reason for review.

Psychiatrists should develop parameters and practices that allow them to inform patients if needed care is unavailable or if qualified specialty providers are unavailable within the limits of their insurance plan. Referrals outside the system may be indicated if needed to ensure appropriate care. Clinicians also need to inform patients of options for treatment that extend beyond their benefits, because most insurance companies have mental health limitations. Furthermore, it is important to appeal adverse managed care decisions, and it may be necessary in some circumstances to provide medically necessary treatment in the emergency department setting even if reimbursement from the managed care organization does not appear forthcoming (Appelbaum 1993). Although a PES clinician may be tempted to alter reports to obtain prior approval, honesty is fundamental to the doctor-patient relationship and should not be compromised (Lazarus and Sharfstein 2002). It is incumbent on psychiatrists and PES clinicians to adapt to the constraints of managed care while maintaining their clinical professional ethics (Lazarus and Sharfstein 2002).

Key Clinical Points

- Clinicians in a psychiatric emergency service need to operate within the boundaries of law, ethics, and regulations and to be knowledgeable about the parameters of these boundaries as they apply to clinical practice.

- Psychiatrists should respect patients' confidentiality by making every effort to ensure the highest degree of privacy possible.

- Psychiatric emergency service staff should ensure proper assessment and formulation of the issues relevant to the requirements for involuntary hospitalization in order to preclude the abuse of power related to civil commitment.

- Determination of capacity to make medical decisions involves respecting the autonomy of patients who are capable of making such decisions and protecting those who do not have the capacity to make such decisions.

- Components of informed consent include disclosure, competence, and voluntariness. Informed consent requires that a physician disclose certain information to a patient and allow the patient to make an informed decision about his or her own care.

- Legislation and policies have been created to protect patients and health care providers from financial, institutional, and political pressures that may interfere with the ability to evaluate and treat patients in a psychiatric emergency service setting.

- Psychiatric emergency service clinicians and psychiatrists can anticipate and prepare for malpractice lawsuits by practicing professionally, seeking consultation in difficult cases, documenting clearly, using adequate risk assessment techniques, and arranging clear follow-up.

- Psychiatrists and psychiatric emergency service clinicians often must balance the need to adapt to the constraints of managed care with their obligation to maintain high ethical standards.

References

Alvarez MJ, Roura P, Osés A, et al: Prevalence and clinical impact of childhood trauma in patients with severe mental disorders. J Nerv Ment Dis 199(3):156–161, 2011 21346485

Appelbaum PS: Legal liability and managed care. Am Psychol 48(3):251–257, 1993 8317777

Appelbaum PS: Clinical practice. Assessment of patients' competence to consent to treatment. N Engl J Med 357(18):1834–1840, 2007 17978292

Appelbaum PS, Gutheil TG: Clinical Handbook of Psychiatry and the Law, 4th Edition. Philadelphia, PA, Wolters Kluwer/Lippincott Williams & Wilkins, 2007

Bazemore PH, Gitlin DF, Soreff S: Treatment of psychiatric hospital patients transferred to emergency departments. Psychosomatics 46(1):65–70, 2005 15765823

Brook M, Hilty DM, Liu W, et al: Discharge against medical advice from inpatient psychiatric treatment: a literature review. Psychiatr Serv 57(8):1192–1198, 2006 16870972

Byatt N, Pinals D, Arikan R: Involuntary hospitalization of medical patients who lack decisional capacity: an unresolved issue. Psychosomatics 47(5):443–448, 2006 16959935

Christopher PP, Pinals DA, Stayton T, Sanders K, Blumberg L: Nature and utilization of civil commitment for substance abuse in the United States. J Acad Psychiatry Law (in press)

Colognori D, Esseling P, Stewart C, et al: Self-disclosure and mental health service use in socially anxious adolescents. School Ment Health 4(4):219–230, 2012 24015156

Cutcliffe JR, Barker P: The Nurses' Global Assessment of Suicide Risk (NGASR): developing a tool for clinical practice. J Psychiatr Ment Health Nurs 11(4):393–400, 2004 15255912

Gutheil TG: Paranoia and progress notes: a guide to forensically informed psychiatric recordkeeping. Hosp Community Psychiatry 31(7):479–482, 1980 7380415

Herbert PB: The duty to warn: a reconsideration and critique. J Am Acad Psychiatry Law 30(3):417–424, 2002 12380423

Heslop L, Elsom S, Parker N: Improving continuity of care across psychiatric and emergency services: combining patient data within a participatory action research framework. J Adv Nurs 31(1):135–143, 2000 10632802

Hoge SK: On being "too crazy" to sign into a mental hospital: the issue of consent to psychiatric hospitalization. Bull Am Acad Psychiatry Law 22(3):431–450, 1994 7841515

Jaffe v Redmond, 518 U.S. 1 (1996)

Knox DK, Holloman GH Jr: Use and avoidance of seclusion and restraint: consensus statement of the American Association for Emergency Psychiatry Project BETA Seclusion and Restraint Workgroup. West J Emerg Med 13(1):35–40, 2012 22461919

Lamberg L: New tools aid violence risk assessment. JAMA 298(5):499–501, 2007 17666664

Lazarus JA, Sharfstein SS: Ethics in managed care. Psychiatr Clin North Am 25(3):561–574, 2002 12232970

Lidz CW, Mulvey EP, Appelbaum PS, et al: Commitment: the consistency of clinicians and the use of legal standards. Am J Psychiatry 146(2):176–181, 1989 2912259

Lindor RA, Campbell RL, Pines JM, et al.: EMTALA and patients with psychiatric emergencies: a review of relevant case law. Ann Emerg Med 64(5):439–444, 2014 24491351

MacArthur Research Network on Mental Health and the Law: MacArthur Coercion Study executive summary. February 2001. Available at: http://macarthur.virginia.edu/coercion.html. Accessed January 5, 2015.

Mermelstein HT, Wallack JJ: Confidentiality in the age of HIPAA: a challenge for psychosomatic medicine. Psychosomatics 49(2):97–103, 2008 18354061

Munetz MR, Roth LH: Informing patients about tardive dyskinesia. Arch Gen Psychiatry 42(9):866–871, 1985 2864030

Murray B: Informed consent: what must a physician disclose to a patient? AMA Journal of Ethics (formerly Virtual Mentor) 14(7):563–566, 2012. Available at: journalofethics.ama-assn.org/2012/07/hlaw1-1207.html. Accessed April 8, 2015.

Pinals DA: Informed consent: is your patient competent to consent to treatment? Curr Psychiatry 8:33–43, 2009

Pinals DA, Mossman D: Evaluation for Civil Commitment: Best Practices in Forensic Mental Health Assessment. New York, Oxford University Press, 2012

Quinn DK, Geppert CM, Maggiore WA: The Emergency Medical Treatment and Active Labor Act of 1985 and the practice of psychiatry. Psychiatr Serv 53(10):1301–1307, 2002 12364679

Saks SJ: Call 911: psychiatry and the new Emergency Medical Treatment and Active Labor Act (EMTALA) regulations. J Psychiatry Law 32(4):483–512, 2004 16018118

Shen JJ, Cochran CR, Moseley CB: From the emergency department to the general hospital: hospital ownership and market factors in the admission of the seriously mentally ill. J Healthc Manag 53(4):268–279, discussion 279–280, 2008 18720688

Simon RI, Goetz S: Forensic issues in the psychiatric emergency department. Psychiatr Clin North Am 22(4):851–864, 1999 10623974

Tarasoff v Regents of the University of California, 118 Cal Rptr 129, 529 P2d 553 (1974)

Tarasoff v Regents of the University of California, 17 Cal. 3d 425, 131 Cal Rptr 14, 551 P2d 334 (1976)

U.S. Department of Health and Human Services: The Health Insurance Portability and Accountability Act of 1996 (HIPAA) privacy rule. Available at: http://www.hhs.gov/ocr/privacy. Accessed January 5, 2015.

Weinstock R, Bonnici D, Seroussi A, et al: No duty to warn in California: now unambiguously solely a duty to protect. J Am Acad Psychiatry Law 42(1):101–108, 2014 24618525

Williams AR, Cohen S, Ford EB: Statutory definitions of mental illness for involuntary hospitalization as related to substance use disorders. Psychiatr Serv 65(5):634–640, 2014 24430580

Zinermon v Burch Z, 494 U.S. 418 (1979)

Suggested Readings

American Medical Association: Informed Consent. Available at: http://www.ama-assn.org/ama/pub/physician-resources/legal-topics/litigation-center/case-summaries-topic/informed-consent.page?. Accessed April 8, 2015.

Appelbaum PS: Clinical practice. Assessment of patients' competence to consent to treatment. N Engl J Med 357(18):1834–1840, 2007

Appelbaum PS, Gutheil TG: Clinical Handbook of Psychiatry and the Law, 4th Edition. Philadelphia, PA, Wolters Kluwer/Lippincott Williams & Wilkins, 2007

U.S. Department of Health and Human Services: The Health Insurance Portability and Accountability Act of 1996 (HIPAA) privacy rule. Available at: http://www.hhs.gov/ocr/privacy. Accessed January 5, 2015.

13

Supervision of Trainees in the Psychiatric Emergency Service

Monique James, M.D.

Erick Hung, M.D.

The psychiatric emergency service (PES) is often an intense, busy environment that provides assessments and care to severely ill psychiatric patients. It has become a main entry point into the mental health system for many patients and is often the only treatment setting for patients who are chronically mentally ill (Allen 1996; Schuster 1995). A busy PES is an excellent setting for trainees of mental health services because it offers many opportunities to view a wide range of acute psychopathology. Beginning in the early 1980s, a number of articles appeared focusing on the exciting learning opportunities in the PES and discussing ways to optimize learning experiences (Accreditation Council for Graduate Medical Education 2007; American Association for Emergency Psychiatry Education Committee 1998; American Medical Association 2002; Brasch and Ferencz 1999; Muhlbauer 1998). Furthermore, several groups, including the American Association for Emergency Psychiatry, have outlined model curricula for emergency psychiatry training (Brasch et al. 2004). As these curricula mature, psychiatric supervisors and educators must tend to how they supervise and teach emergency psychiatry. What makes emergency psychiatry supervision both exciting and challenging for the supervisor is the variety of settings, the vast array of professional interactions, and the diversity of roles that a supervisor must undoubtedly adopt.

Research confirms that the performance of medical students, as measured by knowledge and skills assessments, is directly related to the prowess of their teachers (Paice et al. 2002). Good teachers are recognized not only by their teaching abilities (i.e., organization and clarity of presentation, enthusiasm and stimulation of interest, group interaction skills) but also by their supervisory skills and "doctoring" qualities (i.e., competence, clinical knowledge, analytic ability, professionalism) (Kilminster and Jolly 2000).

Following principles of good supervision has a positive impact on both patient outcomes (Grainger 2002; Kilminster and Jolly 2000; McKee and Black 1992; Osborn et al. 1993) and trainee learning (Luck 2000). When more supervision is provided, patient satisfaction is higher, patients report fewer problems with care, and morbidity and mortality rates are lower. The effect of good supervision is greater when the trainee is less experienced and the cases are more complex (Kilminster and Jolly 2000). Good supervision reduces trainee stress and increases learning (Luck 2000). Trainees do not mind working long hours if they receive good support (Kilminster and Jolly 2000).

Work in medicine has many stressors, and failing to cope well with these stressors can lead to emotional exhaustion and burnout (Luck 2000; Willcock et al. 2004). Trainees who cannot cope with stress make significantly more errors (Jones et al. 1988). Increased stress leads to increased costs as a result of trainee absenteeism and litigation by patients against hospitals because of suboptimal care (Firth-Cozens 2003). The causes of poor performance may lie with the person, the system, or the supervisor (Lake and Ryan 2005). Supervision is often perceived to be inadequate by trainees, and lack of supervisors is one of their greatest stressors (Paice et al. 2002). The concept of supervision is more global than clinicians providing episodes of help with patient care (Kilminster and Jolly 2000). Planning is required to ensure that trainees provide high-quality patient care all the time, that their time in a particular clinical service provides a good opportunity for professional growth, and that

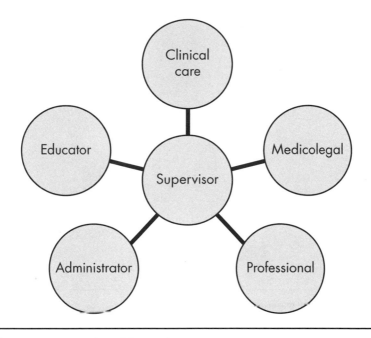

Figure 13–1.   Roles of the psychiatric emergency service supervisor.

potential problems are anticipated and prevented (Busari et al. 2005; Kilminster and Jolly 2000).

Psychiatric emergency settings vary based on 1) type of facility (e.g., independent community facility vs. academic teaching hospital), 2) proximity to medical emergency services, and 3) types of providers (e.g., psychiatrists, other physicians, psychologists, therapists, nurses, social workers, technicians). Consequently, the role of an emergency psychiatry supervisor is broad. As shown in Figure 13–1, a supervisor's duties include providing clinical care to patients, assuring that each patient receives a quality standard of care; abiding by legal statutes; working in complex systems and administration; and modeling professionalism. In addition, and perhaps most important, educating mental health trainees is a core responsibility.

Although the emergency psychiatry supervisor wears many hats, we focus in this chapter on the supervisor's role as an educator in a PES. To be a competent clinician-educator in emergency psychiatry, the supervisor must first

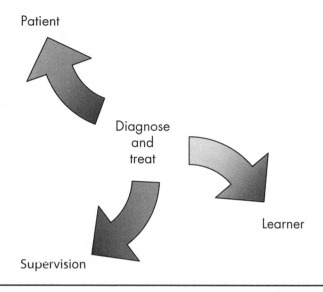

Patient

Diagnose
and
treat

Learner

Supervision

Figure 13–2. Centrality of diagnosis and treatment.

be able to diagnose and treat the patient, then diagnose and treat the learner, and finally diagnose and treat the supervision (Figure 13–2).

Duties include understanding and assessing the learner and then teaching to the learner's level and educational needs. To improve as educators, supervisors must be able to self-reflect, collaborate with colleagues, and solicit feedback from learners. In "diagnosing" the supervision, supervisors need to assess the strengths and weaknesses of the teaching encounter. In "treating" the supervision, supervisors need to clarify areas of confusion, modify styles of teaching, and address any tensions in the learning climate.

Diagnose and Treat the Patient

Other chapters in this book have addressed specific clinical issues in emergency psychiatry relating to the diagnosis and treatment of patients in the emergency setting. The challenge for supervisors in the psychiatric emergency training service is that they must diagnose and treat patients in a learning environment, while tending to the dual and at times conflicting needs of patients and trainees. Consequently, supervision can take a variety of forms.

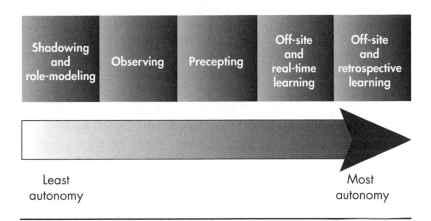

Figure 13–3. Spectrum of supervision.

One organizational schema for forms of supervision is based on the degree of learner autonomy (Figure 13–3).

At the beginning of the spectrum, learners essentially shadow the supervisor as he or she provides direct clinical care in the PES. At this stage, learning is through observation. The learner takes part in a discussion in which the supervisor discloses thoughts about the case, while walking the learner through the decision-making process that led to a particular differential diagnosis or treatment plan. As a learner progresses to being more autonomous, the supervisor may ask the learner, after shadowing a clinical interview, what the learner's impressions are of the case. The supervisor increases the learner's autonomy and potential for learning by moving away from self-disclosure of his or her own thought process and toward questioning the learner to provide thoughts and impressions regarding the case.

Learner autonomy is further increased when the supervisor asks the learner to engage in the interview with the patient. At this stage, the supervisor is more of a direct observer in the room, allowing the learner to conduct the psychiatric interview independently. The supervisor may interject intermittently during critical teaching moments, but ultimately these should decrease in frequency as learner autonomy is maximized. Further autonomy is achieved when the learner independently interviews the patient in the PES and then presents the case to the supervisor immediately following the interview. In this situation, the supervisor is present on the service and is immediately available to precept the case. Removing the supervisor from the physical vicinity of the learner allows the learner to interview the patient, formulate an initial assessment and plan, and then discuss the case immediately with the off-site supervisor. At this stage, the real-time supervision provides opportunities to impact the formulation and direction of clinical care as it progresses, while simultaneously allowing for significantly more learner autonomy. Often, this stage of supervision takes place on call overnight in the PES, where the supervisor discusses the case with the trainee over the phone and collaborates on the diagnosis and treatment plan.

In the final stage of the supervision spectrum, the supervisory experience is disconnected from the direct clinical care of the patient. At this stage, supervision takes place off-site and retrospectively. The supervision may occur the following day, week, or even month after the direct clinical care. Unquestionably, this final stage of supervision maximizes the learner's degree of individual autonomy. It should be noted that learners will not always be interns or medical students in the first years of training. In some cases, the learner may be a senior trainee with years of clinical experience. In other cases, the learner is a professional peer requesting supervision for consultation and self-growth.

Thus, the spectrum of supervision is broad and complex. Teaching and effective supervision inevitably take place at every stage on the spectrum. However, the essential point in creating a successful supervision encounter is not where a supervisor falls on the spectrum, but rather *how* he or she decides where on the spectrum to mold the supervision experience. Several factors influence this choice, including learner needs, clinical considerations, medicolegal considerations, and system constraints (Figure 13–4). The tension between these factors and learner educational needs is always present in a PES with trainees. Because of this tension, it is also necessary to focus on the educational needs of the learner and thereby foster an effective supervision experience, as discussed in the following section.

Diagnose and Treat the Learner

Diagnosing and treating the learner can be a challenging yet exciting experience for the supervisor. How does a supervisor know whether the learner is

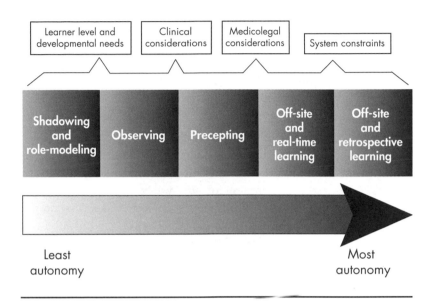

Figure 13–4. Factors influencing spectrum of supervision.

really learning from the teaching session? How does a supervisor assess the learner's needs? Even assuming accurate assessment, how does the supervisor best teach to that learner's level? Supervisors (particularly those who are "natural teachers") may accomplish aspects of diagnosing and treating the learner intuitively, but for many supervisors, clinical teaching skills are not innate. Most supervisors have experienced both effective and poor teaching styles during their own training and need to be sensitive to the impact these styles have on trainees' competence and confidence. The supervisor who is starting out in clinical teaching, however, can be uncertain about what constitutes a successful teaching interaction. Fortunately, over the past two decades, an explosion of research has occurred in medical education. Several easy-to-use models help supervisors elicit learners' educational needs, teach to their learners' level, and provide effective feedback (Neher and Stevens 2003; Neher et al. 1992; Pangaro 1999; Wolpaw et al. 2003). In this section, we highlight some of the most helpful models that can be useful for effective teaching in busy PESs, as well as for providing feedback.

RIME Model

Pangaro (1999) initially described the RIME model as a developmental framework for assessing learners in clinical settings. He described a progressive continuum of four performance levels: reporter, interpreter, manager, and educator. In 2002, Battistone et al. proposed an additional introductory stage for the model—that of observer.

Preceptors can use this model to assess the level of an individual learner's clinical performance during case presentations in the PES. Learners at the observer level (e.g., early first-year medical students) will not yet have the skills to take a pertinent history or present findings about a patient. Learners at the reporter level (e.g., second-year medical students) will be able to reliably, respectfully, and honestly gather information, write basic notes, differentiate normal from abnormal, and present their findings. Interpreters (e.g., early third-year medical students) will be able to present a patient case, select the important issues, offer a differential diagnosis, and support arguments for or against various diagnoses. Learners at the manager level (e.g., most late-third-year medical students) will be able to present the case, offer a differential diagnosis, and formulate diagnostic and therapeutic plans. Learners who have reached the educator level will be able to do all of the above, as well as define important questions, research information regarding the topic, and educate others. Some students attain educator-level skills by the time they graduate from medical school, whereas others may not achieve this level until they are residents.

The value of the RIME model is that it provides a common descriptive terminology that is highly acceptable to learners and preceptors (Ogburn and Espey 2003). The RIME descriptors are nonjudgmental and assist supervisors in giving meaningful feedback. This model could easily be introduced during an orientation to the PES for learners at any level of training and will establish a shared vocabulary for feedback.

Table 13–1 presents an example of the use of the RIME model in a clinical scenario—that of a young woman with an acute manic episode who presents for mental health evaluation and care. This same clinical scenario will be used with subsequent educational models so the various models can easily be compared and contrasted.

Table 13–1. Example of use of RIME model

RIME level	Description	Case presentation by RIME level	Preceptor coaching response
Observer	Understands only what is happening	"The patient is a 26-year-old female. She was brought into the psychiatric emergency service by the police on an involuntary hold."	"Good. Now, go in and ask the patient herself to describe to you what she is feeling."
Reporter	Understands "what" is wrong	"…and the police report that she was running down the main street, half-naked, screaming that God has given her the power to fly.…She endorses feeling on top of the world, racing thoughts, pressured speech, grandiose ideas, decreased need for sleep, and impulsively using street drugs. She denies psychotic or anxiety symptoms."	"Excellent report. Now, 'interpret' these symptoms for me. What do you think could be going on? Let's come up with a differential diagnosis."
Interpreter	Understands "why" it is wrong	"Based on her symptoms and past psychiatric history, I believe she has an acute manic episode in the context of a bipolar illness secondary to recent medication nonadherence. Other possibilities include schizoaffective disorder, substance-induced mood disorder, drug intoxication, or delirium."	"Excellent differential diagnosis. Now, how will we proceed to 'manage' the workup?"
Manager	Understands "how" to address the problem	"I'll complete the workup by ordering a set of baseline labs including lithium level and urine toxicology screen. I'll also assess her orientation by completing the Folstein Mini-Mental State Examination. I plan to treat her with drug X to target her manic symptoms. I also think we should put her in an open seclusion room to minimize stimulation from other patients."	"That sounds like a first-class workup and an excellent plan. Why would you choose this particular drug instead of drug Y?"

Table 13–1.   Example of use of RIME model *(continued)*

RIME level	Description	Case presentation by RIME level	Preceptor coaching response
Educator	Committed to self-learning and education of the team	"This case seems representative of a typical manic presentation. According to the Texas algorithm for acute mania, we should also consider starting an atypical antipsychotic or mood stabilizer. Also, the algorithm suggests that drug X is more cost-effective and efficacious than drug Y."	"Good job. You are right on top of the latest literature. Now let's get you a more complicated case."

One-Minute Preceptor Model

Often, after presenting a patient to a preceptor, learners tend to end their presentations and wait for the preceptor to formulate the case and discuss an assessment and plan for the patient. In a busy emergency care setting, preceptors may be tempted to jump right in and discuss their thoughts and opinions immediately after hearing the case. The unfortunate danger in this approach is that the preceptor does not assess the learner's knowledge or skill level. Because this interaction is typical of many teaching encounters (Irby and Papadakis 2001; Parsell and Bligh 2001; Tiberius et al. 2002; Ullian et al. 1994), preceptors may feel that they are being effective teachers when in essence they have not fully engaged their learners in "owning" the learning process. The one-minute preceptor model, originally developed by Neher et al. (1992) and subsequently modified by Neher and Stevens (2003), is a five-step model that helps supervisors assess the learner and teach to the learner's level. The following are the five parts or microskills of the model: get a commitment, probe for supporting evidence, teach general rules, reinforce what was done right, and correct mistakes.

By asking the learner specific questions based on the model, the preceptor can effectively understand the learner's current knowledge and skill level, tailor training to teach toward specific learning needs, and provide formative, specific feedback to the learner. The model has been studied in outpatient settings in multiple specialties, with both learners and preceptors describing significant improvement and confidence in their teaching skills after using the model (Aagaard et al. 2004; Furney et al. 2001; Irby et al. 2004; Neher and Stevens 2003; Parrot et al. 2006; Salerno et al. 2002).

Using the five steps in the one-minute preceptor model will help the supervisor assess the learner more effectively, provide more targeted teaching, create a culture of positive reinforcement and constructive feedback, and ultimately improve the teaching encounter on behalf of the learner and the educator. The model can easily be delivered in busy PESs with trainees. Table 13–2 provides an example of the use of the one-minute preceptor model in the clinical scenario of the young woman with an acute manic episode who was introduced in Table 13–1.

SNAPPS Model

In busy emergency settings, learners have a tendency to become relatively passive reporters focused on presenting history and objective findings to the preceptor (Wolpaw et al. 2003). Foley et al. (1979; cited in Wolpaw et al. 2003) directly observed teaching encounters and found that students were passive and received a preponderance of low-level, factual information. Learners were seldom asked questions and rarely asked to verbalize their problem-solving efforts. Based on work in cognitive learning and on reflective practice for educators, the SNAPPS model is a collaborative model for case presentations in an outpatient setting that can easily be translated to the emergency setting. The SNAPPS model for case presentations follows a mnemonic consisting of six steps: summarize, narrow, analyze, probe, plan, and select (see descriptions of steps and sample questions in Table 13–3).

The SNAPPS model links learner initiation and preceptor facilitation in an active learning conversation. It focuses on what supervisors can do to empower learners and enable trainees to contribute more to the clinical encounters. Rather than passively awaiting the preceptor's assessment of the learning climate, learners are expected to identify their own learning goals. The learner-driven educational encounter in the emergency setting emphasizes the role of the learner and the supervisor in a collaborative learning conversation. In this teaching and learning "dance," one partner may lead, but each must know the steps. Wolpaw et al. (2003) advocated that the learner can and should be taught to lead. The preceptor or supervisor may coach the learner until the steps become automatic but should avoid taking over the conversation.

Table 13–2.   Example of use of one-minute preceptor model

Microskills	Description	Preceptor questions/comments	Common pitfalls
Get a commitment	After hearing a presentation or seeing a patient together, ask the learner what he or she thinks. *Rationale:* Learners should be involved in processing and problem solving as opposed to just collecting data.	"What do you think is going on with this patient?" "What do you think is the most important issue to address today?" "What would you like to accomplish during this evaluation?" "What do you think led to the patient's current manic episode?" "What do you think has been contributing to this patient's medication nonadherence?"	Quickly offering your own opinion Asking for more data only Jumping straight into a mini-teaching session
Probe for supporting evidence	Ask the learner for evidence that supports his or her opinion. *Rationale:* Asking learners to reveal their thought processes allows you to identify what they do and do not know.	"What were the major findings that led to your conclusion?" "What else did you consider?" "What facts led you away from acute mania"	Grilling the learner Giving away the answer too quickly

Table 13–2.   Example of use of one-minute preceptor model *(continued)*

Microskills	Description	Preceptor questions/comments	Common pitfalls
Teach general rules	Make one or two brief teaching points tied to the case. *Rationale:* Teaching is more memorable and transferable when it is offered as a general rule and when it is tied to a clinical experience.	"Like we see in your patient, most patients with acute mania have these core features:…"	Trying to accomplish too much in a single teaching encounter Providing unsupported, idiosyncratic personal opinions
Reinforce what was done right	Comment on specific work that was done well and what effect it has on patient care. *Rationale:* Skills in learners are vulnerable and become well established with reinforcement.	"You did a good job asking specific and detailed questions about the patient's sleep patterns throughout the night." "Excellent: detailed and nonjudgmental history taking on the patient's recent substance abuse."	Giving feedback that is too general (e.g., "Great job!")
Correct mistakes	Identify mistakes to the learner as soon as possible in an appropriate setting, and discuss how to avoid or correct the error in the future. *Rationale:* Mistakes left unattended have a good chance of being repeated.	"Given the patient's recent suicide attempt, 'we'll need to get more information from a family member and therapist instead of just relying on today's visit for all the information."	Providing judgmental feedback (e.g., "Terrible job—even a high school kid would have known to ask about current suicidality!")

Table 13–3. Example of use of SNAPPS model

Step	Preceptor directive	Example response by learner
Summarize	Summarize briefly the history and findings	"The patient is a 26-year-old woman who was brought into the psychiatric emergency service by the police on an involuntary hold. Her current symptoms include euphoria, grandiosity, racing thoughts, pressured speech, decreased need for sleep, and impulsively using street drugs. She has not been adherent to medications prescribed to her for bipolar disorder."
Narrow	Narrow the differential to two or three relevant possibilities	"The patient's clinical presentation is consistent with an acute manic episode. This episode could be explained by several possibilities: 1) an exacerbation of her bipolar disorder in the context of medication noncompliance; 2) a substance-induced mood disorder secondary to recent stimulant intoxication; or 3) a delirium secondary to electrolyte abnormalities."
Analyze	Analyze the differential by comparing and contrasting the possibilities	"I think that the most likely possibility is an exacerbation of the patient's bipolar disorder in the context of medication noncompliance. The supporting evidence for this possibility is that the patient's family told me that she has not been taking her medications at home over the past month. A substance-induced mood disorder is less likely because the patient denies any recent substance use. A delirium seems less likely because the patient is fully oriented and does not have any medical risk factors for electrolyte abnormalities."

Table 13–3. Example of use of SNAPPS model (*continued*)

Step	Preceptor directive	Example response by learner
Probe	Probe the preceptor by asking questions about uncertainties, difficulties, or alternative approaches	"I am uncertain as to how much I should believe the patient when she says that she has not used any substances recently. I have been mistaken in the past. I do not know what objective clinical examination findings I could observe in patients with stimulant intoxication." "I also am not sure how to structure an interview with a manic patient. In this interview, I feel that the patient controlled the questioning, and I had difficulty redirecting the patient."
Plan	Plan management for the patient's psychiatric issues	"I would like to gather more collateral information from the patient's outpatient mental health clinic. Given that the patient is acutely manic right now, I would like to order a urine toxicology screen and basic labs. Additionally, I would like to minimize the patient's stimulation in the milieu and start an atypical antipsychotic and a benzodiazepine. What do you think about this management plan?"
Select	Select a case-related issue for self-directed learning	"I am not entirely sure what algorithms have been developed for the management of acute mania. I have heard about the Texas algorithm but would like to read more about it. Maybe I will look up a flowchart and present it to you on our next teaching encounter."

SNAPPS makes learners do most of the work, through justifying their thinking and exploring what they do not know (rather than having the preceptor question them on what they do know). A pilot study of SNAPPS showed that learners were more actively involved and readily came up with questions, unlike in more traditional interactions (Wolpaw et al. 2003). Supervisors could respond to learners rather than thinking up novel questions (Wolpaw et al. 2003).

When teaching, clinicians often ask questions aimed at elucidating low-level knowledge. In 1933, John Dewey, one of the most influential thinkers on education in the twentieth century, proposed that thinking and problem solving occurred not when answering a question posed by a teacher, but when attempting to solve a problem important to the learner (Irby and Papadakis 2001). People learn more from what they "don't know" than from what they "do know." Therefore, shifting from asking, "What is the cause of...?" to "What are you uncertain about?" moves away from simple factual recall and promotes thinking. SNAPPS is a strategy to introduce this approach.

Tips for Effective Feedback

Giving feedback is an essential skill for all supervisors, yet techniques for giving *effective* feedback are rarely taught in clinical medical education. By definition, *feedback* is the ongoing appraisal of performance based on direct observation aimed at changing or sustaining behavior (Aagaard et al. 2004). The literature on effective feedback focuses on several strategies, including creating a safe learning environment for feedback, reviewing educational objectives, providing a format for delivering feedback, and dealing with poorly performing trainees (Gordon 2003). The following guidelines, summarized in Table 13–4, can improve a supervisor's effectiveness in providing meaningful feedback to trainees.

1. *Understand educational goals and objectives from the beginning.* Before a trainee begins working in the PES, it is essential for supervisors to give a brief orientation, outlining the educational goals and objectives during the time spent on the service. Educational learning goals and objectives often overlap with the expectations and needs of the service, but to the greatest extent possible, educational goals should be highlighted separately from the service needs. For effective feedback to occur, learners

Table 13–4. Ten tips for effective feedback

 1. Understand educational goals and objectives from the beginning.
 2. Maintain a safe learning environment.
 3. Foster mutual respect.
 4. Provide feedback in a timely manner.
 5. Provide feedback that is specific.
 6. Limit feedback to a few objectives at a time.
 7. Provide feedback in a specific format.
 8. Label feedback as feedback.
 9. Limit feedback to behaviors that are remedial.
10. Solicit feedback rather than impose it.

need to understand what the actual educational goals and objectives are, because these are the markers against which they will be measured.

2. *Maintain a safe learning environment.* Provide a safe setting for students to experience autonomy in data gathering and initial evaluation of patients. For patients on the service whose cases are less acute, learners are encouraged to be the first "clinician" beyond the triage desk. For patients whose cases are more acute (e.g., those requiring emergent medications, seclusion, or restraint), learners are often involved in more peripheral tasks or observer status; however, supervisors must ensure that learning issues and learners' performance are addressed once the patient has been stabilized.

3. *Foster mutual respect.* Supervisors should show learners the respect they would give to any other colleague. Anything that helps the trainee see feedback as an informed, nonevaluative, objective appraisal of performance intended to improve his or her own clinical skills (rather than as an estimate of his or her personal worth) will help in the process. When feedback fails, it is usually because it led to trainee anger, defensiveness, or embarrassment.

4. *Provide feedback in a timely manner.* Feedback should not necessarily be restricted to a scheduled session designed solely for the purpose of performance appraisal. Often, in fact, the most effective feedback occurs on a day-to-day basis, as part of the flow of work on the service and as close to the event as possible. This maximizes both trainee and supervisor capacity to remember specific aspects of the clinical and teaching interaction. Fur-

thermore, it provides ample opportunity for trainees to improve skills and to demonstrate their improvement to the supervisor. Of course, the pace of events in the emergency psychiatry setting can be challenging to seasoned preceptors and daunting to trainees. Despite this challenge, feedback can be effectively done "on the run" as the supervisor reviews a case's progression or the communication skills of a trainee in conveying only essential information.

5. *Provide feedback that is specific.* Feedback should deal with specifics, making use of real examples. Generalizations, such as references to a trainee's organizational ability, efficiency, or diligence, rarely convey useful information and are far too broad to be helpful as feedback. For example, saying, "Gee, what a great job you did," may bolster the learner's self-esteem but does not really provide a meaningful assessment of his or her performance.

6. *Limit feedback to a few objectives at a time.* The supervisor can often give a lot of very useful feedback to the learner after a clinical encounter. However, even the most well-intentioned and informative feedback session can be diminished if the supervisor provides an exhaustive, all-inclusive list. Limiting feedback to a few pearls at a time (generally one to three points) not only allows the learner to digest the information appropriately but also forces the supervisor to establish more frequent feedback sessions. Additionally, limiting feedback encourages the supervisor to actively determine what his or her two or three most important teaching points should be.

7. *Provide feedback in a specific format.* Many educators like the "feedback sandwich" technique: 1) start with acknowledging something that the learner did well, 2) offer constructive critique of an area for growth, and 3) finish with another area of strength. Other educators believe that overemphasis on the positive may undermine appreciation for and attention to the deficiency. Regardless of the specific format, the crucial element in providing feedback is that it should be descriptive and nonjudgmental.

Information that is shared with the trainee should focus on actions rather than interpretations or assumed intentions. Data based on actions not only are more accurate but also allow for psychological distance, a critical component when the feedback is negative or the trainee is insecure. Subjective data are also perfectly appropriate for feedback about clinical skills. When included as part of the feedback, subjective data should be clearly labeled as such. When dealing with personal reactions and opinions, "I" statements should be used. When the supervisor says, for example, "In watching this videotape, I began to feel that you were not comfortable talking about the patient's recent suicide attempt," the trainee is allowed to view the assessment as one person's reaction. Even more preferable are statements such as, "I saw your hand shaking; you abruptly changed the subject," which allow the trainee to interpret the behavior.

8. *Label feedback as feedback.* Unless feedback is explicitly labeled, learners will fail to recognize feedback and supervisors will not be recognized for their efforts. Supervisors need to clearly identify their comments as constructive or formative feedback on the performance for that shift or clinical encounter. Helping learners understand that the comments to come are intended to foster their improvement rather than serve as an evaluation reduces the likelihood that a learner will receive the feedback in an emotionally charged fashion.

9. *Limit feedback to behaviors that are remedial.* The supervisor should limit feedback to behavior that the learner can correct or improve. If observed behaviors are not within the trainee's power to change or are far beyond his or her developmental level, then these should not be included as feedback. Such deficits, if they are substantial, mean that the trainee should alter his or her goals, not the process by which he or she attempts to meet a goal. Preceptors who find themselves frustrated with a trainee should take a 5-minute time-out before providing criticism.

10. *Solicit feedback rather than impose it.* Feedback works best when it is solicited rather than imposed. By first soliciting feedback from a learner on his or her own performance, the supervisor conveys a positive message that both learner and supervisor can improve their communication and performance. Furthermore, the trainee should take an active part in the process, and the supervisor's open-ended questions can help break the ice. If both parties can reach agreement on these questions, they will have an agenda for the remainder of the discussion.

Stop, Keep, Start Method for Feedback

One effective approach for giving concise and specific feedback to learners is the Stop, Keep, Start method (DeLong 2011; DeLong and DeLong 2011). Using this technique, the supervisor chooses to discuss with the learner one thing from each of three categories:

> Stop: What is one thing the learner is doing that is ineffective and should be stopped?
> Keep: What is one thing that is working well for the learner and should be continued?
> Start: What is one new thing the learner should consider doing in the future?

The supervisor should strive to communicate specific points that are attuned to the learner's current knowledge and skill level. Feedback such as "Continue taking great histories" is not specific and therefore not very useful for the learner. Instead, feedback such as "Continue asking about length of time and side effects on previous medication trials" is more specific and invites further discussion about the importance of this particular history taking skill. The supervisor should be careful to adhere to citing only *one* thing in each category. Otherwise, the learner may become overwhelmed, which can lead to difficulty prioritizing change. Also, with this method, the supervisor and learner can easily track the learner's incorporation of specific feedback items.

Diagnose and Treat the Supervision

Supervisors need to assess their own teaching skills. There are times when educational efforts fail, and lack of assessment of the teaching in those moments guarantees that the learner will continue to flounder. This section explores crucial elements of supervision, mechanisms to be reflective in teaching, and ways to troubleshoot an unsuccessful teaching experience by evaluating structural and teacher-learner dyadic barriers to good teaching.

Qualities of a Good Supervisor

A good supervisor does the following:

• Ensures that both supervisor and trainee are clear about their respective roles and responsibilities for the encounter, particularly with regard to patient care.

- Informs the trainee how supervision will occur (e.g., that time will be set aside to observe the trainee's performance).
- Provides feedback in a positive way. Unless weaknesses are tackled in a clear, unambiguous way, trainees will not get the message.
- Makes time to get to know the trainee as a person, as someone who has a life outside medicine as well. It can be interesting and impressive to learn what trainees can do, along with letting them learn something of the supervisor's own life.
- Recognizes that power factors (e.g., age, gender, sexuality, race) may influence the relationship. If any of these cause a problem that cannot be satisfactorily resolved, a different supervisor should be found for the trainee.

Another way of considering the qualities of a good supervisor is to examine the factors that are associated with a happy trainee (Firth-Cozens 2003; Jaques 2003; Jones et al. 1988; Lake and Ryan 2004a, 2004b, 2004c, 2005; Luck 2000; Paice et al. 2002; Willcock et al. 2004). Among these factors are the following:

- Being supported, especially out of hours
- Being given responsibility for patient care
- Being involved in good teamwork
- Receiving feedback
- Having a supportive learning environment
- Being stimulated to learn
- Having a supervisor take a personal interest in him or her

Being Reflective in Teaching

Improvements in a supervisor's teaching can occur only if he or she reflects on how each encounter went (Irby and Papadakis 2001; Wall and McAleer 2000). The supervisor can do this in simple ways, such as these:

- Ask oneself, "How did that go? What went well? If I did it again tomorrow, what would I change to make it better?" Too often supervisors rush on to the next busy task and never do this, then find themselves doing the same thing year after year.

- Ask the learners for both verbal and written feedback. Ask them what they thought went well and what could be improved. Ask them to write down any points that were not clear, then collect and read the comments to find out what still confuses them. Also, ask learners to fill in an evaluation form.
- Review the learners' progress. Next time, consider whether they remembered the lessons taught and whether they performed well in assessments. Don't ask, "What did I teach?" but rather "What did they learn?"
- Ask a colleague to observe one's teaching and provide structured feedback.

Although it may not seem possible, "just-in-time" teaching can be thought of as a planned learning activity (Cantillon 2003; Gordon 2003; Kaufman 2003; Lake and Ryan 2004a, 2004b; Morrison 2003). Supervisors in PESs know that 1) they will be busy, 2) they will be teaching, and 3) certain topics are likely to recur. Therefore, planning is critical for effective "just-in-time" teaching. By being reflective about teaching, an instructor can refine his or her lessons so that each iteration will be better than the one that preceded it. With experience, supervisors build up teaching scripts on common topics (e.g., acute mania), including components related to diagnosis, management, social circumstances, and so forth (Kaufman 2003). Supervisors can then draw on these scripts in the context of assessing the patient, to guide them in covering the essential teaching points. This can be in a 5-minute opportune moment, a 20-minute interactive tutorial, or a 1-hour lecture, as appropriate.

Troubleshooting an Unsuccessful Teaching Event: Structural Barriers

Supervisors cite several factors that can lead to poor teaching encounters, each of which can be overcome with personal efforts, such as reading about education in book chapters such as this one, as well as preparation, such as the tips and suggestions offered in the previous two subsections (see "Qualities of a Good Supervisor" and "Being Reflective in Teaching"). The factors that lead to poor teaching encounters include the following:

- *Lack of time:* The single most important factor clinicians cite is lack of time, due to increased patient and administrative loads. Other contributors to the time problem include shorter hospital stays, sicker patients, and fewer patients that may be appropriate "teaching cases." These pressures are unlikely to be resolved in the near future (Spencer 2003).

- *Lack of training:* Most clinical educators have never been taught how to teach, supervise, or assess, regardless of whether the trainees are students, junior doctors, or other health professionals in training (Gibson and Campbell 2000).
- *Criticism of teaching:* Although most educators diligently try to teach well, they often learn that their trainees rated them poorly, which leads to diminished motivation to improve teaching. Some clinical supervisors have been found to teach by humiliation and sarcasm, provide poor supervision and assessment, teach in variable and unpredictable ways, and provide insufficient feedback (Irby 1995). An inquiry into the clinical services at a tertiary hospital noted poor supervision and training and recommended that all senior doctors should partake in "train-the-trainer" courses (Douglas et al. 2001).
- *Lack of rewards:* Material rewards and recognition for teaching remain inadequate. To cope with these challenges, educators need both knowledge and skills (Spencer 2003; Wall and McAleer 2000) to teach effectively in the clinical setting.

Despite a supervisor's best efforts, there will still be barriers that will diminish the quality of teaching. Supervisors need to recognize that not all "moments" in the clinical setting are good teaching moments. Enhancing the number, length, and frequency of good teaching moments requires the supervisor to consider the following (Douglas et al. 2001):

- Are the learners (or supervisor) distracted by other duties, time constraints, tiredness, or hunger?
- Is the location busy, noisy, too public, or uncomfortable?
- What is the atmosphere? Do the learners feel comfortable demonstrating their lack of knowledge and asking questions, or are they fearful of being humiliated?
- Do the learners feel as though they belong? Do they believe that their opinion is valued?
- Do the patients know what is expected? Have they agreed to be involved? Is their dignity respected?

In the emergency department, where patients may be agitated and dangerous to others, the safety of the environment is a critical factor to assess when determining why an educational effort was less than successful. If the environment is not safe (e.g., in the case of threatening behavior by the patient), then fear will preclude this autonomy and the learner will be less able to engage in and learn from the clinical situation. Assurance of safety may even require specific instruction in how to remain safe in the face of dangerous situations.

Troubleshooting an Unsuccessful Teaching Event: Dyadic Barriers

If the environment was right and the teacher was appropriately positioned to teach but there was still a failure in the educational intervention, then perhaps something in the teacher-learner relationship led to the failure. To address this possibility, the teacher should be aware of two critical theoretical concepts: 1) the psychological distance between a teacher and a learner and 2) basic adult learning theory.

The teacher-learner relationship has an enormous impact on the quality of teaching and learning, with interpersonal variables accounting for half the variance in teaching effectiveness (Tiberius et al. 2002). Positive interpersonal relationships between teachers and learners increase the quality of teaching (Deci et al. 1991). The concepts of psychological size and psychological distance are crucial for understanding what aspects in the interpersonal environment contribute to a successful learning climate (Vaughn and Baker 2004). *Psychological size* is defined as the perceived status that one person has relative to another (e.g., the difference between trainee and teacher). *Psychological distance* relates to the degree of positive and negative emotional connectedness in a relationship. Vaughn and Baker (2004) used these concepts in examining 45 pediatric preceptor-resident pairs engaged in longitudinal continuity training experiences. They demonstrated that both residents and preceptors perceived the residents as having a smaller psychological size than the preceptors, and that residents perceived greater psychological distance in the relationship than did preceptors. This distance was significantly related to both residents' satisfaction with particular preceptors and their perception of the preceptors' effectiveness. Teachers who are able to capitalize on specific strategies to emphasize their interpersonal relationships (i.e., by reducing the psychological size difference and distance in the relationship) can facilitate the learning process in general and simultaneously increase learners' sense of self and their professional and personal competence. Some specific strategies to consider include using

Table 13–5. Questions to optimize the learning climate

Category	Specific questions
Personal motivation	Are trainees interested and eager to learn (internal motivation), or do they want to learn simply to pass an exam (external motivation)?
Meaningful topic	Is the topic relevant to trainees' current work or future plans? Have you made it clear why it is important?
Experience-centered focus	Is learning linked to the work trainees are doing and based on the care they are giving patients?
Appropriate level of knowledge	Is learning pitched at the correct level for a trainee's stage of training?
Clear goals	Have you articulated the anticipated outcome goals so that everyone knows where you are heading?
Active involvement	Do trainees have the opportunity to be actively involved in the learning process and to influence the outcomes and process?
Regular feedback	Do trainees know how they are doing? Have you told them what they are doing well (positive critique), as well as what areas could be improved?
Time for reflection	Have you given trainees time and encouragement to reflect on the subject and their performance (self-assessment)? Shifting from thinking about what you want to teach to what trainees want to learn (e.g., asking what areas they are unclear about) shifts from a teacher-centered to a learner-centered approach.

first names reciprocally, sharing one's own experiences as a trainee, using self-disclosure as appropriate, and taking time to learn about trainees' hobbies or other professional and personal obligations.

The trainees in PESs are adults who want to learn. If it appears that learning is not progressing, supervisors should consider whether their own teaching style and their trainees' learning styles are congruent, as well as whether the clinical setting is conducive to learning. Adults like to have an input into their learning. Adult learning principles are not evidence based but should be regarded as "models of assumption about learning" (Deci et al. 1991; Kaufman 2003; Newman and Peile 2002). Questions to consider in optimizing the learning climate are provided in Table 13–5.

As educators, supervisors in PESs need to be flexible to suit the learners and the circumstances. Learning is about creating knowledge based on integrating new information with old, an active process that challenges the learner's prior knowledge (Peyton 1998; Vaughn and Baker 2001). As each learner progresses, a shift often occurs from being dependent (where the learner needs substantial input and direction) to being interested (where the learner needs some guidance) to being self-directed (where the learner takes personal responsibility for his or her own learning). A supervisor's teaching style needs to take into account trainees' prior knowledge and stage of learning (Hutchinson 2003; Parsell and Bligh 2001; Vaughn and Baker 2001).

Expecting a struggling trainee to define his or her own needs or presenting a mini-lecture to an experienced trainee will discourage both. Nevertheless, a degree of mismatch can challenge a learner and be a good thing. Shifting teaching styles from authoritarian (telling students what to learn) to delegating (getting them to decide what they need to know) shifts the workload away from the supervisor and makes teaching and learning more fun. Also, learners like to learn in different ways at different times; sometimes a didactic presentation is perfectly appropriate. The key is targeting the teaching to the "learning edge"—wherever that may be for each learner and at that specific moment. Figure 13–5 provides a framework to minimize the degree of mismatch between a teacher's style and specific student's stage of learning such that the teaching encounter can be optimal.

Conclusion

The PES provides a rich environment for patient encounters, rapid clinical decision making, and opportunities for trainees to experiment with a variety of interventional strategies. Although emergency psychiatry supervisors take on many roles on a PES, the educator role is crucial in any teaching service. In this chapter, we discussed the three components to being a good supervisor for trainees on the service: knowing how to diagnose and treat 1) the patient, 2) the learner, and 3) the supervision itself. In practicing the strategies and suggestions outlined for each of these three components, supervisors will be able to be effective, meaningful, and influential educators for trainees. Good teaching not only helps satisfy the clinical work in the emergency setting but also is essential in the training of future mental health providers.

Learner stages	Teaching styles		
	Authority	Motivator/Facilitator	Delegator
Dependent learner	**Match**	Mild mismatch	Severe mismatch
Interested learner	Mild mismatch	**Match**	Mild mismatch
Self-directed learner	Severe mismatch	Mild mismatch	**Match**

Figure 13–5.   Matching of learner stages to teacher styles.

Key Clinical Points

- An effective educator needs to be able to diagnose and treat the patient in a supervision framework that matches the clinical demands and the learner's needs.

- Effective teaching involves understanding and assessing the learner and teaching the learner at his or her educational level.

- The RIME model is useful to assess the level of an individual learner's clinical performance.

- An effective educator needs to reflect actively on the teaching method before, during, and after every teaching encounter.

- In assessing the teaching encounter, educators should clarify areas of confusion, modify styles of teaching, and address any tensions in the learning climate.

- The one-minute preceptor and SNAPPS models are methods for efficient and effective teaching.

- Providing effective feedback to learners is an important teaching skill that should be applied in a timely, specific, limited, behaviorally oriented, and learner-solicited manner.

References

Aagaard E, Teherani A, Irby DM: Effectiveness of the one-minute preceptor model for diagnosing the patient and the learner: proof of concept. Acad Med 79(1):42–49, 2004 14690996

Accreditation Council for Graduate Medical Education: Common program requirements: general competencies. February 13, 2007. Available at: https://www.acgme.org/acgmeweb/Portals/0/PFAssets/ProgramRequirements/CPRs2013.pdf. Accessed May 25, 2015.

Allen MH: Definitive treatment in the psychiatric emergency service. Psychiatr Q 67(4):247–262, 1996 8938826

American Association for Emergency Psychiatry Education Committee: A model curriculum for psychiatric resident education in emergency psychiatry. Emergency Psychiatry 4:18–19, 1998

American Medical Association: Graduate Medical Education Directory, 2001–2002. Chicago, IL, American Medical Association, 2002, p 317

Battistone MJ, Milne C, Sande MA, et al: The feasibility and acceptability of implementing formal evaluation sessions and using descriptive vocabulary to assess student performance on a clinical clerkship. Teach Learn Med 14(1):5–10, 2002 11865750

Brasch JS, Ferencz JC: Training issues in emergency psychiatry. Psychiatr Clin North Am 22(4):941–954, x, 1999 10623980

Brasch J, Glick RL, Cobb TG, et al: Residency training in emergency psychiatry: a model curriculum developed by the education committee of the American Association for Emergency Psychiatry. Acad Psychiatry 28(2):95–103, 2004 15298860

Busari JO, Weggelaar NM, Knottnerus AC, et al: How medical residents perceive the quality of supervision provided by attending doctors in the clinical setting. Med Educ 39(7):696–703, 2005 15960790

Cantillon P: Teaching large groups. BMJ 326(7386):437–440, 2003 12595386

Deci E, Vallerand R, Pelletier L, et al: Motivation and education: the self-determination perspective. Educ Psychol 26:325–346, 1991

DeLong T: Flying Without a Net: Turn Fear of Change Into Fuel for Success. Chapter 11: Second Captain First Choose. Boston, MA, Harvard Business Review Press, 2011, pp 199–201

DeLong TJ, DeLong S: The paradox of excellence. Harv Bus Rev 89(6):119–123, 139, 2011 21714389

Douglas N, Robinson J, Fahy K: Inquiry into the obstetric and gynaecological services at King Edward Memorial Hospital 1990–2000. Perth, Australia, Department of Health, Government of Western Australia, 2001

Firth-Cozens J: Doctors, their wellbeing, and their stress. BMJ 326(7391):670–671, 2003 12663377

Foley R, Smilansky J, Yonke A: Teacher-student interaction in a medical clerkship. J Med Educ 54(8):622–626, 1979 469911

Furney SL, Orsini AN, Orsetti KE, et al: Teaching the one-minute preceptor. A randomized controlled trial. J Gen Intern Med 16(9):620–624, 2001 11556943

Gibson DR, Campbell RM: Promoting effective teaching and learning: hospital consultants identify their needs. Med Educ 34(2):126–130, 2000 10652065

Gordon J: ABC of learning and teaching in medicine: one to one teaching and feedback. BMJ 326(7388):543–545, 2003 12623919

Grainger C: Mentoring: supporting doctors at work and play (Career Focus). BMJ Classified 324:s203, 2002

Hutchinson L: Educational environment. BMJ 326(7393):810–812, 2003 12689981

Irby DM: Teaching and learning in ambulatory care settings: a thematic review of the literature. Acad Med 70(10):898–931, 1995 7575922

Irby DM, Papadakis M: Does good clinical teaching really make a difference? Am J Med 110(3):231–232, 2001 11182114

Irby DM, Aagaard E, Teherani A: Teaching points identified by preceptors observing one-minute preceptor and traditional preceptor encounters. Acad Med 79(1):50–55, 2004 14690997

Jaques D: Teaching small groups. BMJ 326(7387):492–494, 2003 12609949

Jones JW, Barge BN, Steffy BD, et al: Stress and medical malpractice: organizational risk assessment and intervention. J Appl Psychol 73(4):727–735, 1988 3209582

Kaufman DM: Applying educational theory in practice. BMJ 326(7382):213–216, 2003 12543841

Kilminster SM, Jolly BC: Effective supervision in clinical practice settings: a literature review. Med Educ 34(10):827–840, 2000 11012933

Lake FR, Ryan G: Teaching on the run tips 2: educational guides for teaching in a clinical setting. Med J Aust 180(10):527–528, 2004a 15139832

Lake FR, Ryan G: Teaching on the run tips 3: planning a teaching episode. Med J Aust 180(12):643–644, 2004b 15200365

Lake FR, Ryan G: Teaching on the run tips 4: teaching with patients. Med J Aust 181(3):158–159, 2004c 15287835

Lake FR, Ryan G: Teaching on the run tips 11: the junior doctor in difficulty. Med J Aust 183(9):475–476, 2005 16274350

Luck C: Reducing stress among junior doctors (Career Focus). BMJ 321(7268):S2–S7268, 2000 11053204

McKee M, Black N: Does the current use of junior doctors in the United Kingdom affect the quality of medical care? Soc Sci Med 34(5):549–558, 1992 1604361

Morrison J: ABC of learning and teaching in medicine: evaluation. BMJ 326(7385):385–387, 2003 12586676

Muhlbauer HG: Teaching trainees in turbulent settings: a practical guide. Emergency Psychiatry 4:28–30, 1998

Neher JO, Stevens NG: The one-minute preceptor: shaping the teaching conversation. Fam Med 35(6):391–393, 2003 12817861

Neher JO, Gordon KC, Meyer B, et al: A five-step "microskills" model of clinical teaching. J Am Board Fam Pract 5(4):419–424, 1992 1496899

Newman P, Peile E: Valuing learners' experience and supporting further growth: educational models to help experienced adult learners in medicine. BMJ 325(7357):200–202, 2002 12142310

Ogburn T, Espey E: The R-I-M-E method for evaluation of medical students on an obstetrics and gynecology clerkship. Am J Obstet Gynecol 189(3):666–669, 2003 14526289

Osborn LM, Sargent JR, Williams SD: Effects of time-in-clinic, clinic setting, and faculty supervision on the continuity clinic experience. Pediatrics 91(6):1089–1093, 1993 8502507

Paice E, Rutter H, Wetherell M, et al: Stressful incidents, stress and coping strategies in the pre-registration house officer year. Med Educ 36(1):56–65, 2002 11849525

Pangaro L: A new vocabulary and other innovations for improving descriptive in-training evaluations. Acad Med 74(11):1203–1207, 1999 10587681

Parrot S, Dobbie A, Chumley H, et al: Evidence-based office teaching—the five-step microskills model of clinical teaching. Fam Med 38(3):164–167, 2006 16518731

Parsell G, Bligh J: Recent perspectives on clinical teaching. Med Educ 35(4):409–414, 2001 11319008

Peyton JWR: The learning cycle, in Teaching and Learning in Medical Practice. Edited by Peyton JWR. Rickmansworth, UK, Manticore Europe, 1998, pp 13–19

Salerno SM, O'Malley PG, Pangaro LN, et al: Faculty development seminars based on the one-minute preceptor improve feedback in the ambulatory setting. J Gen Intern Med 17(10):779–787, 2002 12390554

Schuster JM: Frustration or opportunity? The impact of managed care on emergency psychiatry. New Dir Ment Health Serv 67(67):101–108, 1995 7476804

Spencer J: Learning and teaching in the clinical environment. BMJ 326(7389):591–594, 2003 12637408

Tiberius RG, Sinai J, Flak EA: The role of teacher-learner relationships in medical education, in International Handbook of Research in Medical Education. Edited by Norman GR, van der Vleuten CPM, Newble DI. Dordrecht, The Netherlands, Kluwer Academic, 2002, pp 463–497

Ullian JA, Bland CJ, Simpson DE: An alternative approach to defining the role of the clinical teacher. Acad Med 69(10):832–838, 1994 7916801

Vaughn L, Baker R: Teaching in the medical setting: balancing teaching styles, learning styles and teaching methods. Med Teach 23(6):610–612, 2001 12098485

Vaughn LM, Baker RC: Psychological size and distance: emphasizing the interpersonal relationship as a pathway to optimal teaching and learning conditions. Med Educ 38(10):1053–1060, 2004 15461650

Wall D, McAleer S: Teaching the consultant teachers: identifying the core content. Med Educ 34(2):131–138, 2000 10652066

Willcock SM, Daly MG, Tennant CC, et al: Burnout and psychiatric morbidity in new medical graduates. Med J Aust 181(7):357–360, 2004 15462649

Wolpaw TM, Wolpaw DR, Papp KK: SNAPPS: a learner-centered model for outpatient education. Acad Med 78(9):893–898, 2003 14507619

Suggested Readings

Neher JO, Gordon KC, Meyer B, et al: A five-step "microskills" model of clinical teaching. J Am Board Fam Pract 5(4):419–424, 1992

Pangaro L: A new vocabulary and other innovations for improving descriptive in-training educations. Acad Med 74(11):1203–1207, 1999

Wolpaw TM, Wolpaw DR, Papp KK: SNAPPS: a learner centered approach for outpatient education. Acad Med 78(9):893–898, 2003

Index

*Page numbers printed in **boldface** type refer to tables or figures.*